Advanced Dental Nursing

SECOND EDITION

Edited by

Robert S. Ireland

BDS, MPhil, MFGDP(UK)
Associate Clinical Professor
Postgraduate Dental Education Unit
The University of Warwick

A John Wiley & Sons, Ltd., Publication

This edition first published 2010
© 2010 Blackwell Publishing Ltd

Blackwell Publishing was acquired by John Wiley & Sons in February 2007. Blackwell's publishing programme has been merged with Wiley's global Scientific, Technical, and Medical business to form Wiley-Blackwell.

Registered office
John Wiley & Sons Ltd, The Atrium, Southern Gate, Chichester, West Sussex PO19 8SQ, United Kingdom

Editorial offices
9600 Garsington Road, Oxford OX4 2DQ, United Kingdom
2121 State Avenue, Ames, Iowa 50014-8300, USA

For details of our global editorial offices, for customer services and for information about how to apply for permission to reuse the copyright material in this book please see our website at www.wiley.com/wiley-blackwell.

Library of Congress Cataloging-in-Publication Data

Advanced dental nursing / edited by Robert S. Ireland. – 2nd ed.
      p. ; cm.
   Includes bibliographical references and index.
   ISBN 978-1-4051-9267-5 (pbk. : alk. paper)   1. Dental assistants–Outlines, syllabi, etc.   2. Dental assistants–Vocational guidance–Great Britain.   I. Ireland, Robert, MFGCP.
   [DNLM: 1. Dental Assistants–Outlines.   WU 18.2 A245 2010]
   RK60.5.A38   2010
   617.6'0233–dc22

2009049784

A catalogue record for this book is available from the British Library.

Set in 9.5/12 pt Palatino by Toppan Best-set Premedia Limited
Printed in Singapore by Ho Printing Singapore Pte Ltd

1   2010

Advanced Dental Nursing

Library and Information Services

Littlehampton Road site   Tel: 01903 606213
Broadwater Road site   Tel: 01903 606451

This book must be returned to the library, or renewed, on or before the date last entered below.
Renewal can be granted only when the book has not been previously requested by another borrower.

PLEASE PROTECT BOOKS FROM DAMAGE   D.9304

Contents

Author Profiles

Editor
Robert S. Ireland   BDS, MPhil, MFGDP(UK)
Associate Clinical Professor
Postgraduate Dental Education Unit
The University of Warwick

Bob has been a part-time lecturer at the University of Liverpool and a senior partner in a group dental practice for 30 years. In 1995, he was appointed Professor of Primary Dental Care and Director of the Dental Therapy Course at the University of Liverpool. He has produced three educational videos for the dental team and has been extensively involved in hospital and practice dental nurse training. He is the editor of *A Clinical Textbook for Dental Hygiene and Therapy*. He is currently a presiding examiner for the National Examining Board for Dental Nurses (NEBDN) and formerly external examiner for dental nursing at Trinity College, Dublin.

Mary Cameron   RDN, DipDHE, FEATC, Cert Health Education,
Licentiateship in Dental Nursing
Oral Health Co-ordinator/Educational Advisor –
Community Dental Service
NHS Greater Glasgow & Clyde

Mary qualified as a dental nurse in 1978. She has worked in general practice and hospitals and, in 1998, moved to the Community Dental Service. In her previous role within the CDS she led a team of oral health educators, with a remit to deliver and evaluate oral health programmes throughout Glasgow. She now leads and advises on DCP training programmes. In 1992, she became a part-time tutor delivering the post-qualification certificate in oral health education in Scotland. She is currently an examiner with the NEBDN and former chairperson of the Oral Health Committee. She continues her role as an external verifier for City & Guilds and the Scottish Qualifications Authority.

Ulpee Darbar   BDS, MSc, FDS (Rest Dent)RCS, FHEA
Consultant in Restorative Dentistry
Eastman Dental Hospital and Institute, London

Ulpee is a full time Consultant in Restorative Dentistry and is also on the specialist lists in Restorative Dentistry, Periodontology and Prosthodontics. She was appointed as Clinical Director of the Eastman Dental Hospital in 2006. Her clinical focus lies in the management of patients with complex and multidisciplinary problems including tooth loss and its replacement with dental implants. She is extensively involved in education and training at postgraduate level for dentists and dental care professionals. She has been proactive in running successful training courses for dental nurses in different implant systems and has written the first book on dental implants for dental nurses. She lectures extensively in these areas both nationally and internationally and is on the Specialist Advisory Board for the Royal College of Surgeons (Edinburgh) Implant Dentistry Diploma and is also an examiner for this exam.

Janet Goodwin   BA(Hons), RDN, LCGI
Qualifications Manager
National Examining Board for Dental Nurses

Janet has worked as a dental nurse in general dental practice, dental hospital and the Community Dental Service as an oral health educator. In 1985 she started teaching oral health and the NEBDN National Certificate in local colleges. In 1988, she was appointed as a training officer in a large youth training scheme primarily for underprivileged teenagers. She then returned to Leeds Dental Institute to take up the position of tutor, before being appointed principal dental nurse in 1991, while also working as an external verifier for City & Guilds. Janet is currently qualifications manager for the National Examining Board for Dental Nurses, and a member of the GDC Council. She is on the editorial board of the journal *Team in Practice* and was involved in the *Child Protection and the Dental Team* handbook.

Tina Gorman   RDN, FAETC
Director of Nursing
Dublin Dental School and Hospital

Tina trained at Belfast Dental Hospital and qualified in 1990. She was awarded the Kilner McCourt prize for the highest mark in Ireland in the National Examination. She was the first person in Northern Ireland to obtain the post-certificate in conscious sedation. She moved to work for *Homefirst* Community Dental Service in 1999, where she assisted in the set-up of a new sedation and general anaesthetic service for adults with physical and learning disabilities. She is an NEBDN examiner for the National Certificate and Conscious Sedation qualifications. She also introduced the West Midlands Special Care Dental Nursing Course in 2001 whilst she was a dental nurse tutor. She is currently based in Dublin Dental Hospital managing the Nursing Department. She is the dental nursing representative on the British Society for Disability and Oral Health, member of the editorial board of the *Journal of Disability and Oral Heath* and is the first non-dentist president of the Irish Society for Disability and Oral Health (2008–2010).

Jayne Harrison   BDS, FDS(Orth), RCPS, MDentSci, MOrthRCS, PhD
                          Consultant Orthodontist
                          Liverpool University Dental Hospital

Jayne qualified from Cardiff Dental School in 1985 and subsequently underwent general dental and then orthodontic training in Merseyside and North Wales. She gained her FDS in 1989, MOrth and MDentSci in 1993, FDS(Orth) in 1998 and PhD in 2002. She was appointed as a consultant orthodontist at Liverpool University Dental Hospital in 1998, where she is also programme director for the orthodontic nursing course. She is on the editorial board of the journal of *Orthodontics and Cochrane Oral Health Group* and has had several papers published on orthodontic subjects and evidence-based dentistry.

Patricia Heap   RDN, FETC, Dip DHE, MRSH
                          Principal Dental Nurse
                          University Dental Hospital of Manchester

Pat qualified as a dental nurse in 1963 at the University Dental Hospital of Manchester. Since then she has been employed in all sections of dentistry and in 1972 she returned to the Dental Hospital as senior dental nurse in periodontology, then tutor dental nurse and finally in 1985 to the post of principal dental nurse. She has since gained the City & Guilds Further Education Teachers certificate with credit, RSH Diploma in Oral Health Education, Dental Sedation Nursing Post Qualification certificate and BTEC Safety in Healthcare certificate. She is on the Board of Examiners for NEBDN and is an examiner for both the national and sedation examinations. She currently sits on the sub-committees for Sedation and the independent assessment for the Oral Healthcare NVQ programme.

Lesley Longman   BSc, BDS, FDS RCS(Edin), PhD
                          Consultant in Restorative Dentistry
                          Liverpool University Dental Hospital

Lesley was appointed lecturer in restorative dentistry at the University of Liverpool Dental School in 1984 and gained her FDS (Ed) in the same year. She was awarded a PhD in 1991 and appointed consultant in restorative dentistry in 1997. She is on the specialist register for prosthodontics and restorative dentistry. She has responsibility for organising the teaching of sedation to dental undergraduates. She currently lectures on postgraduate dental courses in sedation and is course director for the University of Liverpool Certificate in Conscious Sedation. She is also currently programme director for the certificate course in sedation for dental nurses.

June Nunn   BDS, MA, PhD, FDS RCS(Edin), DDPHRCS, FDS RCS
                          Professor of Special Care Dentistry and Head of Department
                          Dental School and Hospital
                          Trinity College Dublin, Ireland

June moved from her post as consultant/senior lecturer in child dental health in the School of Dentistry, University of Newcastle-upon-Tyne to the Chair in Special Care Dentistry at Trinity College Dublin in October 2001. She is past president of both the British Society for Disability and Oral Health, and the International Association for Disability and Oral Health, and in 2003 was the President of the Irish Society for Disability and Oral Health. June edits the *Journal of Disability and Oral Health* and edited the IADH textbook on *Disability and Oral Care*. She has been an examiner at the Royal Colleges of Surgeons of England and Edinburgh for the M Paed Dent, MSCD and DSCD, as well as external examiner for both undergraduate and postgraduate students in a number of UK and overseas dental schools. She is codirector for the Postgraduate Diploma in Conscious Sedation in Trinity College Dublin.

Kathleen O'Donovan   FAETC, RDN
Dental Nurse Manager
Liverpool University Dental Hospital

Kath qualified as a dental nurse in 1973 and has since gained the Certificate in Oral Health Education (Nottingham University) and the NEBDN Certificate in Dental Sedation Nursing. She is currently organising the Certificate in Orthodontic Nursing at Liverpool University Dental Hospital. She is on the Board of Examiners for the NEBDN and is an examiner for the Certificate in Dental Sedation and NVQ. She is involved in teaching on dental nurse courses for dental sedation, orthodontic nursing and oral health care. She was formerly Chairman of Council for the British Association of Dental Nurses.

Mike Wanless   BDS, DipPH, DGDP(UK), MSc, PhD
Head and Clinical Director
Greater Manchester School for Dental Care Professionals

Mike is head and clinical director of the Greater Manchester School for Dental Care Professionals (DCPs), based in Salford. He is also an educational programme director for North Western Deanery and is a director of NEBDN, for whom he has examined since 1986. He lectures widely on communicating with dental patients.

Preface

This second edition of *Advanced Dental Nursing* has been produced five years after publication of the first edition. In that time there have been a considerable number of changes in dentistry, both clinical and administrative. This edition has therefore been extensively updated and revised to bring the book up to date with contemporary clinical practice. In addition, a new chapter on implant nursing has been included to reflect the rapid development of this area of restorative dentistry and the acknowledged need for dental nurses who have knowledge, understanding and skills relevant to dental implantology.

Sadly, there are few textbooks published specifically for dental nurses. This book has been written to fill what is perceived to be a significant gap in the continuing professional development of dental nurses. It is primarily aimed at those nurses who are registered with the General Dental Council in the UK or who already have some clinical experience. It is hoped, however, that there is much useful information, particularly in the first two chapters, for any nurse just starting out on a career in dentistry.

Each chapter, apart from the chapter on implant nursing, has been jointly written by a dentist and a dental nurse. This not only provided an opportunity to develop teamwork, but also assured that the contents are both relevant to and appropriate for dental nurses.

Although the reader may choose to read the book from cover to cover, it is primarily intended that they should be able to dip into sections of specific interest for further study or use the book in conjunction with other teaching programmes. To this end it is anticipated that this textbook will form a useful reference source for dental clinics and practices.

Within each chapter, many key words have been highlighted in bold for easy reference and there is an extensive glossary (at the back of the book) of all the abbreviations used.

The reader should be aware that there is considerable reference to current regulations, legislation and accepted clinical practice, and that these are subject to change with the inevitable advancement in all aspects of dentistry. The reader should therefore be prepared to consult other reference sources for changes that may have been introduced since publication of this book.

Robert S. Ireland

Acknowledgements

Chapter 1   The authors would like to thank Anna Ireland for her advice on the structure and scope of the Salaried Dental Service described within the book.

Chapter 5   The authors would like to acknowledge the assistance of John Scholey for his contribution to the section on radiographs, Brian Cannell for his help with the laboratory skills section and John Cunningham for providing information for the medico-legal section.

Figure 5.22   Reproduced by kind permission of The Victoria University of Manchester, England. The SCAN scale was first published in 1987 by the European Orthodontic Society (Evans R and Shaw W (1987) Preliminary evaluation of an illustrated scale for rating dental attractiveness. *European Journal of Orthodontics* **9**: 314–318).

1 Career Development Pathways

Janet Goodwin and Robert S. Ireland

Introduction

This book is intended primarily for dental nurses who have obtained their national certificate or National Vocational Qualifications (NVQ) equivalent and would like to consider changes in their career development or extend their knowledge and skills, particularly in the areas of oral health education, special needs, orthodontic, sedation and implantology nursing. The recently extended remit for dental nurses has not been included as this is addressed in other texts such as the teamwork publication *Changing Roles in the Dental Team* published by the Faculty of General Dental Practice, UK.

Dental radiography has been excluded not only to reduce the cost and size of this book but also because there are a number of useful textbooks covering this area already on the market, such as *Radiography and Radiology for Dental Nurses*, to which the interested reader is referred. Since general anaesthesia (GA) is now not undertaken in a primary care environment and the number of nurses wishing to specialise in this area has significantly diminished, GA nursing has also been omitted.

Legal framework

In May 2001, the General Dental Council (GDC) approved a commitment to regulate all the members of the dental team, now known as **dental care professionals** (DCPs). This term includes:

- dental nurses
- dental technicians
- clinical dental technicians
- dental hygienists
- dental therapists
- maxillofacial technicians
- orthodontic therapists.

This regulation came into force following the amendment by Parliament of the **Dental Auxiliaries Regulations 1986**. The aim of the GDC in this development was to produce caring, knowledgeable, competent and skilful individuals who are able to accept professional responsibility within the framework of their particular area of knowledge and competence, and who contribute to the safe and effective care of the patient. They will appreciate the need for continuing professional development (CPD) that will foster the knowledge, understanding, skills and attitudes that promote effective lifelong learning and support.

The implementation of statutory registration has ensured dental nurse updating on an annual basis to make sure that they are 'fit to practise'. This process makes dental nurses a professional body that must be prepared to abide by the GDC rules and code of conduct. They are liable to disciplinary and misconduct procedures, which could, in extreme circumstances, result in removal from the register. In such circumstances, that person would no longer be able to practise as a dental nurse.

Governing bodies and professional associations

General Dental Council

The GDC was created in 1956 and is currently constituted by the **Dentists Act 1984**, which was amended in 2005. It protects the public by regulating dental professionals in the UK. All dentists and DCPs are required to register with the GDC.

The role of the GDC is to protect the patient by:

- keeping up-to-date lists of properly qualified dentists, hygienists and therapists
- setting high standards of dental practice and conduct
- maintaining high standards of dental education
- requiring dentists and DCPs to take part in CPD
- taking appropriate action if there is concern about whether a dental professional should be allowed to continue to practise dentistry.

The GDC has undergone a modernisation programme following new legislation implemented through a series of amendments (Section 60 orders) to the Dentists Act 1984. The Council is now much smaller, consisting of 24 members made up of eight dentists, four DCPs and 12 lay people. Further information can be obtained from the GDC website (www.gdc-uk.org).

National Examining Board for Dental Nurses

The aim of the National Examining Board for Dental Nurses (NEBDN) is to 'advance the education of dental nurses for the benefit of the public'. This is achieved by:

- providing qualifications for dental nurses
- publishing syllabuses of study
- issuing certificates and badges
- standard setting for the qualifications
- liaising with other appropriate bodies.

The NEBDN was established in 1943 to provide a national certificate in dental nursing. A part-time secretary was employed to undertake administrative and secretarial duties. The head office was established in Leyland, Lancashire, where the secretary shared offices with the British Association of Dental Nurses (BADN). It relocated to Poulton-le-Fylde, Lancashire, in 1963 and then to Fleetwood (also in Lancashire) in 1978, where it remains to date.

The NEBDN consists of registered dental nurses and dentists, with a current establishment of 400 members. New examiners are appointed according to the needs of the Board. These members form the panel of the Board, from whom 12 council members are elected. The Council is responsible for the finance and administration of the Board. Within the Council are five executive committee members who are empowered to undertake the business and strategic planning of the NEBDN.

The NEBDN currently provides:

■ National Certificate for Dental Nurses
■ NVQ Level 2 Oral Health Support Worker
■ NVQ Level 3 Oral Healthcare Dental Nursing
■ Certificate in Oral Health Education
■ Certificate in Dental Sedation Nursing
■ Certificate in Dental Anaesthetic Nursing
■ Certificate in Special Care Dental Nursing
■ Certificate in Orthodontic Dental Nursing
■ Certificate in Dental Implant Nursing.

Further information can be obtained from the NEBDN website (www.nebdn.org.uk).

British Association of Dental Nurses

The British Association of Dental Nurses (BADN) was established in 1943 with the NEBDN and is also based at Fleetwood, but in different premises from the NEBDN. The association is the professional organisation committed to the representation of all dental nurses, whether qualified or unqualified, working in all areas of employment. The BADN represents dental nurses at all levels and has representation on many working groups, including the NEBDN. It negotiates and represents the interests of dental nurses on remuneration and working conditions. All dental disciplines have journals published by their own associations, and the BADN is no exception. The BADN journal is published every three months, highlighting relevant workplace issues, letters of concern/praise, aspects of good practice and employment vacancies. It is an excellent source for keeping up to date. Further information can be obtained from the BADN website (www.badn.org.uk).

British Dental Association

The British Dental Association (BDA) is the trade union and national professional association for dentists. It represents approximately 18,000 dentists in the UK in all dental services, although the majority are from general dental practice. It strives to promote the interests of its members, to advance the science, art and ethics of dentistry, and to improve the nation's oral health. In pursuing its mission the association is guided by the following beliefs and principles.

- Oral health is necessary for general health and well-being.
- Quality oral health should be easily accessible to everyone.
- Quality oral care is best provided by co-ordinated teams led by dentists and with well-trained support staff.
- Research into oral health and the delivery of quality oral healthcare is to be actively encouraged.
- Collaboration between the association and other appropriate dental bodies is to be actively pursued.

Further information can be obtained from the BDA website (www.bda-dentistry.org.uk).

Faculty of General Dental Practice [FGDP(UK)]

Since its inception in 1992, the Faculty of General Dental Practice (UK) has been the academic home of dentists working in the field of primary dental care. The primary aim of dentistry is the oral health and well-being of the patient, and the FGDP recognises that the care of the patient really is a team effort. Dentistry cannot function without the highly capable support of a whole team of dental professionals, and so the Faculty has developed an approach to education and training that increasingly encompasses the whole of the dental team. The FGDP(UK) welcomes dental care professionals (DCPs) and offers affiliate membership to all DCPs, including dental nurses, who are subject to registration with the GDC. The Faculty also offers diplomas in dental hygiene and dental therapy and has recently established an RCS Eng Diploma in Orthodontic Therapy and a route to GDC registration for clinical dental technicians.

Continuing professional development (CPD)

Continuing professional development is often perceived as education that continues if and when required by the individual. It is in fact lifelong learning that should be ongoing throughout a person's working life. It does not always involve formal studies, and can be achieved through various methods of learning.

It is an individual's responsibility to undertake CPD in order to maintain, enhance and broaden professional knowledge already gained. The benefits of this process can include:

- increased job satisfaction
- promotion of awareness of issues or problems
- improved communication with colleagues

- improved efficiency
- improvement in career prospects
- a greater commitment to the workplace.

Following statutory registration, compulsory CPD requirements were introduced in August 2008 by the GDC. All DCPs must keep a record of their CPD activity from the time of their registration. It is necessary to complete at least 150 hours of CPD every cycle of five years, of which at least 50 hours need to be **verifiable CPD**. For CPD to be classed as verifiable it must satisfy four conditions.

- There must be documentary proof of having taken part provided by the activity provider or organiser.
- The activity should have clearly defined, concise aims and objectives.
- The activity should have clearly defined anticipated outcomes so that it is evident what can be gained by taking part.
- The activity should have quality controls: there should be an opportunity to provide feedback so that the quality of future activities can be further improved.

Verifiable CPD should include a specified amount of time in three identified core subjects. These are medical emergencies (at least 10 hours in every CPD cycle); disinfection and decontamination (at least 5 hours in every CPD cycle); radiography and radiation protection (at least 5 hours in every CPD cycle). The GDC recommends that all dental professionals undertake CPD in medical emergencies every year. It also recommends keeping up to date with CPD in legal and ethical issues, and complaints handling.

Non-verifiable or **general CPD** does not have to satisfy the four conditions for verifiable CPD but it does need to be recorded. It can include such activities as reading journals, background research, and private study.

The records that need to be kept should include the date, title and venue of the activity, the name of the person or organisation running the activity, whether it is verifiable or general CPD, and the number of hours spent undertaking the activity. The GDC provides a CPD booklet on the back of which is a form that may be used for recording all CPD activity.

The planning and undertaking of CPD should be given careful thought, and the following points should be taken into account:

- it can be time consuming
- it requires self-discipline
- it needs to be structured and organised
- the appropriate course may be difficult to locate
- it will require searching for CPD outside the workplace.

CPD will help to prepare dental nurses for changing roles or circumstances in the practice or clinic and help make them safer workers who understand the implications of the roles and responsibilities they are undertaking in the workplace. It can also prevent complacency and inertia, which could potentially put patients or staff at risk.

To achieve a high quality standard and appropriateness of CPD, it needs planning thoroughly via **appraisals** or performance review. This process will identify the needs of the individual and the needs of the organisation within the requirements imposed by the GDC. It encompasses the short-term and long-term goals that need to be met, and how these can best be achieved. These needs will be addressed through:

- implementation: what, where, when and how these needs can be met
- evaluation: was the CPD appropriate and of high quality?
- review: where do we go now?

If carried out properly, CPD will produce an efficient, enthusiastic, safe and understanding individual in the workplace who will be a great asset to any employer.

This book covers a number of areas of CPD in considerable detail. However, it should be appreciated that CPD can be obtained from a wide variety of sources, including dental journals, local meetings, conferences, formal courses, postgraduate handbooks, computer-aided learning (CAL) and specialist websites. Some of these sources may be verifiable CPD and some may be general. These will be discussed later in this chapter.

Further activities and resources for CPD

Not all compulsory CPD is based around certificated courses or formal learning. This type of learning does not suit many individuals because they require a more flexible approach to their knowledge/skills updating. There may also not be the opportunity to undertake a formal course for geographical, financial or personal reasons.

Learning can often commence via appraisals and individual performance reviews. This allows the dental nurse an opportunity to discuss with the dentist, practice manager or senior nurse, their own development needs, what development is required to deliver the service effectively, and what activity may be required to help others in the workplace within the boundaries imposed by the GDC for general and verifiable CPD. This can lead to productive discussions around the type of activity that can be undertaken.

Conferences

Each year various conferences are held throughout the UK and abroad. These can take the form of specific areas of interest such as orthodontic conferences, or more wide-ranging conferences such as the annual BADN conference. Conferences can be useful for:

- networking
- updating knowledge by attending relevant lectures
- updating skills by attending specific workshops
- obtaining trade materials and information (usually free).

Publications and journals

Most dental practices, community clinics and hospitals receive copies of various journals. These should be stored where they can be easily referenced and used as a medium to keep up to date with current ideas and issues. Most journals are available in an electronic format, some of which can be accessed free of charge to non-subscribers. Useful journals relevant to dental nurses are *Vital* (British Dental Association), *BADN Journal*, *British Dental Journal* (www.bdj.co.uk), *Primary Dental Care* (www.rcseng.ac.uk/dental/fgdp/pdc) and *Dental Update* (www.dental-update.co.uk).

Projects

Some areas of dental practice requiring attention or review may be highlighted during audit (see below). This could be an area where the dental nurse becomes involved by carrying out a project on the topic in question, such as oral health, white filling replacements or evaluating new materials or products. A project could take just a few hours or may involve a longer review over several months, with a final evaluation process.

Secondments and job swaps

A secondment to another area in a practice, clinic or hospital can be a useful experience for someone unsure of which direction to take in their career. Secondments can not only reinforce a decision to make or not make a career change, but they can also provide a valuable insight into another area of clinical practice. Job swaps, even if only for a few hours, can provide an excellent learning opportunity to find out about new techniques or working practices. These can take place within the same building or may involve travelling to a different location.

Audit

Audit is the systematic analysis of an area of clinical or administrative dental practice with the intention of producing an improvement. It is usual to talk about audit as taking place in a cyclic manner as illustrated in Figure 1.1.

A topic for audit is first identified, e.g. how often gloves are contaminated in the surgery, and then a standard should be set. The standard should, where possible, be one defined by acknowledged authorities rather than those carrying out the audit. The process should then be observed and measured against the standard to see whether the standard is met. If it is not, improvements are made and then the process is observed again. The audit can take some time and it is quite possible that the original standard used is out of date on completion of the audit and so the whole audit process would need to be repeated. This is why it is known as an audit cycle. Any member of the dental team can undertake audit either individually or as a group. Virtually any aspect of a dental practice or clinic can be the subject of an audit. Some examples are the reasons for patients failing to attend, correct mixing of impression and filling materials, aspects of infection control, etc. Audit can be a very important and rewarding part of CPD for the dental nurse.

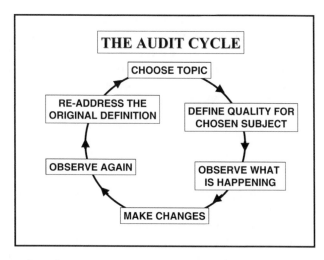

Figure 1.1 The audit cycle.

Distance learning

Distance learning is a form of learning that takes place where the teacher and the student are not in the same place at the same time.

For some people this may be the ideal means of learning on a structured course, and with the advent of registration more of these courses have now become available for dental nurses. They may live in a region where access to the type of training programme they require is unavailable, or they may have no access to transport to get to different locations. Distance learning can overcome the problem of taking time off work or difficulty in attendance due to family pressures.

This type of learning can be very useful, but there may be disadvantages.

- It is not always the most appropriate course.
- It can be expensive.
- Tutors are not always available for support when required.
- It requires motivation and discipline.

It is important to be able to evaluate the quality of distance learning programmes, and some useful guidelines are provided in *Teamwork 6: Changing Roles in the Dental Team* (available from the Faculty of General Dental Practice; www.fgdp.org.uk).

Videos and computer-aided learning (CAL)

Videos and computer-aided learning (CAL) have become a part of modern-day culture and can be very effective tools for learning. They provide an opportunity to build up a personal learning resource, which can be accessed with ease at any time since computers, video recorders and DVD players are now so cheap and widely available. Videos are often cheaper than CAL programs but have the disadvantages that they can become quickly outdated and they are expensive to produce and therefore to buy. Consequently they are tending to go out of fashion. CAL programs can be accessed via the internet and are considered to be of greatest advantage when linked with a structured teaching programme. Many of these programmes include self-assessment and documentary evidence of completion, which is important in contributing to a portfolio of personal CPD.

The internet

Many dental internet sites offer online verifiable CPD on a subscription basis, often linked to a journal such as *Dental Nursing* (a monthly journal specifically for dental nurses) or *Vital* (British Dental Association). The majority of these sites keep an electronic record of verifiable activity, which can be downloaded and submitted to the GDC when requested. Some sites provide online **webinars** using a broadband internet connection, in which a live presentation is given and opportunities are provided for the audience, linked via computers in their own practices, to ask questions. The Dental Channel (dental-channel. co.uk) holds webinars for dental nurses on a monthly basis, usually at times that don't conflict with normal surgery hours.

In-house training

This can be a very flexible approach to learning for both the participant and the deliverer, and is an excellent opportunity for developing teamwork in the workplace. An in-house programme can be a one-off update to a full-length course such as the teamwork programme. Regular practice or team meetings provide excellent learning opportunities. They also provide the possibility of company representatives giving demonstrations or workshops about their products.

In-house training, particularly in hospitals and the Community Dental Service (CDS), can focus on specific areas that are important to the whole team such as fire practice, Control of Substances Hazardous to Health (COSHH) regulations, guidance on lifting and handling, and infection control.

Exhibitions

The largest exhibition in the dental field is 'Dental Showcase', which usually takes place in October each year and features many aspects of dentistry of value to the whole dental team, such as personal protective clothing, materials developments, advances in equipment design and association stands, e.g. BADN.

Many other meetings or conferences have associated trade exhibitions which are usually free to all delegates, e.g. at the BDA annual conference.

There are opportunities for nurses to prepare and display their own exhibition either in the workplace for the benefit of staff or patients or in schools or care homes, etc. This can be very time-consuming because it could involve research and communication with a wide variety of people, but it can also be very rewarding.

Lectures

These are held around the country all year round, and it is a question of deciding which lecture is of interest or relevance and booking a place at the session. The postgraduate deaneries (www.oxdent.ac.uk/links.html) and BDA branches and sections organise a large number of lectures locally, many of which are very relevant to dental nursing. Schools of dental nursing and local BADN groups (www.badn.org.uk) also organise many interesting and relevant lecture sessions.

Special interest groups

Many specialist areas within the dental field have societies primarily focused on the needs of dentists. However, nurses may be invited where it is appropriate for them and where it will help them keep abreast of current trends and changes. Examples of such groups are:

- British Society for the Study of Prosthetic Dentistry (www.derweb.co.uk/bsspd)
- British Society of Periodontology (www.bsperio.org)
- British Orthodontic Society (www.bos.org.uk)
- British Society of Restorative Dentistry (www.derweb.co.uk/bsrd/index.html)
- Armed forces
- British Society of Paediatric Dentistry (www.bspd.co.uk/)
- British Society of Oral Implantology (www.bsoi.org/).

Many of the above groups produce newsletters or hold training/update days to allow nurses to network with others with similar interests and skills. There are also specialised groups specific to dental nurses. They are mainly based within the BADN and can be accessed via its website. Currently the groups are:

- Armed Forces National Group
- Conscious Sedation and General Anaesthetic National Group
- Special Care Dental Nursing Group
- National Teaching Group.

Career opportunities

This section focuses on career and qualification development in the following areas of employment:

- general dental practice
- Salaried Dental Services (including dental access centres)

- Personal Dental Service
- general and district hospitals
- dental teaching hospitals
- armed forces
- industry
- Prison Service
- education sector.

General dental practice

The majority of primary dental care is provided within the NHS General Dental Services (GDS); however, an increasing proportion is now provided within private practice. Additional to their accepted remit, there are a number of areas of responsibility within a dental practice that nurses can undertake:

- additional duties in a specialist practice
- oral health education
- receptionist
- senior dental nurse
- practice manager.

Specialist practice

Recently there has been an increase in the number of practices specialising in certain areas. This includes both existing practices starting to specialise and the establishment of new specialist practices in order to broaden the scope of treatment for patients. Some examples are given below.

Implantology

This is a rapidly growing area where the patient has a metal or ceramic implant inserted into the bone with a fixed or removable bridge or denture attached. Duties of the nurse may include assisting in the surgical placement of the implants or prostheses, patient management and appropriate oral healthcare maintenance. Therefore skills in these areas should be acquired. The NEBDN offers a post qualification Certificate in Dental Implant Nursing. The Dental Nurse Education and Training Centre at Kings College London also offers a Certificate Course in Implant Dental Nursing (www.kcl.ac.uk/schools/dentistry/about/org/acad/dcp.html).

Cosmetic dentistry

These practices specialise in advanced restorative procedures including veneers, multiple crowns and bridges. The nurse needs to attend courses to gain a working knowledge and understanding of the techniques and materials involved. Close support operating skills are essential in this type of work.

Endodontics

These practices specialise in single and multirooted root canal therapy with possible surgical intervention, frequently using clinical microscopes. The nurse needs to be familiar with current endodontic techniques and materials and to be able to assist appropriately at the chairside.

Sedation

With the withdrawal of general anaesthetics from general dental practice, treatment under sedation is often offered as an acceptable alternative. The nurse who is the second appropriate person is required to have undertaken recognised sedation training. The experience and knowledge required for this is addressed in detail in Chapter 4.

Orthodontics

These may be specialist referral practices or general dental practitioners offering orthodontic care using fixed or removable appliances. There is now a new post-qualification certificate for orthodontic nursing, and the knowledge required for this certificate is covered in Chapter 5. Training courses are now available leading to the Diploma in Orthodontic Therapy. These may be particularly attractive to dental nurses who have obtained a Certificate in Orthodontic Nursing (see Interprofessional development, p. 20).

Special care

Special care dentistry is that branch of dentistry that aims to secure the oral health of, and enhance the quality of life for, people with disabilities where an interprofessional approach, supported by appropriate behaviour management techniques, is required to deliver efficacious and effective care in a holistic way. There is a post-qualification certificate for special care nursing, and the knowledge required for this certificate is covered in Chapter 3.

Oral health education

The importance of prevention is now widely accepted, and many practices and clinics have developed dedicated preventive dental units. Delivering effective preventive advice and support to patients of all ages requires both knowledge and great skill. Additional knowledge and training is required, and this subject area is covered in Chapter 2.

Receptionist

In some practices the dental nurse covers both reception and surgery duties, but with the complexity of modern clinical practice it is more common to employ a member of staff specifically as a receptionist. A recent study in southwest England found that 43% of dental nurses also had non-clinical duties (e.g. reception). The duties of a receptionist include:

- patient appointments
- stock control
- office administration
- management of information technology (IT) systems
- patient accounts.

There is a nine-month open learning Business and Technology Education Council (BTEC) level 3 qualification available as part of the Professional Development Award framework leading to an Advanced Diploma in Dental Reception. This diploma includes the role of the dental receptionist, dental reception administrative skills, aspects of patient care and professional development. More information is available from the Dental Resource Company (www.dental-resource.co.uk). Some receptionists obtain customer care or reception qualifications by attending courses provided by local colleges or primary care trusts (PCTs), but the majority tend to learn by means of in-house training provided by more experienced colleagues. The receptionist plays a key role in the smooth and efficient operation of a practice and is therefore a valued and essential member of the dental team.

Senior dental nurse

Due to economic influences, larger practices are now becoming more common, resulting in an expansion of the dental team. This can require an experienced nurse to take on additional responsibilities. This role may involve:

- the allocation of dental nurses to surgeries and specific tasks
- monitoring holiday entitlements
- monitoring sickness absences
- responsibility for continuing professional development
- additional clerical or management duties.

A senior nurse would be expected to be qualified and to have had extensive experience. In the past there has been no formal training in the dental nurse framework for this role, but a supervisor, team leader or management certificate would be advisable to equip a nurse with the skills to cope with these demanding responsibilities.

Practice manager

This new role is becoming very important in general dental practices, particularly within larger practices employing sizeable numbers of staff. Practice managers may be experienced dental nurses who have moved into a management role or they may be recruited from outside the field of dentistry. There are a number of accredited training courses available. Some are specific to dentistry, such as the BTEC Diploma in Dental Practice Management usually delivered in an open learning or workshop format, and the Institute of Leadership and Management (ILM; www.i-l-m.com) Level 5 Diploma in Management. Other training courses that are not specifically dental are available from local colleges or as distance-learning programmes, such as management and leadership qualifications offered by the Management Standards Centre (www.management-standards.org.uk). The non-dental qualifications are either medically, care or generic based and it would be up to the individual to establish if they were suitable for their needs in their practice or clinic.

The **British Dental Practice Managers Association** (BDPMA) was founded in 1993 and its aims are to promote and support all those who are managing dental practices by means of:

- representing the views of dental practice managers at all levels of the profession
- providing support and advice for dental practice managers
- providing a channel of communication and co-operation for all who are active in dental practice management
- encouraging further training and qualifications
- promoting a career structure and pay scale.

Further details can be obtained from the BDPMA website (www.bdpma.org.uk).

Salaried Dental Services

The Salaried (Community) Dental Services and **access centres** were established primarily to provide dental care for patients who are unable to register for treatment in general practice, and to provide care for adults and children in priority groups, including those with special needs. The main areas of activity are paediatric dentistry including school screening and orthodontics, special needs dentistry, health promotion and undertaking epidemiological studies; there is also an increasing role for providing the dental care for 'looked after' children and asylum seekers. Because of the large number of patients seen with special needs, some treatment is carried out under conscious, intravenous, intranasal or oral sedation. A general anaesthetic (GA) service was provided by many salaried dental service clinics. This service has remained under the management of the salaried dental staff, only now the procedures are carried out at a local hospital with critical care facilities to comply with GDC legislation. In some areas the GDC legislation has led to a reduction in the provision of a GA service.

The structure and set-up within the salaried service varies enormously over the whole of the UK. Clinics are managed and run independently within different regions, usually under the control of a clinical director, therefore the dental nurse structure and pay levels may also vary. The career structure within the salaried service is similar to that within general practice, with opportunities for advancement to senior dental nurse, principal dental nurse and dental nurse manager. Some salaried services offer dental nurses the opportunity to specialise in a particular area of dental nursing such as domiciliary care and special needs. Because clinics tend to provide dental services requiring special skills, nurses obtaining or possessing the NEBDN Sedation, Oral Health or Special Care Certificates, or those who have attended a GA course are very much in demand. The pay structure for the Salaried Dental Services is the same across the whole of England with different salary bands being assigned to each specific nurse's role.

Dental nurses in the salaried services are often involved in epidemiological studies, domiciliary visits and nursing home screening. The rural nature of some salaried dental service regions can mean considerable travelling between clinics or the delivery of health-care by means of mobile clinics. With the implementation of the Health and Social Care (Community Health and Standards) Bill which came into effect in 2005, the distinctions between the General Dental Service (GDS), Community Dental Service (CDS) and the Personal Dental Service (PDS) have largely disappeared and they are combined within a Primary Dental Service for which the PCTs have commissioning (purchasing) respon-sibility. Some dental nurses work entirely within the emergency dental service, such as the 'out-of-hours' service, since it can fit in with a family lifestyle and working antisocial hours is often reflected in an increased salary scale.

Personal Dental Service (PDS)

One of the criticisms of NHS general practice has been that because it is delivered in the same way throughout the UK, it is not sensitive to the local needs of different population groups. The **National Health Service (Primary Care) Act 1997** provided the necessary legislation to establish the PDS on a pilot basis in 1998. The aims of the PDS are to:

- provide flexibility to address local needs
- improve access to NHS services
- reduce oral health inequalities
- increase the utilisation of skill mix (including the employment of dental therapists)
- provide more integrated health services for local communities
- provide better value for money.

The PDS pilot schemes were successfully established by dentists working in both the CDS and NHS general practice. These schemes have provided training and employment opportunities for nurses. As stated above, in 2005 the PDS pilot schemes have largely been incorporated into a salaried Primary Care Service administered by the PCTs.

Hospitals

Patients might attend an Accident & Emergency department by self-referral or referral from NHS Direct or from dentists as part of an out-of-hours emergency scheme for swell-ing, bleeding or trauma. Here they would normally be treated only as a medical emer-gency and then referred back to their general dental practitioner for ongoing longer-term care or a more appropriate hospital. There are three types of hospital that undertake the delivery of dental treatment:

- district/general hospitals
- dental teaching hospitals (schools)
- postgraduate teaching hospitals.

District and general hospitals

These hospitals specialise in orthodontics and oral and maxillofacial surgery. They usually employ a fairly small specialised workforce. Nurses working in these hospitals would be expected to undertake post-qualification training in the appropriate discipline.

Dental teaching hospitals/schools

Following a recent expansion in the number of undergraduate dental schools, there are now 13 dental hospitals/schools in the UK, located as follows:

Northern Ireland – 1
Scotland – 2
Wales – 1
England – 11

Their primary roles are the provision of dental care and the teaching and education of undergraduate and graduate dental students, together with the education of DCPs, i.e. dental nurses, dental hygienists, dental therapists and dental technicians. Dental hospitals are linked to university dental schools, which may be responsible for the teaching and the assessment of diploma or degree courses.

Not all hospitals provide training for every category of DCP. The training of dental nurses can also vary, with some hospitals taking on 20–30 students per year while others take only six per year. Some hospitals provide part-time training for dental nurses working in general dental practice. Most hospitals now deliver courses leading to one or more of the post-qualification certificates, although this is dependent on the demands within their geographical area. The structure for training dental nurses in teaching hospitals is subject to wide variation.

Trainee or student nurses receive a salary while undertaking a two-year training programme. They receive day or half-day release for their off-the-job training, and receive assessments and procedural instructions while working in the departments. They now work towards the NEBDN Certificate or the NVQ level 3 dental nurse qualification, but may also receive a hospital certificate or other in-house qualification.

Hospitals are usually split into different departments, such as periodontal, restorative, paediatric dentistry, etc. Qualified dental nurses tend to be assigned to certain departments and they only move due to nurse shortages. This consolidates their skills and they are able to gain additional qualifications to suit their working environment.

Some nurses act as co-ordinators and are employed in a certain field, such as sedation or implantology. Their role is to co-ordinate the clinical and administrative element of these treatment specialties. They undertake patient allocation and organise their own workload. These posts not only demand experience and post-qualification training in the specialist area, but also the ability to take initiatives and additional responsibility.

A **senior dental nurse** takes overall responsibility for the running and day-to-day management of a specific department. They are responsible for staff allocation, ordering supplies and regulating patient throughput, in addition to health and safety issues and Control of Substances Hazardous to Health (COSHH) regulations. They are required to liaise with the clinician or consultant to establish good relationships to help with the efficient running of the department. They are normally required to be qualified for at least a three-year period and preferably have a supervisor, leadership or teaching qualification.

Most hospitals have a **principal dental nurse** or dental nurse manager who may have responsibility and professional accountability for either just the qualified dental nurses working in the departments or for both the qualified staff and the staff within the school of dental nursing. There are also hospitals where the manager is responsible specifically for the school of dental nursing. Post-qualification management experience would be an essential criterion for employment in this role.

As can be appreciated, roles are different and varied throughout the country, as are the criteria for appointment. A candidate for one of these posts would have to demonstrate considerable dental nurse experience, preferably in a wide range of work areas, and possess additional qualifications, especially in management.

A new post, that of **director of dental nursing**, has been developed within the dental nurse workforce. Such an appointee would have overall responsibility for dental nurse training and education within the hospital, and in addition would have responsibility for the delivery of external certification and post-certification courses.

Postgraduate teaching hospitals

These hospitals are usually slightly smaller than traditional teaching hospitals and specifically undertake research and the training of postgraduate students and DCPs to diploma or degree level. They do, however, recruit and maintain similar dental nurse staffing grades to the teaching hospitals described above.

Armed forces

The employment of dental nurses in the armed forces is different from that in civilian life. Personnel assisting the dentist are termed **dental clerk assistants**. They are graded into three categories.

Class III standard
This category can perform the following duties:

- select the appropriate instruments for any dental procedure and present them to the dental surgeon
- routine maintenance of dental equipment
- sterilisation of instruments
- taking of x-rays, and processing and mounting of films
- give emergency treatment for fainting, cardiac arrest, etc.
- carry out a range of clerical duties.

Class II standard

This category can perform the following duties:

- as for class III but with more experience and knowledge
- oral hygiene instruction
- carry out first aid
- handle classified documents.

The person holding this post usually holds the rank of lance corporal or corporal. They are responsible for supervising other dental clerk assistants and will be able to effect office management to a reasonable degree of competence.

Class I standard

The duties this category can perform are the same as for class II, with the following additions:

- have knowledge of relevant anatomy and pathology
- understand the principles and methods of sterilisation
- able to repair fractured plastic dentures
- able to undertake office management of a dental group headquarters.

This person may hold one of several different ranks, such as:

- sergeant or staff sergeant, who may be the senior dental clerk assistant in a multi-surgery dental unit
- company quartermaster sergeant in a dental unit
- warrant officer, who may be a chief clerk in a dental unit
- warrant officer class I, who could be a superintending clerk at the Ministry of Defence, administrative warrant officer of a dental group or a staff assistant in the dental branch of a formation headquarters.

The armed forces also provide facilities for hygiene, therapy and dental technology training. More information about employment can be found at the Dental Defence Services website (www.mod.uk/DefenceInternet/AboutDefence/WhatWeDo/HealthandSafety/DDS/).

Industry

Approximately 30–50 years ago saw the introduction of dental practices within industry. Many companies and large departmental stores such as Marks & Spencer saw the benefits in on-site dental and medical facilities, thereby relieving the need for employees to take time off for appointments that included additional time for travel.

The service is usually manned on a part-time basis, by dentists who work mainly in general dental practice. Nursing staff are either employees of the company or are employed by the dentist. Changes in industry have seen a marked reduction in industrial-based dental practice. Industrial practice provides an opportunity for nurses to become employees and enjoy the benefits of large organisations.

Bodies corporate

The term *bodies corporate* is used to refer to a particular group of dental organisations that share the same type of legal entity, although their philosophy and approach to dental care can vary considerably. The number of bodies corporate was restricted to 27, but following changes to the Dentists Act, any corporate body can now carry out the business of dentistry provided that it can satisfy the conditions of board membership set out in the amended Dentists Act. Employment opportunities can be explored by contacting these bodies corporate directly via their advertisements in the dental press, e.g. in the *British Dental Journal*. Examples of bodies corporate are Oasis Dental Care Ltd, Integrated Dental Holdings and Whitecross Dental Care Ltd.

Prison Service

The Prison Service does not provide its own dentists and nurses, but as with the industrial-based practices it contracts part-time staff to form the dental team. However, some prisons, e.g. Birmingham, have a full-time dentist. Recruitment may be problematic in view of the environment and the limited range of treatment provision. In some instances the salaried dental services hold contracts with the Prison Service for the delivery of primary dental care. Prison healthcare, including dentistry, is now also the commissioning (purchasing) responsibility of the primary care trusts. Dental nurses working within the prison service need to acquire additional skills, such as security awareness.

Interprofessional development

Dental hygienists

Under the Dentists Act 1957 a class of ancillary dental workers called *dental hygienists* was established. Hygienists are permitted to work in all sectors of dentistry. In addition to their health promotion role, they help to treat and prevent periodontal disease by scaling and polishing teeth, applying prophylactic and antibacterial materials, and applying topical fluorides and fissure sealants. A hygienist works to the written prescription of a registered dental surgeon. As from July 2002, following legislative changes and subject to appropriate training, hygienists are permitted to take impressions, administer inferior dental block analgesia, replace dislodged crowns with temporary cement, and carry out dental work on patients under conscious sedation.

Most dental schools are currently offering a two-year full-time diploma course and some, e.g. Manchester University, are offering a three-year degree course. Most of these courses are extended by an additional three months to include the Diploma in Dental Therapy. Entry requirements for training for dental hygiene vary between different schools, but normally two A-level passes are required, although applicants may be considered if they possess a nationally recognised dental nursing qualification. Further details can be obtained from the British Dental Hygienists Association website (www. bdha.org.uk).

Dental therapists

A dental therapist can undertake the full remit of the dental hygienist with the addition of simple restorative treatment in both deciduous and permanent teeth, and the extraction of deciduous teeth under local infiltration anaesthesia. Since 2002, following legislative changes and subject to appropriate training, therapists are permitted to take impressions, undertake pulp therapy on deciduous teeth, place preformed crowns on deciduous teeth, temporarily replace crowns and administer inferior dental nerve block analgesia. They are also permitted to treat patients under conscious sedation.

The number of dental schools offering courses leading to the Diploma in Dental Therapy linked with the Dental Hygiene Diploma has recently greatly increased. Further information can be obtained from the British Association of Dental Therapists website (www.badt.org.uk).

Dental technicians

Dental technicians are responsible for constructing a range of oral and facial appliances to the prescription of a dentist. They require a high degree of manual dexterity, problem-solving skills and the ability to use their skills across a wide and varied range of tasks.

Training can be achieved by full-time study within a dental hospital, college of further education or university. Trainees can also study on a part-time day-release basis from dental laboratories. The entry requirements are five GCSE grades C or above, or BTEC 1st in science. The qualifications they can achieve are:

- BTEC National Diploma
- BTEC Higher National Diploma
- BSc(Hons) Dental Technology (A-level entry only).

The disciplines covered in dental technology are prosthetics, crown and bridgework, orthodontic and maxillofacial appliances. The career opportunities include working in dental hospitals, community clinics, private commercial laboratories and laboratories attached to dental practices. Following changes to the Dentists Act, all dental technicians now have to be registered with the General Dental Council. Further information can be obtained from the Dental Technicians Association (DTA), formerly the Dental Technicians Education and Training Advisory Board, website (www.dta-uk.org or from www.nhscareers.nhs.uk/nhs-knowledge_base/data).

Clinical dental technicians

The GDC has approved the introduction of a new class of PCDs called *clinical dental technicians* who are able to undertake the clinical aspects of the construction of prosthetic appliances. Following new legislation, they have to be registered with the GDC and are able to practise subject to post-technician training in sciences, clinical and interpersonal skills. Further information can be obtained from the Dental Technicians Association (www.dta-uk.org).

Oral health education/promotion

The majority of oral health educators/promoters are employed within the salaried dental service, Personal Dental Service or in hospital settings, although some are now employed in general dental practices. Within the salaried service they not only work on an individual patient basis but also visit schools, care homes, Scout/Guide groups, and give oral health advice and messages to various target groups.

Within teaching dental hospitals oral health educators can have an oral health role for patients on wards in the main general hospital who have chronic illnesses or for those who have illnesses that have side effects affecting the teeth, gingivae or oral structures, such as cancer patients. They may also advise special needs patients visiting the hospital on an outpatient basis.

The National Oral Health Promotion Group is a forum for all professionals interested in the promotion of oral health. The group holds an annual conference and details can be obtained from www.nohpg.org

Nationally recognised oral health courses available for dental nurses include the following:

- The NEBDN post-qualification course, the contents of which are covered in more detail in Chapter 2. This course predominately focuses on one-to-one teaching and applicants must be qualified and registered to undertake this course. A number of centres in the UK offer this course.

- The Royal Society for the Promotion of Health Foundation Certificate in Oral Health Promotion. This is a 13-week course with approximately 32.5 hours of teaching held in Stoke-on-Trent. Details can be obtained from www.hpromo.northstaffs.nhs.uk/pdfs/RSH_Info.pdf

Orthodontic therapists

In 1999 the General Dental Council agreed to establish a new type of PCD known as an *orthodontic therapist*. This PCD classification is not to be confused with the remit of the orthodontic nurse described in Chapter 5. The orthodontic therapist is trained to undertake more specialised and complex tasks, details of which are available in the teamwork publication *Changing Roles in the Dental Team*.

Training for orthodontic therapy is available to nurses holding the NEBDN National Certificate, NVQ level 3. Several training programmes have now been established, either associated with existing dental schools or as outreach programmes. The courses are of approximately 12 months duration, a considerable part of which involves practical chair-side clinical experience. The training programme leads to a Diploma in Orthodontic Therapy, currently awarded by either a university or the Faculty of General Dental Practice.

Teaching and training

The NEBDN has offered the national certificate in Dental Nursing since the foundation of the Board in 1943. There is now the alternative of obtaining competence and qualifications via the NVQ route. It is not the purpose of this book to provide details of NVQ level 2 and level 3 qualifications, but an overview of the NVQ process can be found in *Changing Roles in the Dental Team*.

The introduction of the NVQ level 3 dental nurse qualifications has seen the development of many new and diverse appointments. The main areas of progression within the teaching area are discussed below.

Dental tutor or trainer

This role is primarily involved in the setting up and delivery of either a syllabus for the National Certificate or knowledge evidence and performance criteria for the NVQ. The main qualification tutors usually hold is the City & Guilds 7404/6 teaching qualification. This allows a person to teach the subject in which they are qualified and occupationally competent. Within the NVQ framework tutors or trainers can also hold the D32/33 Award, which enables them to assess their students' progress. Additionally, tutors or trainers can obtain the Certificate of Education, which allows them a broader scope within their teaching. Tutors or trainers are employed in teaching hospitals, colleges of further education, training centres, large practices that deliver their own training and the armed forces.

Assessors

This role is encompassed within the NVQ framework. The assessor's role is to act as an independent unbiased person to ensure the trainee dental nurse is competent in their area of work. They assess the performance criteria within the workplace that the students must undertake. The assessor carries out this assessment and makes the decision as to whether the student is safe and understands what they are doing. The assessor should hold a **D32/33 Assessors Award**. In January 2003 this qualification was upgraded and replaced by the **'A1 and A2' Assessors Award**. The qualification takes from three to nine months to complete depending on access to students, motivation and time constraints.

Assessors can be employed on a full-time, part-time time or peripatetic (as and when required) basis by centres delivering the NVQ qualification. Initially, NVQ centres planned to train and qualify assessors working within general dental practices to assess their own student dental nurses working with them. This resulted in a number of difficulties, such as the time required to undertake the assessment, particularly for remote rural practices, funding issues and the lack of independence of the assessors. It has therefore been found to be more effective to train enthusiastic dental nurses to be assessors but employ them on a peripatetic basis and send them to other practices to assess trainees they do not know who are undertaking the qualification. This has proved to be a more successful solution.

Internal verifiers

This is a completely new role within dental education. The role of the internal verifier is to sample portfolios of students who are undertaking the NVQ to determine whether the assessor has made a valid decision on their work. They are checking to ensure there is sufficient evidence, it is authentic, current and reliable, and signatures and dates are valid. It is one of the many quality assurance mechanisms within the qualification.

The internal verifier must posses a D34 Internal Verifier qualification. In January 2003 this qualification was upgraded and replaced by a 'V' unit qualification. They are also required to be qualified and occupationally competent in the dental field. They can work full time (although there are very few centres large enough to warrant full time), part time, peripatetically or can be subcontracted by centres that require this facility but have no one suitably qualified.

External verifiers

External verifiers are employed by the awarding bodies, i.e. City & Guilds and the Scottish Qualifications Authority. Their role is to provide support and advice to centres and act as the main quality assuror for the course. They visit the centre twice a year and check that systems are in place to offer a fair, equitable qualification.

The external verifiers are usually employed on a yearly contract for a minimum of 20 days per year and they are allocated centres around the region in which they reside. While verifying centres, they are expected to complete the **D35 qualification** which is delivered by the awarding body. They must be occupationally competent in their field of expertise and hold the D32/33/34 qualifications.

Centre managers/NVQ co-ordinators

The establishment and delivery of the NVQ and the complex funding structures involved have led to the development of managers/co-ordinators to manage the areas. Most are employed on a full-time basis and possess all the above qualifications (barring D35), including a management qualification.

Post-qualification courses

Currently, the most widely accepted post-certification courses are those awarded by the NEBDN. The first of these courses was the Certificate in Conscious Sedation introduced in 1989, followed by the Oral Health Education Certificate in 1991. The success of these qualifications led to the development of the General Anaesthetic Certificate in 1996, the Special Care Dental Nurse qualification in 1998, the Orthodontic Dental Nurse qualification in 2000, and in 2010 the Implant Nursing qualification.

The delivery of these courses in many instances is based at the large teaching hospitals, due to the depth of training and resources required to deliver the course, although the Oral Health Education Course has been delivered successfully for many years at local colleges or training centres.

Attendance certificates

In the past, dental nurses have been encouraged to attend courses relevant to either their work environment or to develop their own interest. These were delivered either by marketing companies, BADN training days or teaching hospitals. On some occasions attendance certificates were issued for the nurse to retain or display in the practice.

Statutory registration and CPD has changed this concept, and now registration is mandatory, dental nurses are required to attend relevant courses to keep up to date in order to maintain their annual registration. The provision of attendance certificates has become obligatory for those delivering the course and an essential requisite for dental nurses in enabling them to build up a portfolio of CPD.

There are a number of core areas in which dental nurses will need to keep up to date on a regular basis including:

- cardiopulmonary resuscitation
- first aid
- health and safety
- infection control.

References and further reading

Department of Health (1999) *Continuing Professional Development: quality in the New NHS*. London: Department of Health.

Faculty of General Dental Practitioners (2002) *Teamwork 6: Changing Roles in the Dental Team*. London: Faculty of General Dental Practitioners (UK).

General Dental Council (2008) *Continuing Professional Development (CPD) for Dental Care Professionals*. Available for downloading from www.gdc-org.uk

Whaites E (2005) *Radiology and Radiography for Dental Nurses*. London: Churchill Livingstone.

2 Oral Health Education

Mike Wanless and Mary Cameron

Promoting oral health

Introduction

The role of the dental nurse is constantly developing. In promoting oral health this can vary from translating the hard to hear or understand words of a dentist to active involvement in dental and general public health programmes. *Scope of Practice* (General Dental Council, 2009) has stated that dental nurses can undertake further oral health education and promotion activities subject to appropriate training and competence. It has also enabled dental nurses to undertake a range of other duties, such as the application of fluoride varnish in a programme overseen by a consultant or specialist in dental public health, and other activities, such as using plaque indices. These provide direct opportunities for further involvement in oral health promotion. It also enables dental nurses to perform other patient care duties, which will give them more oral health education opportunities. There is now opportunity for nurse-led clinics in dental practice and community settings. The scope for oral health education and promotion is expanding.

Health education and health promotion

Health education can be defined as any learning activity that aims to improve an individual's or community's knowledge, attitude and skills relevant to their health needs. However, until the mid-1980s the term *health education* had been used widely to describe intervention by health professionals who decided there was a health need. Health education is an integral part of health promotion offering relevant information to individuals or groups. The recipients can then make an informed choice about their health.

The *Our Healthier Nation* (Department of Health, 1999) document highlighted the following health education responsibilities in its contract for health.

- Government and national players can raise awareness of health risks clearly to the public, e.g. smoking, oral cancer.
- The public and others should have the information they need to improve their health.
- People can take responsibility for their own health and make healthier choices about their lifestyle.

The **World Health Organization** (WHO) defines health promotion as a process of enabling people to increase control and improve their health. To reach a state of complete physical, mental and social well-being, an individual or group must be able to identify and realise aspirations, to satisfy needs and to change or cope with the environment. Health is therefore seen as a resource for everyday life and not the object of living. Health is a positive concept emphasising social and personal resources as well as physical capacities. Oral health is certainly encompassed within this definition because a healthy, functioning dentition throughout life will ensure that an individual is free from dental pain, able to eat properly and has a socially acceptable smile.

PUBLIC POLICIES	HEALTHY SURROUNDINGS
• Codes of practice, e.g. on tobacco advertising • Legislation on water fluoridation, seat-belts • Food hygiene regulations • Taxing 'unhealthy products', e.g. tobacco and subsidising 'healthy products', e.g. fruit in schools • Wider availability of sugar-free foods, drinks and medicines and provision of sweet-free checkouts	• Improved housing • Environment safety measures such as safe disposal of sewage • Safe drinking water • Workplace health policies • Provision of safe equipment and protective clothing at work
HEALTHY LIFESTYLES	HIGH-QUALITY SERVICES
• Mass media campaigns, e.g. breast feeding awareness, National Smile Week • One-to-one patient education • Health education/promotion in schools and workplaces, e.g. healthy choices awards • Training for health professionals to enhance their knowledge and skills in health education, e.g. nursing/care staff	• Screening programmes, e.g. cervical and breast cancer • Immunisation programmes • Access to affordable dental services to all groups

Figure 2.1 Examples of general health and health promotion.

The **Ottawa Charter** set out at the first international conference on health in 1986 recognised that health promotion is not just the responsibility of the health sector but goes beyond healthy lifestyles to well-being. Figure 2.1 illustrates some examples of general health and health promotion.

Oral health promotion

Who is involved in oral health education and promotion?

A wide range of professionals and agencies outside dentistry have a key role to play in improving the oral health of the nation. Figure 2.2 illustrates some of these professionals and agencies who are involved in oral health education and promotion.

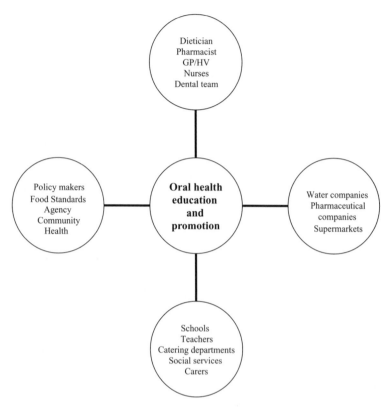

Figure 2.2 Who is involved in oral health education and promotion? GP, general medical practitioner; HV, health visitor.

Definitions

There are many different terms that are used to describe the ways in which people work together to promote health. Although these are often used interchangeably, it is possible to distinguish between them.

- **Multi-agency** refers to organisations that belong to the same sector, such as health, social services or education, and who are all statutory providers of public services.
- **Partnership** refers to joint action between partners (national and local agencies and the public). It refers to equal sharing of power.
- **Inter or multidisciplinary working** is sometimes used to describe joint working of people with different functions or roles within the same organisation or across sectors.
- **Intersectoral** goes beyond any one sector and may include the public, voluntary groups, public and private business and commerce.
- **Collaboration** is a term often used in health promotion. It requires the active participation of a wide range of agencies at national and local levels.

Primary healthcare team

Health visitors have a duty to all parents, carers and new infants. Their public health role is expanding. It is now integrated into the child health surveillance programme which covers weight, height and the oral health status of each child. This programme enables the health visitor to offer advice and support to new parents. There is the opportunity to encourage toothbrushing as soon as the first tooth erupts, weaning advice and, of course, early registration with a dentist.

Community nurses visit people in their own homes and are therefore able to build a strong relationship with their patients over a period of time. This enables them to carry out extensive one-to-one education, such as encouraging a patient to remove and clean dentures to prevent oral infections, and this may in turn affect the eating habits of the patient.

General medical practitioners

General practice has traditionally been a private consultation between doctor and patient. Health promotion may consist of opportunistic advice or information relating to oral health care. However, it has been recognised that the general practitioner has a lead role to play in the screening process for oral cancer, especially with high-risk patients who may be attending for medical reasons other than a dental problem. The general practitioner, whenever possible, should also be prescribing sugar-free medication for patients.

Salaried dental services

Primary care trusts (PCTs) and health boards have salaried dental services (sometimes known as the Community Dental Service or CDS) that may offer specialised oral health promotion services. Sometimes such oral health promotion expertise may lie within the local department of dental or general public health.

Pharmacists

There are nearly 12,000 community pharmacists in the UK, who thus provide an ideal and accessible location for the provision of opportunistic oral health promotion advice. Many pharmacists, when possible, will alter a prescription for a sugar-free preparation if this has not already been prescribed by the general practitioner. Pharmacists also engage in National Smile Month campaigns at a local level to promote the key oral health messages.

Local authorities

Some authorities are major providers of housing. Most are major employers. Individual departments also have key roles in the promotion of health, which includes oral health. This may be incorporated into 'health at work' award schemes across the departments.

Local authorities may also provide a range of services for the community, which may include breakfast clubs and after-school care. Within both these settings toothbrushing programmes and a healthy snacking policy will influence positive oral health.

Residential care workers

Residential care workers have a key role to play in the care of older people. A healthy mouth will greatly assist in the nutritional status of a patient, which will in turn minimise illness. Care workers are often the people who clean dentures and when necessary call on the services of a dentist to visit a residential home. It is important that the correct techniques and materials are used and therefore appropriate training should be offered to all new staff.

Local education authorities

Local education authorities have the responsibility for health promotion in schools, colleges and youth clubs. Oral health is now integrated into the school curriculum and should also be reflected in the tuck shop, which many children will access throughout their school life.

Health Development Agency

The Health Development Agency has the task of leading and supporting health education in England. In Scotland, the Health Education Board carries out this function. In Wales, it is carried out by the Welsh Assembly and in Northern Ireland by the Northern Ireland Health Promotion Unit.

Food Standards Agency

The Food Standards Agency is an independent food safety watchdog set up by an Act of Parliament in 2002 to protect the public's health and consumers' interests in relation to food. One of the aims of the agency is to promote honest and informative labelling to help consumers. Clarity in labelling will assist in the selection of healthier food and drinks, which will impact on oral health in the future. Currently ingredients are listed in weight order, with the main ingredient being listed first. While many manufacturers and retailers provide additional nutritional information, the differences in presentation and the use of small print often make comparison very difficult. It is not realistic for a consumer to read all the labels while shopping.

Supermarkets

Supermarkets are key players in the availability of affordable fresh fruit and vegetables that encourage parents to purchase healthier options for the family. Reducing the number of sweets sold at checkouts, where young children often see and ask parents to purchase on their behalf, is perhaps an area that needs to be addressed. Many supermarkets still have large numbers of checkouts with sweets on show.

In order to guide a patient through changes in their lifestyle to improve health one must consider past and current influences and behaviours. This information enables the dental team to target their advice appropriately, making it relevant and realistic to patients.

Socialisation

Socialisation is the direct or indirect effect of social norms on an individual's attitudes, beliefs, values, knowledge and behaviours.

What are attitudes, beliefs and values?

Attitudes

These are learned feelings that influence a person's particular circumstances. This learning does not have to be based on personal experience; it may be the result of social, cultural or economic influences. These are extremely influential both in terms of **primary socialisation**, which occurs within families, and **secondary socialisation**, which takes place as people learn behaviours that help them to be accepted into a wider social group. This is reflected in popular culture, family, social status, peer groups and the media.

When attitudes are being challenged it is essential that this is done in a non-threatening manner, as health professionals' values may well be resented by those from other backgrounds.

People's attitudes are made up of two components:

- **cognitive**: the knowledge and information they possess
- **affective**: their feelings and emotions, and their evaluation of what is important.

Beliefs

These determine preference based on current knowledge. They can be changed more easily than attitudes, because to change whatever knowledge the belief is based on alters the belief. However, beliefs alone are unlikely to change behaviour. Health beliefs are built on information collected from a wide range of sources. Some of these will be scientifically accurate and some inaccurate and potentially harmful messages, which are motivated by commercial ends rather than health gains. The dental team can lessen the damage of inaccurate messages by offering patients the information they require to make a valued judgement in their decision making.

Values

These are vitally important in forming the rules by which we live. They are an integral part of how we make judgements. To make people change, oral health educators need to identify a person's values because they are a powerful force in shaping behaviour. Values give an individual a positive or negative attitude towards someone or something.

Attitudes, beliefs and values are embedded within primary and secondary socialisation stages. These are explained below in relation to the stages of life and influencing factors.

Primary socialisation

Primary socialisation takes place in the pre-school period. The most important influences on the child at this time are the immediate family, especially the mother. The attitudes, beliefs and values of parents are demonstrated in their behaviour patterns. A good role model in terms of regular, thorough toothbrushing will greatly assist the dental team in reinforcing the oral health messages.

Most parents are motivated to provide the 'best' for their children and therefore should have a positive attitude towards good oral health. Unfortunately there are many barriers to achieving the positive outcome of a healthy mouth. Confused beliefs (toothbrushing prevents decay) and contradictory attitudes (visiting a dentist is expensive, time-consuming and not worth the effort) all have a negative impact on good oral health.

A parent may believe that grandparents may be offended if they are not allowed to give the grandchildren sweets. Many grandparents as well as parents need to be offered support to recognise the hidden cost of using sweets to control or reward children; the dental team can play a valuable role in helping them first to understand and then to find alternatives.

Secondary socialisation: the formal process

Secondary socialisation begins when the child goes to school. This is when the child learns to relate to the outside world away from the security of the family. The influences in secondary socialisation are teachers, friends, classmates and the media. The process continues throughout life, so that later on neighbours, work colleagues and others will be important influences. Behaviours learnt in this stage are much more rational. They are based on decisions that are much less reliable than habit and routine. An example of this is toothbrushing where a patient may make a rational decision to start to brush their teeth more often. However, laziness, forgetfulness and shortage of time may influence the subsequent behaviour.

Changing behaviour

The work of Prochaska and DiClemente (1984, 1986) highlighted that any change we make is not final but part of an ongoing cycle of change. Their work has focused on encouraging change in addictive behaviours, although the model can be used when trying to change or acquire behaviours. This process is illustrated in Figure 2.3 and identifies the following stages.

Precontemplation

Those in the precontemplation stage have not considered changing their lifestyle or become aware of any potential risks in their health behaviour. When they become aware of a problem, they may progress to the next stage.

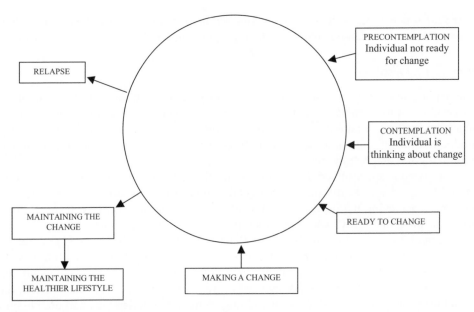

Figure 2.3 The stages of change model (after Prochaska and DiClemente, 1984).

Contemplation
Although individuals are aware of the benefits of change they are not ready and may be seeking information or help to make that decision. This stage may last a short while or several years. Some people never progress beyond this stage.

Ready to change
When the perceived benefits seem to outweigh the costs and when the change seems possible as well as worthwhile, the individual may be ready to change, perhaps seeking some extra support.

Making a change
The early days of change require positive decisions by the individual to do things differently. A clear goal, a realistic plan, support and rewards are features of this stage.

Maintenance
The new behaviour is sustained and the person moves into a healthier lifestyle. For some people maintaining the new behaviour is difficult and the person may revert or **relapse** back to any of the previous stages.

It is not perceived to be a failure on the part of the patient who relapses but recognition that the individual can go both backwards and forwards through a series of cycles of change.

Prochaska and DiClemente argue that while few people go through each stage in an orderly way, they will go through each stage. This has proved helpful for health professionals, who find it reassuring that a relapse on the part of their patient is not a failure, but that an individual can go both backwards and forwards through a series of cycle changes – like a revolving door. Thus a patient with periodontal disease may initially improve their oral hygiene after a visit to the hygienist, but after a period of time may lapse into neglecting flossing or brushing regularly. Nevertheless, the patient is still aware of the benefits of improved oral hygiene and the hygienist may be able to focus on small changes, which can provide the hygienist and the patient with a sense of achievement and identifiable progress.

While individuals may not have an awareness of contemplating, actioning and maintaining change, the intention will be based on individuals deciding it is in their best interest to change. The key to successful intervention is for the patient to be motivated. In oral health education, motivation for a long-term lifestyle change is challenging unless the patient is also aware of short-term benefits. It is difficult to maintain enthusiasm for restricting intake of sugar or for thorough daily oral hygiene for better teeth in later life. Feeling better or being more attractive now rather than later may be more influential in promoting the desired behaviour. Recent anti-smoking campaigns have started to include a greater emphasis on short-term improvements such as the reduction in blood pressure and heart rate after just 20 minutes. If a patient does not make the short-term change, there will be no long-term change either.

Oral health education

Before targeting any oral health promotion activities it is important to consider the ways in which people learn, levels of understanding and the skills they will need to carry out any behavioural changes.

Types of learning

There are three types of learning.

- **Cognitive**: learning that takes place in the head and deals with thinking skills.
- **Affective**: learning that comes from the *heart* and deals with attitudes and behaviours.
- **Psychomotor**: learning that involves the hands and deals with physical and practical skills.

When asking a patient to make changes in their or their child's lifestyle it is necessary to consider the depths of learning that this change requires. Different depths of learning will have the effect of using different verbs to measure the levels of knowledge required.

This can be illustrated by using an example such as toothbrushing. When asking a patient to list or state a fact, you are relating only to *rote learning* which involves solely the memory, therefore you have no assurance that someone can actually explain what something means.

It is important to measure a patient's level of understanding before they leave to ensure they know why they are carrying out a particular task or purchasing a specific type of toothbrush. This type of activity can be measured using verbs such as *explain* and *describe*, and on this occasion both memory and understanding are being used. When asking a patient to select an appropriate toothbrush and demonstrate their toothbrushing technique you are now able to measure all three levels:

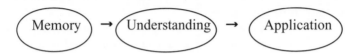

Aims and objectives

Once the level of knowledge required has been established it is necessary to have specific aims and objectives to measure the effectiveness of any activity. Aims and objectives help to identify what someone is hoping to do and how they are going to achieve it.

An **aim** is a general statement of intent. Examples might be:

- to promote oral hygiene
- to promote safer snacks.

Umbrella statements like these are useful as they help to give a broad overall view before specialising in introducing objectives. There are, however, limitations in solely using aims as one is never certain whether aims have been achieved and therefore they are of no use without objectives.

Objectives are what one is trying to achieve, reach or capture; they are much more specific than aims and therefore can be identified as a means of achieving an aim. Objectives will always contain a key verb which will give evidence of behavioural change having taken place.

Objectives should be **SMART**:

Specific
Measurable
Achievable
Realistic
Time-related.

Examples of objectives are:

- to **state** the reason for flossing regularly
- to **list** four sugar-free snacks
- to brush teeth and gums effectively

- to **identify** three types of sugar on food labels
- to **select** the correct fluoride supplement for their child
- to **describe** the early carious lesion.

Some further examples of aims and objectives linked together are shown in Figure 2.4. It is necessary to consider carefully what is being asked of someone and is it achievable. Using the checklist illustrated in Figure 2.5 can help in this process.

As well as setting aims and objectives it is necessary to identify the target group. If a practice nurse is invited to speak to a local group about oral health it is necessary to consider the following points.

- How much do you know about your target group?
- How many will be in your target group?

AIM:

To provide an overview of periodontal disease

OBJECTIVES:

1. Understand the formation of plaque

2. Identify the role of plaque in periodontal disease

3. Describe the stages of periodontal disease

4. Classify the types of inflammation related to periodontal disease

5. Identify the role of calculus in periodontal disease

AIM:

To provide an insight into the caries process

OBJECTIVES:

1. Identify the factors involved in the caries process

2. Understand the acid attack theory

3. Describe the Stephan curve

4. Understand the role of demineralisation/remineralisation

Figure 2.4 Examples of aims and objectives in oral health education.

AIMS AND OBJECTIVES: CHECKLIST

- What are your aims?

- Are they clear and understandable by other people?

- Do your objectives agree with your aims?

- Are your aims and objectives consistent with what your target group might want to learn about?

- Have you checked with your colleagues that these aims make sense?

- Have you set realistic targets for your aims and objectives?

Figure 2.5 Checklist for aims and objectives in oral health education.

- What is the age range of the group?
- What sex/race are they?
- How will their culture, social or environmental background affect the way they will understand your presentation?
- What will they expect from your presentation?
- What do they already know about your topic?
- What misconceptions might you have to correct?

Planning an oral health education session

To assist in the delivery of oral health education (OHE) a formal lesson plan should be written. Before this can be done the following questions need to be answered.

Information required before a lesson

- **Number in group**: this will determine the number of resources required, e.g. tooth-brushes, leaflets, etc.
- **Age and ability**: this will influence the type of activity and resources that can be used, e.g. games, disclosing tablets or solutions, etc.
- **Any previous instruction or prior knowledge**: this prevents duplication. New information will maintain interest.
- **Location**: size of the room, access and availability of the location, e.g. church hall.
- **Time of lesson**: this may be, for example, before or after lunch. Children react differently at different times of the day.
- **Length of time available**: this will reflect in the objectives set – SMART (see Aims and objectives).
- **Power supply available**: this is necessary when using additional resources.

- **Use of additional resources**: these may be overhead projector (OHP), screen, sink, video recorder. These are all useful resources to maintain interest with groups and expand activity, e.g. sinks are needed when disclosing with individuals.
- **Blackout facilities**: necessary when using slides or OHP.
- **Chalkboard**: particularly important if no electrical supply is available.

Why have a lesson plan?

A lesson plan makes it possible to do the following.

- **Provide an analysis**: a structured lesson plan allows each section of the lesson to be reflected upon and any alterations made for the future.
- **Establish realistic achievable objectives**: in considering the age, ability, resources and the methodology it will become apparent if the objectives set are achievable.
- **Establish what has to be taught**: defining the topic will assist in formulating the lesson.
- **When and to whom methodology**: this information ensures the lesson is pitched at the right level.
- **Establish a logical sequence invoking the principles of learning**: introduction and developments incorporate different levels of activities aimed at the group. The summary and conclusion brings the lesson to a natural closure.
- **Determine resources/materials required**: it enables the resources to be clearly identified, indicating when and where they will be used.
- **Avoid teaching from memory since this is not dependable**: a written lesson plan will assist on returning to the right section if you are disturbed or interrupted.

It should always be remembered, however, that a plan is a plan and not a straitjacket and should be altered accordingly.

Information to be included in a lesson plan

- Aims and objectives
- Target group
- Topic and duration
- Time and evaluation process

Sample lesson plan templates are shown in Figures 2.6 and 2.7. Examples of how these might be completed for a typical lesson are shown in Figures 2.8 and 2.9.

Evaluation

Evaluation is needed to assess results, determine whether objectives have been met and find out if the methods used were appropriate and efficient. It should be carried out for the following reasons.

LESSON PLAN						
LOCATION DATE DURATION AIM OBJECTIVES TOPIC EDUCATOR'S NAME						

	TIME	KEY WORDS	CONTENT	METHOD		AIDS
INTRODUCTION						
DEVELOPMENT 1				TEACHER ACTIVITY	STUDENT ACTIVITY	

Figure 2.6 Sample: lesson plan 1 template.

	TIME	KEY WORDS	CONTENT	METHOD		AIDS
DEVELOPMENT 2				TEACHER ACTIVITY	STUDENT ACTIVITY	
DEVELOPMENT 3	TIME	KEY WORDS	CONTENT	METHOD		AIDS
				TEACHER ACTIVITY	STUDENT ACTIVITY	
CONCLUSION						
SELF-EVALUATION						

Figure 2.7 Sample: lesson plan 2 template.

LESSON PLAN					
LOCATION DATE DURATION AIM OBJECTIVES TOPIC EDUCATOR'S NAME	Surgery 1 3 April 2004 30 minutes Highlight the importance of effective oral hygiene The patient will be able to: 1. Understand the role of plaque in gum disease 2. Identify signs of poor oral hygiene 3. Highlight areas of plaque accumulation using disclosing solution 4. Brush teeth and gums effectively A. N. OTHER				

	TIME	KEY WORDS	CONTENT	METHOD		AIDS
INTRODUCTION	3 mins	Introduction	Reason for visit	Friendly, informal welcome		Name badge
DEVELOPMENT 1	7 mins	Plaque	Describe plaque Relate to photographs 1–3 on flip charts	OHE ACTIVITY Demonstrate Discussion Q & A	PATIENT ACTIVITY Observation	Flip chart Pages 1–3 Stages of plaque formation Bacteria involved

Figure 2.8 Completed example: lesson plan 1. OHE, oral health education.

- To assess what has been achieved. Did the intervention have its intended effects (**efficiency**)?
- To measure its impact and whether it was worthwhile (**effectiveness**).
- To judge its cost effectiveness and whether the time, money and labour were well spent (**economy**).
- To inform future decisions and plans
- To justify decisions to others perhaps for funding or future support.

Evaluation of health programmes is usually concerned with identifying their effects. The effects of an intervention may be evaluated according to its:

- **impact**: immediate effects such as increased knowledge or shifts of attitudes
- **outcome**: the longer-term effects such as changes in lifestyle.

Outcome evaluation
What is assessed and how it is assessed depends on the aims, objectives and methods of the programme. As has previously been described, any objective should be **SMART** (see Aims and objectives).

	TIME	KEY WORDS	CONTENT	METHOD		AIDS
DEVELOPMENT 2	8 mins	Healthy gums	Relate to: Page 4: photograph pink, firm, healthy gums	TEACHER ACTIVITY	STUDENT ACTIVITY	Flip chart Pages 4–6 Healthy gums
				Discussion Q & A		
		Inflamed gums	Pages 5–6: bleeding, shiny gums Relate to patient's mouth	Demonstrate	Observation	Inflamed gums
				Demonstration Q & A		Mirror
DEVELOPMENT 3	TIME	KEY WORDS	CONTENT	METHOD		AIDS
	10 mins	Disclosing tablets	Explain role of disclosing solution Use disclosing tablets Systematic approach to brushing on models Patient brushes own teeth and gums	TEACHER ACTIVITY	STUDENT ACTIVITY	Flip chart Page 7 Disclosing tablets Mirror Vaseline Models Toothbrush and paste
				Observation	Practical	
				Discussion Q & A		
		Effective brushing		Demonstrate	Observation	
				Observation	Practical	
				Q & A		
CONCLUSION	2 mins	Consolidation of objectives Positive reinforcement with patient				
SELF-EVALUATION		Forward planning assisted in positive feedback from patient Objectives 1–4 achieved. However, need for reinforcement at future visits if necessary				

Figure 2.9 Completed example: lesson plan 2.

Changes in **knowledge** can be assessed by:

- interviews and discussions
- pre- and post-questionnaires
- short answer tests.

Changes in **attitudes** can be assessed by:

- pre- and post-questionnaires with a rating scale.

Changes in **behaviour** can be assessed by:

- pre- and post-questionnaires
- records of behaviour, e.g. diet sheets.

Changes in **skills** can be assessed by:

- pre- and post-clinical examination, e.g. plaque scores and gingival indices.

Process evaluation

This is concerned with assessing the process of the programme/session implementation. It addresses the participants' perceptions and reactions to the intervention and identifies the factors that support or limit these activities. Process evaluation is therefore a useful tool to assess the appropriateness and acceptability of the intervention.

The following methods may be used in the evaluation process.

Self-evaluation/reflective practice: this should always be done to assess positively what was well done and what could be improved. Self-evaluation can be undertaken as an ongoing process for reflective practice. It may, however, be carried out at a specific point in time immediately after the event or days or weeks later. There are a number of useful questions that can be asked.

- Prior to presentation:
  - ☐ Who is your intended target group?
  - ☐ How will you decide what should be evaluated?
  - ☐ How will you carry out the evaluation, e.g. questionnaires, demonstrations etc?

- After the presentation:
  - ☐ How happy are you with its effectiveness?
  - ☐ What have you learned from giving the presentation?
  - ☐ What would you most like to change?
  - ☐ How durable is your presentation; will you or could you use it again?

Peer evaluation: feedback should be obtained from a colleague who has observed or participated in the lesson. An observer may have a different, more independent, less emotionally involved perception of the presentation. They can observe the presenter's body language, speech pattern and how the audience behaves when eye contact is not made with them. They can concentrate on the content and presentation of the session without the distraction of having to deliver it.

Target group evaluation: This can be assessed by:

- verbal and non-verbal feedback
- active participation
- questionnaires, rating methods
- reviewing the content and presentation of the programme.

It may be carried out immediately after the event or deferred for days or weeks. Deferred evaluation can result in a poor response or inaccuracies due to memory loss of the participants, but it provides an opportunity to assess any long-term changes in knowledge, attitudes or behaviour.

Questionnaires are very powerful evaluation tools but require great skill to design if they are to be useful or effective. All questionnaires should first be piloted using a small number of respondents who are not going to participate in the final evaluation. This will help to eliminate simple design errors. The types of questions used reflect the quality of data obtained. Closed questions (see Ways to improve communication, below) are easy to analyse but give limited information. Open questions allow great variation in the answers but make analysis more difficult and can be a disincentive since they take longer to complete. Some common faults are spelling errors, poor grammar, poor layout, illogical ordering of questions and making the questionnaire too lengthy. Generally speaking, anonymous questionnaires will result in a greater response rate and will probably provide more honest answers. Further information on questionnaire design can be found in Oppenheim (1999).

Cost-effectiveness

- Time spent
- Number of staff employed in activity
- Cost of resources, e.g. room hire, equipment, materials, etc.

Evaluation is only worthwhile if it will make a difference. This means that the results of the evaluation need to be interpreted and fed back to the relevant parties. An indication in advance that this is going to take place will often improve the response rate of the participants.

Principles of communication

There are many aspects to consider when communicating with individuals or groups. In oral health education much communication involves face-to-face contact with an individual, a family unit or a group. Face-to-face communication is a two-way process in which all participants transmit information about what they know and feel. Effective communication involves being aware of what we are saying, how we are saying it and how it is being interpreted by other people. Everyone makes judgements about the person with whom they are communicating and there are skills that the oral health educator can use to convey messages and recognise how they are being interpreted.

Research has shown that we rapidly make judgements about the person with whom we are communicating. This applies whether we are talking, listening or observing. The judgements made can help or hinder communication.

It has been shown that when an individual makes a judgement on what sort of person is communicating with them or on how that person feels, the decision is based on a combination of factors. These can be classified as verbal, paralinguistics and non-verbal communication. **Verbal communication** relates to what the person says. **Paralinguistics** relates to how they say it and includes voice tone and volume, speed of speech and the uhms and ahs they say. **Non-verbal communication** includes gestures, facial expression, eye contact, body language and clothes.

Research has indicated (Mehrabian, 1981) that value judgements on the person communicating with us are based on these three factors in the following percentages:

- verbal – 7%
- paralinguistics – 38%
- non-verbal – 55%.

These figures are only approximate but indicate the relevance of the adage 'It isn't what you say, but the way that you say it'. Further, they show that non-verbal communication is the most important factor in assessing the person with whom we are communicating. Oral health educators should therefore be aware of the signals they are transmitting non-verbally and those of the patient or group with whom they are communicating.

If the oral health educator is to address the needs of their patients, the first and most important communication skill is listening. Unless the patient's needs can be identified they cannot be met. It is important that the oral health educator should both listen and show that they are listening.

Active listening is a term used to indicate the skills that show one is listening. It involves appropriate verbal responses, but again paralinguistics and non-verbal communication are the more important features. The acronym **SOLER** is useful for the non-verbal demonstration of listening:

Square
Open
Leaning
Eye contact
Relaxed

Square. For effective demonstration of listening skills the oral health educator should face the client squarely. Otherwise they might seem uninterested.

Open. Open body position involves avoiding crossing arms and legs, as these are often interpreted as a defensive or shutting-out action.

Leaning. A slight forward lean indicates an eagerness to hear more.

Eye contact. When listening, most people maintain good eye contact and this encourages speakers to continue.

Relaxed. A relaxed posture is important, as otherwise the communication will seem very artificial.

It should be remembered, however, that overdoing these powerful signals can be confusing and therefore discretion is necessary.

The educator should also be aware of the effects of height and distance. Height is often associated with power. Patients may feel vulnerable if they have to look up at the person with whom they are communicating. For discussion as equals, both parties should be at an equal height. Shy people may feel more confident speaking if the other person is lower than they are. All people have an area of personal space and feel threatened if a person with whom they are not intimate invades it. The oral health educator should look for non-verbal clues to check they are not too close to the person they are trying to help. They should also look for similar clues to indicate that they are not too distant. If they are too far away, communication will be lacking any sense of working together and is not likely to be effective. Some people need more personal space than others. City dwellers are used to having people around them and will tolerate the close proximity of strangers better than country dwellers. The appropriate distance varies with their relationship to the person with whom they are communicating. The closer the relationship to the other person, the closer they will be tolerated. Because of the individual nature of personal space it is worth asking if the patient is comfortable with the standing or seating arrangements and moving either nearer or further apart if they are not.

Barriers to communication

It is also useful to be aware of potential barriers that may impact on the delivery of oral health education/promotion. **Social** and **cultural barriers** include:

- ethnic/cultural and religious beliefs
- socioeconomic groups
- family values.

All of the aforementioned must be carefully considered in order not to offend or set objectives that perhaps cannot be achieved due to pressures outside the control of the individual or group.

It may be the case that an individual may not wish to or cannot communicate because of learning disabilities or may be too busy or preoccupied and does not see oral health as important in their list of priorities. On some occasions negative communication may be influenced by:

- a bad past experience of dental treatment
- the patient thinking the oral health educator will pass judgement or criticise
- the patient thinking they know it all in relation to the advice being offered
- objectives being set too high; a patient may feel they cannot comply
- financial constraints; these will have an impact on the availability to purchase toothbrushes, toothpaste, etc.
- social constraints that relate to lifestyle; a patient may not want to give up sweets as they are used as a comforter or bribe with children.

Limited understanding or memory, poor English and the use of jargon or dental terminology will all have an influence on communication. Therefore knowing the target group will assist in the correct information being delivered in the most appropriate way. Reinforcement of messages will reduce the possibility of *information fade*. It is important that contradictory messages between other health workers offering conflicting advice or 'experts' changing their minds is minimised to enable the individual delivering or receiving information to have confidence and credibility. It is also important to be realistic and acknowledge that some deeply held beliefs may be contrary to current oral health education messages and extremely difficult to change.

Ways to improve communication

Communication is a two-way process that involves listening as well as talking. By using some simple techniques it is possible to improve the interaction between individuals or groups. The following need to be considered.

Respect
By identifying the patient's needs and expectations and involving them in decision making it is more likely that a positive outcome will be achieved.

Listening skills
Listening to patients is essential for an oral health educator to be able to help them. Until patients have been listened to, the oral health educator can not be sure that the patients' needs are being met nor can the best way to help be decided. Listening itself is a good starting point, but the patient also needs to know that they have been listened to. This is known as active listening. Active listening involves showing by body language, responses and questioning that we have truly heard and understood what the patient has said.

Questioning skills
Patients can be helped to talk by adopting a careful questioning technique. The following are examples of some of the different types of questions that may be used, although some are best avoided.

- *Closed questions*
  These invite a short response usually 'yes' or 'no'. Questions such as 'Do you like visiting the dentist?', 'Do you know what plaque is?' or 'Are you going to do this now or later?' are examples of closed questions. They fail to open up the conversation and allow the patient to give a reply without necessarily having given it much or any thought. Closed questions should be avoided. They can, however, be used to clarify what the patient has said, but give only limited information.

- *Open questions*
  These provide no guidance to the patient as to what might be the correct answer and cannot be answered by either 'yes' or 'no'. They require the patient to give some thought to the response. Examples are: 'What type of toothbrush do you use?', 'How often do you attend the dentist?', 'What is plaque?'.

- *Leading questions*
  These give the patient an indication of the answer that is expected. 'Surely you don't brush your teeth only once a day?' or 'You don't have more than one fizzy drink a

day do you?' are examples of leading questions because they give clues as to the answer that the questioner wishes to hear. The answers will therefore not necessarily be truthful.

- *Multiple questions*
  'Do you brush and floss your teeth?' is a multiple question. If the person questioned answers 'Yes', it would be impossible to determine whether the reply is yes to brushing, flossing or both. This type of question only serves to confuse everyone.

- *Offensive questions*
  It is all too easy to antagonise a patient by using an ill-conceived question. Saying to an overweight person 'Do you eat a lot of chips or doughnuts?' is likely to be interpreted as being offensive even if it is true.

- *Ambiguous questions*
  'Do you go to the dentist for regular check-ups?' is an ambiguous question since 'regular' to one patient might be once every six months whereas to another it might mean a visit every five years.

Encouragement should be offered, as this in turn will enable the patient to feel positive about changes that are suggested.

Non-verbal communication should also be considered when interacting with patients, for example:

- physical appearance, i.e. uniform or casual clothes
- facial expression – welcoming smile
- posture – relaxed rather than crossed arms
- eye contact – shows interest
- hand and head movements acknowledge responses
- non-verbal behaviour – yawning indicates a lack of interest!

The environment in which oral health advice is offered can have an impact on the patient's receptiveness to advice. A comfortable, non-clinical setting in which the seats are carefully positioned at the same height to prevent a non-threatening approach is desirable. This format will enable the patient to feel more comfortable.

Language should also be carefully considered as follows.

- Tailor messages to the needs of the individual.
- Talk at the same level.
- If there are communication problems, speak clearly and simply.
- Do not use jargon.
- Use a logical sequence when explaining key messages.
- Check understanding by asking the patient to confirm knowledge.
- Gain feedback to improve the next session, if necessary.
- Reinforce the message to ensure retention.

Relevant visual aids will assist in retaining the interest of the patient.

- Demonstrations are always a useful tool to tell and show techniques.
- Patient involvement – active participation will allow the patient to feel included.

Levels of preventive intervention

The type of preventive message needs to be related to the relative stages of the disease process that the target group is experiencing. This can be considered under the headings below.

Primary prevention

This is the stage where there is no disease present and any information or advice is related to potential health threats. Offering appropriate dietary advice to mothers of very young children even though the primary dentition has not erupted will reduce the caries risk. Similarly, offering fissure sealants as the permanent molars erupt is another preventive regime.

Secondary prevention

Secondary prevention relates to changing the behaviour of a person who is at risk of a disease but has not yet developed it, such as a smoker who is still healthy. This does not fit well with the main dental diseases, which are extremely common and of insidious onset. The dental profession usually interprets secondary prevention as being concerned with the prevention of the development of existing disease, minimising its severity and reversing its progress. Some behavioural change is necessary. For example, patients with gingivitis may be able to return to a healthy gingival state if they improve their oral hygiene regime.

Tertiary prevention

Tertiary prevention is concerned with preventing deterioration, relapse and complications associated with a disease process. A patient with dentures will never regain their own dentition, but it is important to offer advice on denture care and the need for regular dental attendance to monitor the health of the oral tissues and the fit of the denture.

Identifying the stage that a patient is at before intervention will greatly assist in the delivery of an oral health message specific to that individual or group.

Evidence-based prevention

It is important that the dental nurse is able to assess the evidence that supports the advice and preventive measures being given to the patient. The strength of evidence indicates the level of confidence that we can have that our information is correct and therefore unlikely to change. This is often presented in the form of a hierarchy such as the following.

- **Level 1** Systematic review of a number of well-designed random controlled trials (RCTs).
- **Level 2** Evidence from at least one well-designed RCT. The evidence is not as strong, as it has not been replicated by other researchers on different populations.
- **Level 3** One or more studies where bias has not been controlled by randomisation, such as a cohort or case control study.
- **Level 4** Evidence from well-designed non-experimental studies from more than one research group or centre.
- **Level 5** Opinion of respected bodies or organisations based on clinical studies, reports of expert committees or descriptive studies.

As the hierarchy is descended the information available is less robust and is more likely to change as new evidence becomes available. A systematic review is a very thorough review of the available evidence, which states the criteria by which studies were included and excluded and details of the assessment criteria on which its findings are based.

There have been a number of systematic reviews of oral health education and promotion. Most notably that of Kay and Locker (1998) indicated the lack of high-quality evidence in both domains, to the extent that it is generally unclear what activities are effective in producing significant long-term change. They did find strong evidence that indicated the utilisation of fluoride as being effective in reducing caries incidence.

Prevention of dental disease

The main dental diseases are preventable. Individuals who can control their frequency of sugar intake can prevent themselves from developing caries. Those who can clean their teeth thoroughly every day can prevent themselves from suffering from periodontal disease. Restriction of alcohol intake and not smoking reduces the risk of oral cancer. Prevention relies mainly on the person looking after their own oral health with the support of their family, carers and peers. The dental team can help by giving scientifically correct messages in a way that the person can understand and act on. They can also help through the application of preventive agents such as fluoride. As discussed earlier in this chapter empowering the individual is far more effective than reliance on professional help.

The *Scientific Basis of Dental Health Education* can be downloaded from the Business Services Authority website (www.nhsbsa.nhs.uk/dental). It is also available in print format. It gives excellent guidance to an oral health educator to give to patients. Clear and simple messages are backed up by scientific information and advice. Comprehensive knowledge of this document is essential for any oral health educator.

Formation and structure of plaque

Plaque is involved in both dental caries and periodontal disease. It is a soft bacterial deposit that forms on the surface of the teeth. The first deposit to form on a cleaned tooth is the acquired pellicle. This is a film of glycoproteins from saliva formed within a few minutes. Bacteria can stick to this film and within about three hours there will be considerable colonisation. Unless removed, the bacteria will multiply.

Plaque changes in nature as different organisms start to grow within it. The plaque, however, will be composed almost entirely of bacteria (70%) and the substance they have produced, the **matrix**. Food is not a main component of plaque.

If left, the plaque can absorb minerals from the saliva to become **calculus**. This is physically hard and has a high inorganic content (70–90%). It is partly crystalline and partly amorphous calcium phosphate.

Dental caries

Dental caries is caused by the action of acids on the surface of the tooth. Bacteria in plaque, especially *Streptococcus mutans*, metabolise sugars and some other carbohydrates. They produce acid, which attacks the tooth. The plaque also holds this acid in contact with the tooth. As the acid attacks the tooth, calcium and phosphate ions leach out of the tooth into the plaque. This is known as **demineralisation**.

If the plaque is not fed with sugars, the calcium and phosphate ions slowly return to the tooth, repairing it. This is called **remineralisation**. If, over time, demineralisation continues more rapidly than remineralisation, caries will occur and progress.

Many mothers believe that their teeth are weakened when they have a baby. There is no evidence that calcium and phosphate ions leave the teeth during pregnancy to aid the growth of the baby. Even if this did happen the teeth would remineralise. Some mothers also blame themselves unnecessarily for their children's weak teeth as they think they did not consume sufficient calcium in pregnancy. Again there is no evidence that this is a factor in developing caries. In the UK there is no evidence that a lack of calcium in the diet increases susceptibility to caries. While these suppositions have become accepted wisdom in some societies, they are 'old wives' tales' and should be discouraged. They may prevent people taking the action for themselves to look after their oral health and that of their family.

Progress of caries

Many books describe the carious process but the importance of the surface layer of enamel is not always indicated. The surface is so resistant to caries that in the early stages the main area of demineralisation is beneath the surface. Because of its colour, this is known as a **white spot lesion**. At this early stage caries is reversible – the tooth can fully recover. If the caries continues to progress the surface will break down and the tooth will not be able to repair itself completely. Caries can then either become **arrested** (i.e. stops progressing) or it may continue.

Frequency of sugar consumption

There is a very strong association between the frequency of sugar consumption and caries. The most important sugars are the **non-milk extrinsic (NME) sugars**. These are the sugars added to food and drinks during their manufacture and in the home. They include sucrose, the type of sugar with which we are most familiar. Others are dextrose, glucose, glucose syrup, maltose, invert sugar, fructose, hydrolysed starch and lactose. Lactose is a sugar found in milk and is less likely to cause caries.

Fruit contains naturally occurring sugars known as **intrinsic sugars**. Intrinsic means that the sugar is part of the cell wall. These sugars are not so rapidly broken down by the bacteria in plaque and are not likely to cause caries. Fruit juices, even without added sugar, can cause caries as the sugar has been separated from the cell walls and is easily metabolised. Juices have NME, not intrinsic, sugars.

Each time an NME sugar is consumed the plaque produces acid within one to two minutes. This is when demineralisation starts. It usually continues for about 20 minutes but can take up to two hours, depending on the salivary flow and the buffering ability of the saliva. Salivary flow may be reduced in the elderly, while people sleep and in conditions affecting the salivary glands and ducts. **Stephan's curve** is the name given to a graph that depicts the fall in pH in plaque following the intake of a 10% glucose solution into the mouth. A similar fall is seen with other concentrations and other NME sugars in foods and drinks. When the pH drops below the critical level of pH (5.5) demineralisation takes place; above this remineralisation occurs. Stephan's curve for someone taking sugar at mealtimes only and someone having frequent sugar intakes between meals is shown in Figure 2.10. As can be seen, with frequent sugar intake the pH remains below 5.5 for a considerable time. Sugar between meals increases the number of acid attacks and therefore also reduces the opportunity for remineralisation. This is the basis for the advice to restrict the frequency of intake of sugar-containing foods and drinks. Sugar at mealtimes only is not damaging as there are long repair periods and there will be increased salivary flow and therefore increased salivary buffering. Sugar intake between meals is relatively easily controlled. Most people can realistically control their diet sufficiently to ensure they get no further caries.

A similar demonstration of the importance of sugar intake frequency can be given using a **sugar clock**. Shading a 30-minute block on a drawing of a clock gives a visual indication which can be recognised by many patients. A sugar clock with a low number of acid attacks on the teeth is illustrated in Figure 2.11, whereas Figure 2.12 shows the increased number of acid attacks produced by the more frequent intake of sugar. This also reduces the length of time of enamel repair between intakes.

The progression of dental caries and its treatment is described in a number of books. It is important that the dental nurse can explain the process and procedures to patients in a simple, non-threatening way. Children and some elderly patients may well be at high risk of developing caries and if so, preventive advice should always be given. Many adult patients may only require repair to existing restorations. They may not develop new carious lesions.

Dietary advice should always be specifically tailored to meeting the health needs of the patient. For example, restriction of the frequency of sugar intake by young children can involve parental advice and practical tips to:

OCCASIONAL SUGAR INTAKES

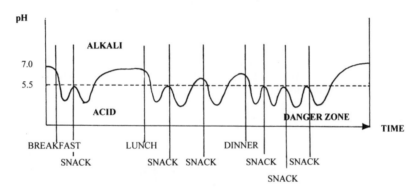

FREQUENT SUGAR INTAKES

Figure 2.10 Stephan's curve: the effect of the frequency of sugar intake on the pH level in tooth surface plaque.

- avoid sugared dummies or juices in a feeder cup or night comforter
- discourage the use of a bottle after 12 months – a cup is better
- restrict fruit juices and other acidic drinks to mealtimes and dilute well
- ask for sugar-free medicines.

For dietary advice to be effective it should be SMART – specific, measurable, achievable, realistic and time-related – in the same way as when an oral health educator is teaching a group (see Aims and objectives). Realistic objectives are more likely to be achieved than difficult or complex tasks. Small behaviour changes are more likely to be adopted than major ones. For example reducing the number of sugar intakes from 10 per day to six is more feasible than the total elimination of sugar. This could be a suitable objective for a person whose diet record indicates they have a particularly high frequency of sugar intake. If the patient achieves the objective they have agreed with the oral health educator they should be praised. A further objective may then be set, such as four intakes per day

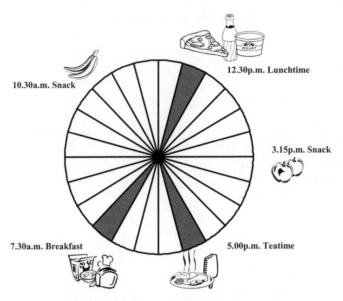

Figure 2.11 The sugar clock: a good day for teeth (reproduced with permission from Fuller S and Harding M (1991) The use of the sugar clock in dental health education. *British Dental Journal* 170, 414–416).

Figure 2.12 The sugar clock: a bad day for teeth (reproduced with permission from Fuller S and Harding M (1991) The use of the sugar clock in dental health education. *British Dental Journal* 170, 414–416).

if this is considered to be beneficial and achievable. Other advice may be to substitute a sugar-free cola for a sugary one. While erosion may continue to be a problem, caries will not be supported. Such a small behaviour change is more likely to be adopted and maintained than the advice to drink only water or milk.

The final target may be for patients to consume only those foods and drinks between meals that are safe for the teeth, but for many patients this is most successfully achieved in instalments rather than all at once. The small changes are likely to be supported by peers, friends and family, whereas a sudden dramatic change may make the individual feel isolated from those around them. In such isolation the behaviour change is unlikely to be adopted and even less likely to be maintained. Some people find the best way is to eliminate the behaviour completely, such as a smoker who may feel the need to quit completely at once, but for others a gradual alteration is more acceptable.

Some foods are alkaline and help neutralise acid. Hence peanuts and cheese have been recommended either as dentally beneficial snacks or a good food with which to finish a meal. However, as both contain a large amount of salt and fat, they are likely to be detrimental to general health if eaten excessively. Also if it is dentally acceptable to consume sugar at mealtimes, there appears to be no real reason to rapidly neutralise the plaque after meals.

Sugar-free chewing gum, fruit and vegetables stimulate salivary flow and thus aid remineralisation. For many individuals these are likely to provide a healthy alternative to sugar-containing foods and drinks.

Fluoride

The application of fluoride to the enamel surface increases the tooth's resistance to caries. The topical effect is more important than the systemic value of swallowing fluoride. This is because the important surface zone is being continuously attacked and repaired and, as discussed earlier, it is the integrity of this part of the tooth that decides whether complete repair is possible. A fuller description of the various mechanisms by which fluoride protects teeth can be obtained from the British Fluoridation Society website (www.bfsweb.org).

Toothpaste

All children should regularly use a correctly formulated toothpaste according to the manufacturer's and dentist's instruction. To reduce the risk of opacities children under six years who are at low risk of developing caries should use a toothpaste containing no more than 600 parts per million fluoride (F). Those with a higher risk of developing caries should use a standard 1,000 ppm F paste. In Scotland a 1,000 ppm F paste is recommended for all children as the caries rate is so high. Children under six years of age should use only a small pea-sized amount of paste. Children over six years should be encouraged to use a toothpaste of between 1,000 and 1,450 ppm F. An adult should supervise the amount of toothpaste used and the toothbrushing technique, up to at least seven or eight years of age.

Fluoride supplements

Fluoride supplements are of limited value as a public health measure but may be considered for those at high risk of caries. Factors that affect caries risk in children are shown in Figure 2.13.

The recommended levels of daily supplement in areas where there is no more than 0.3 ppm fluoride in the drinking water are:

- less than 6 months – nil
- 6 months–3 years – 250 micrograms F
- 3 years–6 years – 500 micrograms F
- over 6 years – 1,000 micrograms F.

Where there is between 0.3 and 0.7 ppm fluoride in the drinking water the recommended levels are:

GENERAL	LOW RISK	HIGH RISK
Social	Mother's education: secondary, tertiary. Good attendance pattern Family: nuclear, employment, social class I,II,IIINM	Mother's education: secondary only. Poor attendance pattern Family: single parent, social class IIIM, unemployment
General health	Good health No sugar-containing medication	Poor health/chronically sick Medication containing sugar
LOCAL	**LOW RISK**	**HIGH RISK**
Oral hygiene	Good oral hygiene, regular brushing twice per day with assistance	Poor oral hygiene, irregular brushing without assistance
Diet	≤ 3 sugary intakes per day	≥ 3 sugary intakes per day
Fluoride experience	Regular brushing with fluoride toothpaste Optimally fluoridated water	Irregular use of fluoride toothpaste No fluoridated water supply
Past caries experience	dmft ≤ 1, DMFT ≤ 1 No initial lesions Caries-free first permanent molars at 6–8 years of age 3 year caries increment ≤ 3	dmft ≥ 5, DMFT ≥ 5 ≥ 10 initial lesions Caries in first permanent molars at 6 years of age 3-year caries increment ≥ 3
Orthodontic treatment	No appliance therapy	Fixed appliance therapy

Figure 2.13 Factors affecting caries risk in children.

- less than 3 years – nil
- 3 years–6 years – 250 micrograms F
- over 6 years – 500 micrograms F.

Supplements are not recommended in areas with above 0.7ppm fluoride in the drinking water.

Sucking fluoride tablets until they dissolve in the mouth maximises the topical benefit. They are best taken at a different time from toothbrushing to increase the topical effect further and to reduce plasma levels of fluoride which peak after ingestion.

Professionally applied fluoride

Topical fluoride varnishes are effective and help arrest **nursing bottle caries** and cervical decalcification. The recommended dose should not be exceeded. Fluoride gels (e.g. acidulated phosphate fluoride containing 12,300ppm F) can also be effective. They are applied to the teeth in trays. They are not recommended for use in small children, as if swallowed, there will be high plasma levels of fluoride. They may also remove the glaze from porcelain crowns. They are less pleasant for the patient and not as safe as fluoride varnish.

Fluoride varnish application by dental nurses

Fluoride varnish can now be applied by appropriately trained and competent dental nurses. It can reduce the incidence of caries in children and adolescents by 33% (Marinho *et al.*, 2007). The varnish can be applied twice a year to the teeth of all children and young people, except those with a history of hospitalisation for asthma or who have the very rare allergy to colophony. Those at greater risk can have it applied three or four times each year. Fluoride varnish can also be used in the prevention and control of root surface caries in the elderly or those with reduced salivary flow. It also relieves the symptoms of dentine hypersensitivity experienced by patients suffering from tooth surface loss through abrasion, attrition or erosion. *Delivering Better Oral Health: an evidence based toolkit for prevention* (Department of Health/BASCD, 2007) provides guidance on recommended frequencies of application for different patient types.

Fluoride varnish can be applied in the dental surgery or in outreach situations such as children's centres, schools, residential and nursing homes. It is suitable for outreach situations as it is relatively simple to apply and does not need complete moisture isolation. As with many agents it is important not to exceed the recommended dose, which for a 2.26% varnish is:

- 0.25ml for the primary dentition
- 0.40ml for the mixed dentition
- 0.75ml for the permanent dentition.

If there is a small overdose the patient should be encouraged to vomit and be given a drink of milk as the fluorine in the varnish reacts with the calcium in the milk to form a stable compound so that less is available for absorption. If a large overdose is taken then the ambulance service should be contacted.

Role of toothbrushing

For a long time many dentists told patients that clean teeth do not decay and many people believe this to be so. It is incorrect. The use of a fluoride toothpaste reduces caries susceptibility as fluoride is applied to the surface of the teeth. The actual removal of plaque is relatively unimportant in caries control. It is the too frequent consumption of sugar that causes caries so it is best prevented by reducing the frequency.

Erosion

Frequent or prolonged contact between teeth and acidic foods or liquids may cause loss of enamel by chemical erosion. Erosion affects the tooth surfaces without the presence of plaque. While acidic drinks are the most common cause, some foods such as yoghurt are also acidic. Vomiting or gastric reflux also causes erosion. Conditions resulting in gastric reflux and vomiting are more extensively described in Chapter 3.

There has been a large increase in the consumption of **carbonated 'fizzy' drinks**, which are acidic. Any acid-based drink, such as cordials, squashes or fruit juices, can cause erosion. These are best well diluted and taken in moderation. Ribena Toothkind appears less damaging than other fruit-based drinks. Some drinks have what is called a high **titratable acidity**. This means that they are hard for the saliva to neutralise and are particularly damaging to teeth. Pure fruit juices have high titratable acidity. Carbonated water is acidic but has a low titratable acidity and so is less likely to cause severe erosion. Erosion is usually painless but there may be sensitivity to hot and cold stimuli. It is difficult to diagnose until well advanced. There is often a widespread loss of enamel affecting the labial and lingual surfaces of the anterior teeth and the occlusal surfaces of the lower molars.

Erosion may be reduced or prevented by:

- restriction of the frequency of acidic foods and drinks
- referral for investigation for frequent vomiting, as in bulimia, or gastric reflux
- the use of a straw to reduce erosion of anterior teeth
- avoiding holding or washing fizzy drinks round the mouth
- not brushing the teeth for about half an hour after drinking acidic drinks as more tooth substance will be brushed away.

There is lack of evidence that fluoride is effective in combating erosion, although its well-documented role in reducing demineralisation indicates it may be beneficial. Specialised toothpastes are available.

It is essential to identify the cause before restoration is attempted. Just covering eroded teeth would leave others exposed to continuing damage. Treatment can involve covering the teeth with porcelain veneers and metal casings, although restoration with composites and glass ionomers is becoming more commonplace.

Periodontal disease

Gingivitis may be considered to be the first stage of chronic periodontal disease. The gingival margin becomes red and swollen and bleeds when brushed. This can be reversed completely by effective oral hygiene. If allowed to progress, **chronic periodontitis** may develop. In periodontitis the bone and fibres that support the teeth are destroyed. Although this usually happens gradually, in some people it progresses rapidly.

There are several theories about how plaque causes periodontal disease. It is widely accepted that the bacteria in plaque release toxins which cause the inflammation. *Aggregatibacter actinomycetemcomitans* and *Porphyromonas gingivalis* are among the organisms that appear to be associated with periodontal disease.

The prevention of the disease is by the effective removal of plaque. Once-a-day plaque removal is sufficient so long as all the plaque is removed. A thorough cleaning twice a day is recommended as it gives two opportunities to ensure all the plaque has been eliminated. This fits in with most people's lifestyles and is a realistically achievable objective. Thorough cleaning is far more effective in preventing periodontal disease than more frequent but incomplete brushing to make the mouth 'feel nice'.

Smoking and diabetes are also important risk factors in periodontal disease. People vary widely in their susceptibility to periodontal disease. There are also considerable differences in the pattern of the disease. **Early onset aggressive periodontitis** is uncommon, affecting about one person in 1,000 in the UK. This term covers a range of disorders.

- **Pre-pubertal periodontitis**: which is usually associated with an immune system defect.
- **Localised** and **generalised juvenile periodontitis**: where there is severe disease before the age of 25 years.
- **Rapidly progressing**: in which most destruction happens in less than one year, usually before the age of 35 years.

Chronic adult periodontitis usually starts in the late teens or early twenties. It progresses slowly and is more common than the other forms.

Sub- and supragingival calculus contributes to the progress of periodontal disease. Calculus forms a rough surface onto which the plaque can stick. Calculus itself is inert and would be harmless if the plaque did not adhere to it. Orthodontic appliances, poorly contoured fillings and partial dentures can also contribute to plaque retention.

Prevention

Toothbrushing is the most important oral hygiene measure. A simple, short backward and forward scrubbing action is the simplest and most effective technique for most people, especially children. The more complex a technique is, the more difficult it is for the patient to learn and to maintain over weeks, months or years. Toothpaste has a detergent effect and some toothpastes also contain an anti-bacterial agent such as triclosan. A fluoride toothpaste should be recommended for its caries prevention properties.

A variety of other oral hygiene aids are available. For a patient with poor oral hygiene the first advice should be to develop a methodical, thorough brushing technique that causes no damage. This should then be established as a daily routine. When this has been achieved it can be supplemented with a variety of aids such as floss, tape and interdental brushes. It is good practice to concentrate on achieving oral health by helping patients learn one skill at a time.

Not all patients have good manual dexterity. Some will need a toothbrush adapting so they can grip it properly. Flossing is not suitable for young children. Wood sticks can cause damage if misused. While most people need encouragement to clean their teeth effectively, some patients will do so excessively. A heavy-handed enthusiast may cause tooth abrasion and gingival damage. Such a patient could be encouraged to use only small backward and forward actions. Holding the brush in a pen grip reduces the pressure with which the brush is applied.

There are many mouthwashes available for purchase. Some have little demonstrable effect. The most effective mouthwashes against plaque formation contain 0.2% chlorhexidine gluconate. If this is used for two minutes every 12 hours it prevents plaque accumulating on a clean tooth surface. It is not a replacement for toothbrushing as it should only be used for up to one month. It also tends to form brown stains on the teeth especially if red wine, tea or coffee are consumed. Chlorhexidine gluconate is also less effective if sodium lauryl sulfate, which is an ingredient of many toothpastes, is present in the mouth. Because of this the mouthwash should not be used until at least half an hour after toothbrushing.

The establishment of good oral hygiene is essential for success in both the prevention and treatment of periodontal disease. Unless patients clean their teeth effectively, established periodontal disease will progress despite the best efforts of the dental team. Many patients expect a six-monthly scale and polish. There is no evidence that this produces any significant health benefit. As calculus makes plaque removal difficult it should be removed, but the most important measure is the patient's daily oral hygiene routine. Any patient who needs regular scaling does not have a high enough level of oral hygiene to ensure any periodontal disease does not progress.

Dental nurses are permitted to use plaque indices to monitor patients' oral hygiene, so long as they are trained and competent to do so. There are many different indices which can be used. They use specific surfaces on selected teeth in various parts of the mouth which represent the whole dentition so that the operator does not need to measure how much plaque there is on all surfaces of all teeth. Most are used following disclosing of the teeth with a vegetable dye and record the amount of the tooth surface which is covered with plaque. Some indices measure the thickness of plaque at the gingival margin. The findings are converted into a numerical score. There is always some subjectivity in recording plaque levels but the operator should try to be as consistent as possible. The patient should agree realistic objectives with the operator and should be praised for any improvement seen. The amount of plaque varies with the length of time since toothbrushing and so a poorer score may be seen in afternoons than in the mornings.

Anti-bacterial chips can be placed by a hygienist, therapist or dentist. They are placed in periodontal pockets to prevent further progression and may be associated with limited repair in some patients. Periodontal surgery should be undertaken only once the patient has demonstrated that they can clean their teeth effectively and will maintain this, otherwise any surgery will be doomed to failure.

Once effective oral hygiene has been established and obvious plaque and calculus removed, **root surface planing** has been shown to be effective in resolving inflammation, reducing pocket depth and improving clinical attachment. A patient having root planing or other forms of periodontal surgery should be forewarned about the prospect of sensitivity (although this usually reduces with time) and gingival recession which may leave the margins of previously fitted crowns visible or give the appearance of 'being long in the tooth'.

Systemic antibiotics are of limited use in the treatment of chronic periodontal disease. Tetracyclines may help in early onset periodontitis as they may help to reduce the breakdown of collagen. Metronidazole may be used in slower adult forms. Such use of antibiotics is only in addition to other measures and on its own is ineffective and should be avoided.

Osseointegrated implants can be used to replace lost supporting tissues. Once the implant has successfully integrated with the remaining tissues it can be left for about six months and can then be used as a base for a denture, crown or bridge.

Acute necrotising ulcerative gingivitis

Acute necrotising ulcerative gingivitis (ANUG) is a much less common form of gingivitis. It is caused by anaerobic organisms (i.e. they thrive in the absence of air). Poor oral hygiene and stress may contribute to the disease. It is characterised by destruction of the interdental papillae of the gingivae, which become covered by a grey slough. The gingivae become painful and there is often noticeable halitosis. The pain will initially prevent effective toothbrushing. Anti-bacterial therapy is commenced initially to control the infection until the condition settles sufficiently to permit thorough oral hygiene. Metronidazole is an effective antibiotic. Oxygenation can be achieved using hydrogen peroxide or sodium perborate mouthwash. Effective daily oral hygiene should be encouraged as soon as the pain has subsided sufficiently to permit it. A chlorhexidine mouthwash will not have a marked effect on ANUG but may help to control plaque levels during the initial treatment. Following severe ANUG there may be cratering of the interdental papillae, which looks unsightly and makes oral hygiene difficult. Surgical recontouring may be necessary.

Denture stomatitis (denture sore mouth)

Many people who wear their dentures throughout the day also like to wear them at night. The continuous warm, damp environment in the mouth provides favourable conditions for the growth of the fungal organism *Candida albicans* (thrush). The area under the denture may become inflamed, or there may be painless white plaque which can be wiped off with some gauze. The area under the upper denture is most often affected. Prevention is best achieved by leaving the dentures out at night and stressing the importance of regularly brushing the fitting surface of the denture.

Angular cheilitis

If either of the dentures, or the teeth, are worn down there is a reduction in the height of the face. As the jaw overcloses, folds develop at the angles of the mouth that can become infected. This is known as angular cheilitis. It is characterised by soreness, redness and cracking at the corners of the mouth. Both *Candida* and bacteria (β-haemolytic streptococci or *Staphylococcus aureus*) are often involved. In addition to treating any underlying causes of overclosure, the patient should be advised to use an antifungal agent, such as miconazole, and hydrocortisone cream or nystatin ointment. For staphylococcal infection, the dentist can prescribe sodium fusidate ointment. Prevention usually involves restoring the vertical height of the face by building up the dentition or providing dentures of the correct vertical height.

Oral cancer

Each year about 3,000 people in the UK develop tumours in their mouths. Most are elderly, but the number of middle-aged people developing tumours has increased. Causative factors include smoking and alcohol consumption. Prevalence increases in patients who both smoke and drink, and with the frequency and amount. First signs may be symptomless ulcers, often on or near the tongue. They may be surrounded by a thickened area of tissue. Non-malignant ulcers usually heal rapidly when the cause is removed. Those associated with malignancy do not heal and should be referred without delay to a maxillofacial surgeon. This is described in more detail in Chapter 3.

Recommended tasks

(1) Write down what the term socialisation means. Thinking of patients, friends or relatives, who are the most important influences on a three-year-old child? Who are the most important influences on a 13-year-old child? Write down how an oral health educator can use this knowledge to help a patient adopt and sustain a healthy lifestyle.

(2) Identify a patient with whom you communicate well. How do you know that the two of you communicate effectively? Think of a patient with whom communication is difficult. Why is it difficult? What could you and the patient do to make it better?

(3) Refer to the record card of a child patient you know who has arrested caries. Can you identify when the caries stopped progressing? What caused the caries? Why did it stop? What role did the parent, patient or dental team play in stopping it?

(4) Refer to the record card of a child patient you know who has been referred for a general anaesthetic because of dental caries. Use your knowledge of the patient and the record card to see which of the risk factors apply to this patient. What could the family have done to avoid the extractions? What part did the dental team in the practice play? Check in the *Scientific Basis of Dental Health Education* to see if any other preventive measures could realistically have been used.

(5) Refer to the record card of a patient who has recently had teeth extracted for periodontal reasons. What indications are there that the periodontal status had been worsening? What could the patient have done to keep their teeth? What has the dental team done to help? Realistically what more could have been done?

Care of appliances and advanced restorations

Dentures

Full dentures

Ill-fitting dentures can damage tissues. This often appears as ulcers at the edges of the flange of the dentures. Treatment usually involves trimming and smoothing the denture or adding a soft lining. Where the denture is badly fitting or worn down a new denture is usually advisable. Sometimes the irritation may cause an overgrowth of the soft tissues. Such **hyperplasia** can be excised if it is not possible to adjust the denture to accommodate it. Malignancy is a possibility at such sites.

Dentures should be removed at night. This will help prevent **thrush**, a fungal infection caused by *Candida albicans* as described in the previous section. Thrush may be painless and appears as a red area, typically conforming in shape to the upper denture. It may also present as white patches on any surface within the mouth. These white patches can easily be identified as they can be wiped off on some gauze. Treatment consists of anti-fungal agents such as nystatin, amphotericin or miconazole.

Bleaching of dentures is popular with patients who want particularly white teeth. Some patients also use abrasive pastes or toothpastes. Patients should be strongly discouraged from using household bleaching agents. Soap, water and a toothbrush provide a cheap and effective cleaning mechanism which rarely causes damage. Patients should be encouraged to clean their dentures over a bowl, part-filled with water, so that the denture will not break if dropped. Proprietary denture cleaners can also be used, but may cause soft linings to harden.

Many denture wearers do not visit the dentist regularly. Even those with no natural teeth should be encouraged to visit the dentist once a year so that their mouth can be examined for any abnormalities such as early signs of malignancy.

When patients are first fitted with full dentures they should be shown how to clean them, and advised to cut up food well before eating, to eat soft foods if necessary, to remove their dentures at night and to return to the dentist for any adjustment.

Partial dentures

Partial dentures can be made from a variety of materials. Some proprietary cleaners are not suitable for some materials. For example, acidic cleaners may corrode certain metals. Soap, water and a toothbrush are appropriate for all dentures so long as they are well rinsed.

Particular attention needs to be paid to cleaning the teeth which abut the denture. Plaque stagnation may lead to periodontal disease and contribute to caries of the crown or root. The patient should be advised to remove the partial denture for cleaning as this makes cleaning the denture and teeth easier.

Patients should be instructed to return to the surgery if the denture is damaged or becomes ill fitting. They should not attempt to adjust it themselves.

Immediate dentures

There are two types of immediate denture, flanged and socket fit. **Flanged** immediate dentures help compress and protect sockets from which the teeth have been extracted. **Socket fit** dentures have no flange and may be a somewhat looser fit initially, especially if there is swelling, such as at the injection site under the denture. Patients should be warned to expect this. The denture should initially be worn continuously. The patient should return to the dentist for the removal and refitting of the denture for the first time. This is to make sure that the bony plates do not spring open preventing refitting in the case of a flanged denture, and that the replacement teeth are refitted back into the socket without displacing the gingival tissue in the case of a socket fit denture. Hot salt mouthwashes may be recommended.

Before the patient decides to have this course of treatment they should be informed that immediate dentures only have a short lifespan. The dentures will need relining or replacing after a few months, as there will be resorption of the periodontal tissues and loss of bone following the extraction of the teeth.

Orthodontic appliances

Removable orthodontic appliances

The patient should be instructed when to wear the appliance. This is usually all the time except when cleaning. It is important to clean the teeth and rinse the appliance after eating. The appliance should be worn when eating, as otherwise the forces on the teeth being moved tend to interfere with the treatment, which may prolong the treatment time. The patient should be instructed to pay particular attention to oral hygiene, control of sugar intake and also to avoid eating hard and sticky foods which may damage the delicate clasps and springs. The patient should also be told to contact the orthodontist immediately if there is any damage to the appliance or if the appliance cannot be worn for any reason.

Fixed orthodontic appliances

The patient should be advised to avoid eating sticky foods such as chewing gum and toffees which can damage arch wires or lead to debonding. The patient should not attempt to adjust the appliance or repair it themselves. They should contact the orthodontist straight away if it is damaged. Thorough oral hygiene with a fluoride toothpaste is important as demineralisation around the brackets can lead to caries. A fluoride mouth rinse should be recommended if the patient is at high risk of developing new caries. Chapter 5 on orthodontic nursing provides further guidance on the care of these appliances.

Crowns

Crowns need special attention. It is important for the patient to pay special attention to plaque removal from the gingival margin. Any further gingival migration may make the cervical margin of the crown visible. This can seriously impair the aesthetics of an anterior tooth. Even with a well-fitting crown there is always the possibility of stagnation around its margins. Oral hygiene aids, such as floss, tape or interdental brushes can be recommended. If flossing, care should be taken not to remove the crown inadvertently.

Bridges

Care needs to be taken not to damage bridges. They are susceptible to trauma and if the patient is involved in contact sports a mouth guard should always be worn. The periodontal health of the abutment teeth is particularly important. Any loss of attachment will increase forces on the remaining tissues and may lead to fracture or mobility of the bridge. Oral hygiene is again of great importance. Superfloss is suitable for cleaning under many pontics.

Implants

Thorough daily oral hygiene is essential to maintain the integrity of implants. Care must also be taken not to damage any part of the implant that protrudes into the mouth. While patients might consider metal studs to be robust they can easily be abraded or scratched.

Dental public health

Epidemiology

This is the branch of medicine concerned with the incidence and distribution of disease in populations. It involves looking at the relationship between disease and socioeconomic, geographic, environmental and other factors. Several factors may make someone more susceptible to a particular disease. The more common ones include:

- age
- sex
- social group
- smoking
- drinking
- diet.

Epidemiological data are important if preventive programmes are to be effective. If a particular group of people is more likely to be affected by a disease then preventive resources should be focused on the 'at risk' group rather than being spread thinly over the whole community.

Terms used in epidemiology

Experience: The cumulative effect of a disease past and present, up to the date of examination, i.e. caries experience includes decayed, filled or extracted teeth, where the extractions were due to caries.

Incidence: Concerns new disease occurring in a period of time, e.g. one year.

Prevalence: The amount of active disease present at any one time.

Epidemiological indices are used to assess either the prevalence or severity of disease.

National dental surveys

Standardised surveys are undertaken on randomly selected children and adults. These surveys enable health authorities and boards to compare their own results with other areas across the UK. National dental surveys are carried out by the **Office of Population Census and Surveys** (OPCS). Adults and children are surveyed every 10 years. The most recent adult survey was conducted in 2009 and the next child survey will be in 2013. **Scottish Health Boards' Dental Epidemiological Programme** (SHBDEP) takes place annually for five-year-olds. The NHS National Epidemiology Programme co-ordinates studies in England, Wales and the Isle of Man. These surveys are essential for monitoring progress towards the targets set out in oral health strategies.

Different ages are studied in different years. This gives a national picture of the distribution of caries in children. In general, caries rates are lowest in England, higher in Wales and Scotland, and highest in Northern Ireland. The studies also show reduced caries rates in areas with fluoridated water.

Fluoride in the community

Water fluoridation

In 1931, Trendley Dean started to investigate mottling of enamel in the USA. This had first been identified in Colorado Springs in 1902. He identified fluoride as the cause. He also noted the low caries incidence in people who lived in areas where the water was naturally fluoridated. He found that where the level of fluoride in drinking water was 1ppm there was nearly maximal reduction in caries experience and little noticeable mottling. Further information on fluoride and the fluoridation of water supplies can be obtained from the British Fluoridation Society (www.liv.ac.uk/bfs). This website gives details of the safety and general health effects of fluoridation.

Fluoridation of water supplies is the most important dental public health measure. A systematic review of the literature by the University of York in 2000 was critical of the quality of some studies but concluded that fluoridation is both safe and effective. The results can be viewed at www.york.ac.uk/inst/crd/fluorid.htm. The substantial reduction in caries levels outweighs the slightly increased risk of enamel opacities. Fluoridation is also effective in reducing health inequalities. The optimum level of fluoride in drinking water is 1ppm. Lower concentrations give less protection. The consultant in dental public health will be able to supply details of the fluoridation status in the area they cover.

Fluoride in food

In some countries, e.g. Switzerland, fluoride is added to basic products such as salt or bread, but it is not readily available in such a form in the UK. Schemes whereby schools are supplied with fluoridated milk have proved to be acceptable and provide a mechanism by which fluoride can be accurately targeted to those in need in communities where caries is prevalent.

Fluoride tablets have been tried as a community health measure. While they can be of considerable benefit to the individual patient they are less successful on a community basis. Few parents remember to give them to their children on a daily basis. This is not surprising as it is an extra behaviour they are being asked to do and there is no obvious immediate benefit. The parents most likely to comply are those whose children, in general, are least likely to need such measures.

Erosion

The epidemiological evidence of erosion is rather lacking. This is largely because it is only in recent years that dentists have become aware of how prevalent it is. It is also more difficult to diagnose than caries as it can affect many surfaces without being obvious. It is also difficult to standardise its recording by a group of dentists. Considerable work is being undertaken in this area.

Periodontal disease

Gingivitis is uncommon in young children but becomes widely present during adolescence. By puberty almost all children have gingivitis, probably as a result of hormonal influences. Chronic periodontal disease is irreversible and therefore the prevalence increases with age. In many individuals it starts in adolescence and the majority of the population are affected by the age of 30 years.

There are a number of indices that can be used to measure periodontal disease. The most widely used is the **Community Periodontal Index of Treatment Need** (CPITN). This is now also known as the Community Periodontal Index (CPI). It is similar to the **Basic Periodontal Examination** (BPE) score, but applied to populations rather than individuals. It is measured by gently placing a specially designed probe (WHO probe) into the gingival margin and measuring the depth of pocket, observing bleeding and the presence of calculus. For scoring, the mouth is divided into sextants. A CPITN score of 0 indicates healthy periodontal tissues, with no active treatment being necessary. Primary prevention includes reinforcing the existing good practice. If the gingivae bleed on gentle probing a score of 1 is given, indicating that oral hygiene instruction is necessary. A score of 2 is given if supragingival or subgingival calculus is present. The appropriate treatment is scaling and oral hygiene instruction. The same treatment is required for a score of 3, the probed pocket depth being 4–5mm. A score of 4 is given if the pocket depth is 6mm or more. This requires more complex treatment, including root planing and perhaps periodontal surgery.

Caries

Vipeholm study

Gustaffson led a large study into the relationship of sugar consumption and dental caries from 1945 to 1953. Such a study would now be considered unethical as it led to damage in vulnerable adults. The Vipeholm study demonstrated that:

- consumption of sugar at meals is associated with only a small increase in caries
- frequent consumption of sugar between meals is associated with a large increase in caries
- the increase in caries activity disappeared when high sugar snacks were stopped.

The study was undertaken at the Vipeholm Hospital in Sweden. This housed a large number of adults with learning difficulties. These patients were allocated to various test groups and a control group. The test groups had a basic diet supplemented with sucrose, which they were given in a variety of forms. Some were given these supplements at meals only and some were given snacks. The supplements were as drinks with meals, bread, chocolate, caramel, eight toffees per day and 24 toffees per day. In the 24 toffees per day group the increase in caries was so great that the issue of toffees was stopped. Further details are available in Murray's *Prevention of Dental Disease* (1996), which also gives details of other notable epidemiological studies into caries, including the Hopewood House and Tristan da Cunha studies.

There are many indices to measure caries experience. The most common one is DMF (also known as **DMFT**). This measures the number of **D**ecayed, **M**issing due to decay and **F**illed permanent teeth. It is written as **dmf** (i.e. lower case) when used for deciduous teeth.

Other studies have shown a strong correlation between the level of dental caries and the deprivation status of the population. The level of caries is higher as deprivation increases.

Dental services

Knowledge of the functions of different dental services is important so an oral health educator can inform people where they and their acquaintances can most appropriately access oral healthcare and advice. These services are described in Chapter 1.

Other providers of oral health education

It is important that the dental team works with other providers of oral health education. Consistent, scientifically correct messages need to be given by all. The dental team is in a good position to educate those who attend regularly for dental care. Irregular attenders are frequently those with the greatest need and have little contact with the dental team.

People other than the dental team may be even more important sources of oral health education advice. The mother is the most important influence on a pre-school child. A carer may be the most important influence on a disabled or elderly person. Key healthcare workers at various times in people's lives may be doctors, nurses, school nurses, health visitors, district nurses, carers, speech and language therapists, and indeed many others. Nursery nurses, teachers, classroom assistants, social workers and caterers can be very important in promoting oral health. The dental team can learn from colleagues in other roles and professions, just as much as they can learn from the dental team. Together, more can be achieved than by working in isolation.

The Ottawa Charter discussed earlier in this chapter indicated the importance of the community in promoting the health of its own members. The more people who are close to a person to support their health improvement, the more likely it is that the healthy choice will be an easy option and the more likely they are to be able to maintain a healthy lifestyle.

The greatest likelihood of healthy options being the easy ones are when policy makers, those who implement policies, health, education and social care professionals work in a co-ordinated way with the society for which they provide care.

Recommended tasks

(1) Find out the dmft of five-year-olds in the area where you work. Find out how this figure has changed over the past 10 years. How does the current figure compare with data from the 1970s? What do you think are the reasons for any changes?

(2) Look at the record cards of the last five five-year-old patients seen in your practice. How does their dmft compare with the mean in your area? Why might it be different?

Planning and setting up a preventive dental unit

Design

When designing an area for preventive use the basic function must always be kept clearly in mind. It is a place in which to motivate and communicate with patients effectively. Thus the surroundings and layout must be conducive to a relaxed atmosphere in which the patient will really listen and take on board the information that is being offered. It is most desirable that this area is entirely free from any clinical look or feel.

Consideration should be given to the needs and age of the patient who will be using this area, e.g. it is no good having a room entirely decorated with nursery-rhyme characters and then expecting to communicate effectively with a 12-year-old child or an adult. Material aimed at the youngest age groups can be restricted to one wall of the area which can be screened when the unit is being used by older age groups.

The ideal preventive dental unit (PDU) is one that is also perfectly suitable for preventive teaching of adults. Where there is a hygienist, it may be decided that adults needing plaque control guidance should receive this from the hygienist. However, even with adults there is a case for conducting these sessions in the completely non-threatening atmosphere of the PDU.

One of the biggest challenges encountered with any motivational activity is that of keeping the message constantly fresh as time goes by. Therefore, a set-up where the motivational material and resources can easily be changed and updated is extremely important.

There are several characteristics that contribute to a well-designed PDU or preventive area:

- fittings and furniture need to be robust
- worktops should be at a standard uniform height with no fixed fascia board underneath to enable access for people in wheelchairs
- all surfaces should be smooth and easy to clean to reduce the risk of cross-infection
- worktop space can be used for displays and flipcharts
- large size mirrors with an overhead light will give the illusion of extra space in small locations
- a well-lit room with a good level of background lighting will be needed for oral hygiene instruction
- small sinks with at least cold water should be available
- the layout should not place the dental professional in a dominating or confrontational position, therefore careful consideration to the choice of seating is necessary.

Barriers

In considering the aspects of a good PDU, barriers such as those listed below should be removed:

- the sight of drills or other dental instruments
- the noise of work going on in other surgeries such as air rotors, aspirators, etc
- the clinical smell of the surgery environment
- the nurse preparing for another patient as the dentist offers advice (or other staff causing distraction when the nurse is offering advice)
- appointments being made while the dentist/hygienist/nurse is offering advice
- advice offered in a hurried manner as the patient is leaving the surgery.

Recommended tasks

(1) You have been asked to plan a PDU where you work. Decide where it should be and what alterations you would need to make. How would the other members of your team be affected by these changes? Prepare how you would present the case for the PDU at your next team meeting.

Planning and preparing an exhibition or display

Questions to consider

Target group, topic, location, time, resources and cost all need to be considered in the planning stage of any promotional activity. The following specific questions need to be considered when preparing an exhibition or display.

- **Who will be viewing your work?**
  - ☐ What will be the age range and will the audience be the general public or health professionals?
  - ☐ Collect material appropriate to the target group, which may include text, diagrams, photographs, cartoons and slides.

- **How large a group will you be catering for?**

If large numbers are viewing use larger text or rotate the numbers attending at any one time.

- **How will your material be laid out?**

When creating your poster:

  - ☐ measure out available size
  - ☐ enlarge text on a photocopier
  - ☐ photographs can be enlarged or scanned
  - ☐ variations in colour, shape and size can make a display more interesting
  - ☐ stick the photographs onto a cardboard background to provide a frame
  - ☐ check the size that has been allocated and measure up posters beforehand
  - ☐ ensure poster is straight before framing
  - ☐ remember you do not have to fill all the available space.

- **Is the light adequate around your display?**

Selecting a bright area or locating the display beside a window will enhance the content of it. Care should to be taken to ensure that reflections from windows and lights do not obscure the images.

- **How long will your display be on show?**

If you are required to leave a display up for a long period of time it is worth having posters laminated. Make sure the display doesn't start to look tired and tatty.

- **Would you be able to use your display again?**

By carefully setting up and dismantling a display many aspects will be able to recycled for future exhibitions.

Location

Location checklist

- How big is the venue?
- Is there sufficient space for people to access and view the display?
- How many people will be present?
- Is your display part of a larger health promotion activity, e.g. nursery, residential home?
- What equipment and facilities are there available?
- If the display is manned all day it is useful to know if there are catering facilities.
- What problems might you encounter due to your location?
- What car parking facilities, lifts, janitorial services are available?
- Are there any limits to availability (when is the venue open)? A church hall or youth club may have restricted access which will impact on the set-up time available.
- How easy is it for wheelchair users to gain access to the venue?
- Access for all patient groups should be a priority.
- Floor space available should always be considered when measuring up for appropriate display boards.
- Seating (is there adequate seating for everyone who needs it?).
- Health and safety regulations should be adhered to at all times.

Resources

Resources checklist

- Have you identified all the material you could use as part of your presentation? Resources or promotional material includes display boards, notice boards, display items such as packaging, oral hygiene aids, leaflets, handouts, videos, flipcharts, colouring sheets, diagrams, models, games and stickers.
- What resources will you use? Consider the age and number in the group.
- Which of these will you use? Consider the cost and availability of material.
- How much freedom do you have to decide on what you will use?
- What resources are already available that you could make use of or adapt?
- What budget limitations are there on the resources you can use?
- Have you checked that the equipment you might need is available and working?
- How much time do you have to prepare yourself within the time available?
- Have you checked that the time, cost, etc. taken to prepare certain types of more technical material isn't going to detract from other cheaper and more easily created methods of presentation?
- You should not decide on what resources you are going to use before you have thought through your learners' needs, objectives and the topic you are going to cover.
- Make sure that your presentation is driven by the educational needs of your target group, rather than by what technology can do for you.

- Remember that a picture is worth a thousand words.
- Make sure that your choice of graphics is as self-explanatory as possible. Some graphics are much easier to understand than others.
- What graphics do you have already in your practice, clinic or at home which you could use?
- How can you adapt these to use in your presentation?
- Where else could you get hold of new material? Dental suppliers are often very helpful.
- What other graphics do you need or might you find useful?
- Identify how much you can do yourself and where you will need extra help.
- Remember that computers can produce graphics cheaply, quickly and efficiently.

When assessing either your own poster or leaflet or one produced by someone else there are some criteria that give guidance on how effective a communication tool it is likely to be. The following questions should be asked.

- Is the target group clearly indicated? People need to have evidence that the resource is of interest to them.
- Is the information scientifically correct? Incorrect information will confuse rather than help people.
- Is the aim evident? People like to know how they will benefit from looking at the display or reading the leaflet.
- Does the material address an oral health problem relevant to the target group? If the people do not perceive the resource as benefiting themselves or those close to them it will be ineffective.
- Does the material present a positive image? Fear arousal or any form of victim blaming can reduce the impact of the material. To empower people to look after their own oral health they should be encouraged with positive presentation of the benefits of the health behaviour.
- Is it understandable to the target group? Messages should be simple and short if possible. Written text needs to be understandable by those at whom it is aimed and presented so that it is likely to be read.

Readability

There are a number of different tools available to assess the readability of text. The **SMOG** (Simple Measure of Gobbledegook) index (see Table 2.1) is a simple measure of how readable text is. Ease of reading also depends on other factors, including design. The following points should be considered.

- It is important not to cram too much information in a leaflet or poster.
- Too little space between lines makes reading difficult.
- Space around 'chunks' of text is better for those who have difficulty reading. Fancy typefaces or lettering are difficult to read. Simple is easier!

Table 2.1 SMOG index: assessing the readability of a poster or leaflet.

1. Select a block of text
2. Select 10 sentences from the block of text
3. Count the total number of words in the 10 sentences which have three or more syllables
4. Multiply this number by 3
5. From the numbers below, circle the number closest to your answer:
   1   4   9   16   25   36   49   64   81   100   121   144   169
6. Select the square root of the number you have circled from the numbers below:
   1   4   9   16   25   36   49   64   81   100   121   144   169
   Square root: 1   2   3   4   5   6   7   8   9   10   11   12   13
7. Add 8 to the square root number to give the readability level
   The number of the readability level indicates the anticipated age range of the reader

- Lower case is easier to read than upper case.
- Overuse of capital letters to emphasise is counterproductive.
- Dark backgrounds make the words harder to read.
- Long sentences are confusing to those with limited reading ability.
- Long words are difficult to read.
- Even small amounts of jargon or words the reader does not know cause considerable loss of meaning.
- Writing as though speaking to the target group is helpful.

Recommended tasks

(1) Write down the information that you would give to a patient who is about to receive an upper partial denture for the first time. Check if your practice gives out this information in writing. Compare your advice with the information currently being given to patients. Should the information given to the patient be changed? Check the SMOG index (Table 2.1) for the readability of the written information.

Resources and information

There are readily accessible sources of information for dental nurses wishing to expand their knowledge of oral health, education, promotion and evidence-based practice. The Scientific Basis of Oral Health Education (Levine and Stillman-Lowe, 2004) gives an excellent account of current knowledge of oral health and disease, and contains a brief summary of levels of supporting evidence at the time of publication. Clear and simple messages are backed up by scientific information and advice. Comprehensive knowledge of this document is essential for any oral health educator.

The Scottish Intercollegiate Guidelines Network (SIGN) produces an extensive range of guidelines some of which are relevant to oral health promotion (www.sign.ac.uk). In England, copies of the joint Department of Health/British Association for the Study of Community Dentistry publication *Delivering Better Oral Health: an evidence-based toolkit* have been distributed to all practices (Department of Health/BASCD, 2007). It contains a comprehensive summary of the evidence-based procedures that can be used by all practices to ensure that they are being effective in the prevention of oral disease. It is to be updated regularly and can be downloaded from www.dh.gov.uk/en/Publicationsandstatistics/Publications/PublicationsPolicyAndGuidance/DH_102331. It provides superb guidance about preventive pathways that can help all the dental team.

The useful references listed below are published by NHS Scotland:

NHS Scotland – Action Plan for improving oral health and modernising NHS dental services in Scotland, www.scotland.gov.uk
NHS Quality Improvement Scotland: Scottish Intercollegiate Guidelines Network (SIGN) Guidelines
47: Targeted prevention of dental caries in the permanent teeth of 6–16-year-olds presenting for dental care.
83: Prevention and management of dental decay in the pre-school child.
Both are available on line at www.SIGN.ac.uk

The following are useful sources of further information.

- Local health promotion departments
- Commercial companies and their representatives
- British Dental Health Foundation (BDHF) – www.dentalhealth.org.uk
- Health Scotland (formerly Health Education Board for Scotland [HEBS]) – www.healthscotland.com
- The National Oral Health Promotion Group (formally the National Dental Health Education Group [NDHEG]) – www.nohpg.org
- General Dental Council – gdc-uk.org
- British Association for Dental Nurses (BADN) – www.badn.org.uk
- Childsmile (Fluoride varnish programme) – www.child-smile.org
- National Fluoride Information Centre – www.fluorideinformation.com
- British Fluoridation Society (BFS) – www.bfsweb.org
- Action for Information on Sugars (AIS)
- Food Standards Agency – www.foodstandards.gov.uk
- Her Majesty's Stationery Office (HMSO) – www.hmso.gov.uk
- British Nutrition Foundation – www.nutrition.org.uk
- The Health Development Agency (formally the Health Education Authority)
- The Institute of Health Promotion and Education – www.ihpe.org.uk
- Many intraoral pictures can be downloaded from the Image Library at – www.sciencecentral.com

Recommended tasks

(1) Think of a group of patients at your practice who have dental problems. What do they need to know to be able to look after their dental health? Think of SMART objectives (see p. 36) for what you want them to know or do. Design a simple display to achieve these objectives in a positive, easy way using words and pictures. If any of your objectives could not be achieved by the display, how else could they be attained?

References and further reading

Blinkhorn AS (ed.) (2001) *Notes on Oral Health (3e)*. Manchester: Eden Bianchi Press. This gives excellent guidance on oral health promotion. It offers considerable information at a reasonable price. Details can be obtained from helen.draper@man.ac.uk.

Department of Health (1999) *Our Healthier Nation. A Contract for Health*. London: The Stationery Office.

Department of Health/BASCD (2007) *Delivering Better Oral Health: an evidence-based toolkit for prevention*. London, DoH

Downer MC, Gelbier S, Gibbons DE and Gallaher JE (1994) *Introduction to Dental Public Health*. London: FDI World Dental Press. This gives useful information about measuring dental disease, the role of health promotion and contains a summary of considerations for questionnaire and interview design.

General Dental Council (2009) *Scope of Practice*. www.gdc-uk.org

Kay E and Locker D (1998) A systematic review of the effectiveness of health promotion aimed at improving oral health. *Community Dental Health* 15: 132–144.

Levine R and Stillman-Lowe C (2004) *The Scientific Basis of Oral Health Education*. London: BDA Books.

Marinho VCC, Higgins JPT, Sheiham A and Logan S (2007) Combinations of topical fluoride (toothpastes, mouthrinses, gels, varnishes) versus single topical fluoride for preventing dental caries in children and adolescents. Cochrane database of systematic reviews. Issue 2. Art.no: CD002781. DOI;10.1002/14651858.CD002781 pub2.

Mehrabian A (1981) *Silent Messages: implicit communication of emotions and attitudes (2e)*. Belmont, CA: Wadsworth.

Murray JJ (1996) *The Prevention of Oral Disease*. Oxford: Oxford University Press.

Oppenheim AN (1999) *Questionnaire Design, Interviewing and Attitude Measurement*. New York: St Martins Press. This gives detailed information on questionnaire design and gaining information from patients.

Prochaska JO and DiClemente CC (1984) *The Transtheoretical Approach: crossing traditional boundaries of therapy*. Homewood, IL: Dow-Jones/Irwin.

Prochaska JO and DiClemente CC (1986) Towards a comprehensive model of charge. In: Miller WR and Healther N (eds) *Treating Addictive Behaviour: process of change*. New York: Plenum Press.

SIGN guidelines at www.sign.ac.uk (under dentistry) give direction on the targeting of prevention to 6–16-year-old patients at risk of caries who present for dental care.

3 Special Care Dentistry

June Nunn and Tina Gorman

Introduction

Definitions

Special care dentistry is the branch of dentistry that aims to secure the oral health of, and enhance the quality of life for, people with disabilities where an interprofessional approach, supported by appropriate behaviour management techniques, is required to deliver efficacious and effective care in a holistic way. The people it serves have been defined as those who by virtue of illness, disease and/or its treatment, disability, lifestyle or cultural practices are at greater risk of poor oral health or for whom the management of dental care poses other health risks or who experience barriers to the access and receipt of dental care.

There has been a move away from the 'medical model' definition (divided into impairment, disability and handicap) which focuses on what a person *cannot* do, to the social model that focuses on an individual's impairment relative to the external environment in which they are situated and the obstacles thus imposed on them. It is thus society that disables people with impairments and the way to reduce disability is to change society, not the individual. More recently, the World Health Organization has moved to an International Classification of Functioning Disability and Health which is much more focused on functional aspects, that is what a person *can* do.

Social model of disability

Impairment: Is the functional limitation within the individual caused by physical, mental or sensory impairment. For example, having quadriplegic (all four limbs affected) cerebral palsy and being reliant on wheelchair to move around is a physical limitation.

Disability: Is the loss or limitation of opportunities to take part in the normal life of the community as an equal with others due to physical and social barriers. For example, a person who needs to use a wheelchair is restricted on where they can go because of lack of ramps.

Epidemiology

Numbers

It is estimated that there are 500 million people worldwide with a disability. In the UK there are 6.5 million disabled people, equivalent to one in eight of the population.

Among younger people, there are more males than females with disabilities, with the exception of specific impairments such as spina bifida and some syndromes, e.g. Rett's syndrome. The causes of the majority of disabilities can be divided into: (i) genetic, e.g. Down syndrome; (ii) acquired, e.g. brain injury; and (iii) a combination of these, e.g. cleft lip and palate. However, in many conditions the cause is unknown.

Demography

As the survival rate of very premature babies increases, so does the number of people with disabilities. Currently, a baby born at 24 weeks has a 25% chance of survival, at 26 weeks 50% and at 28 weeks 90%. Such young, small babies need to be ventilated and they are prone to brain haemorrhage. For the survivors, there is a 5% chance of severe disability and a 10–15% risk of impairment. Survival into adulthood is also increasing. About 70–80% of people with spina bifida reach their twentieth birthday and many live well into adulthood; the average life expectancy for people with cystic fibrosis is 26 years and with lung/heart transplants even longer. There has been a 400% increase in survival from leukaemia since 1960. Most people with Down syndrome live to 55 years and older. Survival is not without other, acquired impairments. Two-thirds of the people with disabilities in the UK are over the age of 65 years. Of those over 85 years of age, 20% are house-bound and 12–14% of these people are bed-bound.

Barriers to care

Barriers fall broadly into two main categories: physical and attitudinal. Examples of **physical barriers** include stairs for people with mobility problems and inadequate communication systems for those with sensory impairments (visual and hearing). **Attitudinal barriers** are those imposed by prejudice and as with physical barriers, mean that people are discriminated against when it comes to accessing services such as dentistry. It also excludes people from educational and employment opportunities as well as the right to self-determination. There are also significant cultural differences in acceptance or otherwise of disability.

Barriers can also be divided into people-centred (patients and carers) and professional (oral healthcare team). For the former, fear and anxiety, a lack of perceived need often by parents or carers, and an inability to make needs known are crucial. In relation to professional barriers, the failure to recognise and accept difference, failure to see oral health in the context of illness and disability, ignorance of inter-professional support, failure to prioritise, inadequate staff training and professional reluctance to offer care or arrange appropriate services maintain the disadvantage suffered by people with disabilities.

In part this is due to reluctance on the part of dental practitioners to take responsibility for care, based on the misconceptions of dentists:

■ treatment will be too time-consuming/expensive
■ difficulties of access to the surgery
■ challenging behaviour
■ waiting room disturbances
■ need for special facilities
■ lack of training and experience.

Abuse

Children and vulnerable adults with disability are at greater risk of abuse because:

■ they are dependent on others for needs and may not be able to tell someone that abuse is happening
■ they have a lack of control or choice over their own life
■ to be co-operative is seen as desirable (because it is rewarded)
■ they have a lack of knowledge about sex and may be unable to differentiate different types of touching
■ the severely impaired person may be shunned by the family, seen as less human and thus becomes the target for abuse.

Children with disabilities are twice as likely to be sexually abused, and conversely, abused children are five times more likely to be intellectually impaired. Females are more vulnerable than males.

The dental team has a role to play in recognising abuse, since they may see patients on a regular basis, and must be familiar with the local policy on management of suspected abuse, whatever the patient's age.

Characteristics of service use by people with disabilities

People with disabilities have a different history of use of dental services compared with others in the population:

- fewer visits and longer intervals between care
- limited access to buildings
- difficulties communicating pain and distress
- financial difficulties (payment for services as well as time lost from work, travel)
- history of extractions rather than prevention and restoration
- emergency hospital care rather than planned community care
- treatment with sedation/general anaesthesia (GA).

Dental care staff in the salaried services are more often in a position to ensure that dental care is provided for people with disabilities since the additional time needed by some disabled people makes it difficult for their routine care needs to be provided in the more demand-led general dental service.

Recommended tasks

(1) Think about all the different people you see each week. What proportion of your patients have an impairment? What broad groups, if any, do they fall into?

(2) In the clinic/practice where you work, think about the 'barriers' that people with disabilities may face; divide them up into physical barriers and attitudinal barriers. Start outside the surgery, even in the car park, and follow the entire patient's journey through the clinic/practice.

(3) Non-accidental injury or abuse is not confined to children. Read your local guidelines and then rehearse how you would approach the carer of a person whom the clinical team suspected was being abused. How would you phrase your request to obtain records or photographs in a suspected case of elder abuse?

Legislative framework

Normalisation

The move to **normalisation** started in Sweden in the 1950s and enabled many people with disabilities to live outside institutions with greater autonomy over their own lives. In the UK, people with disabilities, a significant number of whom are elderly people, live in their own homes. Increasingly, residents of long-stay institutions live in sheltered housing in communities with carers. The opportunity for respite care still exists in residential care.

Special schools provide education and training for many children and adolescents from 2 to 19 years of age, although increasing numbers are taught in mainstream schools with close support from specialist teachers. Sheltered workshops give employment to some disabled people and others combine this with paid employment. It is a requirement that businesses employing more than five people must offer work opportunities to a disabled person.

The **Disability Discrimination Act 1995** has far-reaching consequences across all sectors of society in the UK. In dentistry, practices have had to make reasonable provision for access to people with disabilities, such as ramps, lifts and communication aids. It is illegal to discriminate against such persons on the grounds of their disability alone. The **Human Rights Act 2000** also imposes a duty of care on health professionals with respect to care offered to disadvantaged groups.

Consent

Before a person gives consent for dental care, the dental team has to confirm that that person:

- is competent to make a decision
- has been informed – reasons, options, consequences
- has understanding – demonstrates ability to weigh up pros and cons
- is not to be coerced – respect autonomy, respect a person's right to choose and self-determination.

There are other considerations in relation to the capacity to consent. It may be task specific: to consent to have teeth cleaned is one thing, but to have third molar surgery is quite another. Capacity to consent may be variable from one occasion to another and allowance ought to be made for this. A person may be temporarily or permanently impaired; for example it may be anticipated that a brain-injured person will make a good recovery, and elective treatment can be deferred until that time. It is, however, the responsibility of the clinician to decide – can the patient understand, reason, recall and apply information? The help of carers, or even an advocate who can act as an intermediary, is helpful. The dentist's duty of care to the patient means that treatment planned will result in oral health gain and will be in the best interests of the patient.

The practicalities of obtaining consent are not straightforward; the law varies from country to country and is often reliant on case law as well as the legislation in each place. For children, the parent or legal guardian is usually the person who can give consent. If it is judged that a young person below the age of consent is **Gillick competent**, then they may be free to consent to, or refuse, treatment.

In the UK, an adult is defined as someone over 16 years of age, which is the legal age of consent. No one else can consent on their behalf, not even if the patient has an intellectual impairment. In Scotland, for example, healthcare professionals have the right to sign adults with incapacity certificates for treatments that they are authorised to carry out within the bounds of their clinical practice. It is wise to involve parents/carers in the discussions and decision making and advisable to get the agreement of a second clinician on any proposed treatment plan, especially where GA or sedation are involved.

Physical intervention

The 1994 American guidelines on the use of physical intervention are sensible; physical interventions should only be used in situations where:

■ it is necessary for safe and effective treatment
■ it is not for punishment or for the convenience of staff
■ it is the least restrictive intervention used
■ it will not cause physical trauma and minimal psychological trauma
■ it is expected that reasonable benefits will result from the treatment
■ there is consent for treatment
■ there is consent for physical intervention
■ the intervention is specific to the planned treatment
■ dental staff are trained in safe physical intervention
■ there is clear documentation of type, duration and reason for use of physical intervention.

The **British Society for Disability and Oral Health** has formulated guidelines on physical intervention for dental care, to include the indications above, and these can be accessed via its website (www.bsdh.org.uk).

Recommended tasks

(1) Consider the Disability Discrimination Act and how it affects where you work. What modifications will be desirable for your clinic/practice to meet the requirements of the Act?
(2) A carer comments that they are not prepared to undertake physical intervention for a patient in order to clean his teeth. Think of ways to persuade the carer that appropriate physical intervention for the task is in the patient's best interest.

Working principles

Guidelines for care

Clinical governance dictates that high-quality care is delivered in an effective and efficient way. To that end, working to clinical guidelines is essential particularly when resources (money, manpower and facilities) are scarce. The British Society for Disability and Oral Health has a number of clinical guidelines and these are available on the Society's website (www.bsdh.org.uk).

Voluntary sector

Oral healthcare can be optimised by a good working relation with the voluntary sector. Many organisations have dental advice leaflets (Parkinson's Disease Society, www.parkinsons.org.uk) and work as advocates to facilitate the setting up of dental care for individuals (e.g. Ectodermal Dysplasia Society, www.ectodermaldysplasia.org) as well as lobbying politicians to bring about improvements in services, benefits and the education of others, such as the **Disability Partnership** (www.disabilitypartnership.co.uk).

Carers

Carers play a vital role in the lives of many people with disabilities when parents are no longer directly involved in day-to-day living (www.carersuk.org). For more dependent people, carers are responsible for oral hygiene practices as well. Such individualised instructions need to be incorporated into the care plan of people in residential care. They need close support from the dental team to ensure that oral hygiene measures are clinically effective. The turnover of carers is high and training in oral hygiene skills needs to be part of the induction procedures. There are training packages to help in training carers in oral hygiene measures.

Facilities for oral and dental care in the UK

People with disabilities are able to access care through the General Dental Service (GDS) either as National Health Service (NHS) or private patients, or under recently introduced arrangements for Personal Dental Service, where most dentists work under a salaried contract with primary care trusts (PCTs). Alternatively, the Community Dental Service (CDS) provides a range of care for people unable or unwilling to access care through the GDS and where more specialised services, such as sedation and dental care teams with the skills to provide care to disabled people, are available. Healthcare is delivered by dental teams with additional training and experience in the care of people with disabilities. The hospital dental service from district general or dental teaching hospitals offers secondary or tertiary care for people whose impairments are such that dental treatment needs to be provided in a hospital with access to special facilities, equipment or expertise. Some patients will require dental care to be delivered to them as inpatients, e.g. patients who are severely medically compromised, such as people with a complex heart defect or unstable epilepsy, so that they can be monitored and their dental treatment provided safely. Dental care under general anaesthesia (GA) can only be provided in hospitals.

Domiciliary services are provided in a limited way by general dental practitioners as well as dental hygienists and by staff in the CDS who hold a bank of mobile equipment. This may be loaned from the PCT to general dental practitioners providing such a service.

Depending on the resources available, services may be offered to special groups such as homeless people, those in psychiatric units and people in prisons.

Recommended tasks

(1) What are the voluntary organisations with which you have most contact in your area? What dental information should they have to help clients and carers?

(2) A patient who has unstable diabetes is being referred to a local hospital for dental treatment under GA. How do you explain to the parents/carers why this treatment needs to be undertaken in hospital?

(3) A patient who lives at home needs new dentures; list the things you would need to prepare for a domiciliary visit to take impressions.

A practical approach

Clinical holding skills for dentistry

It is important when providing dental treatment for this group of patients to ensure that all staff have had suitable training in appropriate clinical holding techniques, whether the patient is having treatment within a clinical environment or in a domiciliary setting. This training should be devised in accordance with the **Manual Handling Operations Regulations 1992**. All activities should have a **risk assessment** carried out to help identify the most appropriate method of moving or handling for that task.

When setting up a 'new' clinical environment to provide treatment for special care patients, these risk assessments will aid in the laying out of the surgery, taking good ergonomics into consideration to promote health and safety, and to give comfort and ease of use which equates to an efficient workforce.

Once the risk assessments are carried out protocols/guidelines should be documented and training implemented, so that all staff are aware of correct manual handling procedures. This training should be mandatory and updated at regular intervals. Guidelines on clinical holding skills for dental services is available on the BSDH website (www.bsdh.org.uk).

Alternative delivery systems

Surgery equipment

Dental surgeries need to be able to accommodate wheelchairs and walking frames. There are building regulations governing the dimensions of a surgery or theatre where care needs to be provided.

The sight of dental equipment evokes fear in many people and efforts should be made to place equipment behind cabinetry where technically possible. In principle, side delivery for handpieces, 3-in-1 syringes, curing light guides and ultrasonic scalers are preferable, particularly for disruptive patients. Surgeries should have facilities to transfer patients safely from wheelchairs, either with a hoist or in a purpose-built chair. There are dental units that allow a patient's wheelchair to be bolted onto the base unit in place of the conventional chair. The alternative is to use a special wheelchair ramp to allow a wheelchair to be reclined so that the operator and assistant are able to sit down to work.

Facilities for piped gases for inhalation sedation as well as for emergencies are desirable. Portable equipment allows the dental team to carry out a limited range of restorative work as well as preventive care, extractions and most routine prosthetic work away from a surgery. There are significant health and safety issues in relation to domiciliary care, not least of which is safety in unfamiliar houses/areas, carrying heavy equipment and safe disposal of waste.

Special mouldable supports are available on the market to accommodate people in the dental chair who have, for example, scoliosis. There are also cushions available that hold patients without physical intervention where there is a behaviour management problem.

Prefabricated finger guards (www.dental-directory.co.uk) can be helpful in avoiding being bitten when examining patients who have uncontrolled movements. Non-breakable mirrors are advantageous with such patients, as are hand-held intra-oral lights or head lamps.

Aids and adaptations

There are commercially available mouth-cleaning aids such as modified tooth-brush handles, powered toothbrushes and modified brush heads, e.g. Superbrush (www. dentocare.co.uk), to help carers with oral hygiene routines. Custom-made devices may need to be made in conjunction with a technician. For example, appliances to help with drooling, occlusal splints to protect teeth for patients who have bruxism (clenching or grinding of the teeth) or gastro-oesophageal reflux, and exercise devices for patients with restricted opening, e.g. arthrogryposis, hemifacial microsomia and juvenile idiopathic arthritis.

Diet

Food may be liquidised for patients whose impairment affects their ability to chew and swallow. Such consistency means that the food item is often retained around the mouth for prolonged periods, and even lodged for days in a high-vaulted palate. Carers need to be made aware of the potential for this to happen and a suitable means of clearing old food residues from more inaccessible places needs to be identified. Using a toothbrush handle or a smooth, rounded spoon handle can be relatively efficient and less traumatic than toothbrush bristles. Patients who are on prescribed food supplements because of growth failure are given nutrients that are often high in non-milk extrinsic sugars (NMES) and the way and frequency with which these are consumed make such patients vulnerable to dental caries. However, the need for adequate nutrition outweighs the disadvantages of dental caries and this needs to be managed with aggressive dental prevention.

Tube-fed patients or those who are fed via a **PEG** (percutaneous endoscopic gastrostomy) often accumulate large quantities of calculus when they take nothing by mouth. Removal of calculus from surfaces adjacent to the gingivae is important since gingivitis and halitosis can be significant problems. Calculus covering occlusal surfaces is less of a problem. Scaling needs to be undertaken with good, high-speed suction to avoid calculus being inhaled by a patient whose airway is vulnerable because of impaired swallowing.

Suction brushes are available for carers to use with patients who may not be able to swallow well and in whom managing toothpaste and oral secretions during toothbrushing would be a problem and an inhalation risk.

Patients who have a PEG often have had, and some continue to have, gastro-oesophageal reflux, and the aspiration of stomach contents into the mouth puts the patient at risk of, among other things, dental erosion. The dental team needs to be aware of the potential for this to happen.

Prevention with fluorides

It is desirable that all patients, particularly those vulnerable to dental caries and/or its treatment, should have optimal protection with fluorides.

Young, high-risk children should use a smear of fluoride toothpaste, a children's version with up to 550 parts per million fluoride (ppm F), until they are six years of age, when the risk of fluorosis to anterior teeth is negligible. If they do not live in a fluoridated water area, consideration should be given to using fluoride supplements or a smear of a higher concentration (1,000 ppm F) toothpaste. The risks of dental caries should be weighed against the threat of dental fluorosis. In the clinic, Duraphat varnish (2,300 ppm F) (www.colgateprofessional.co.uk) can be applied to vulnerable areas; this is better tolerated in the unco-operative patient than topical fluoride gels (12,000 ppm F) that require co-operation for placement over a number of minutes. For those over 12 years of age who are at high risk for the development of dental caries and/or its treatment, prescription of a more concentrated fluoride toothpaste (2,800 ppm F) is advisable. For high-risk individuals over 16 years of age a toothpaste containing even higher concentrations of fluoride (5,000 ppm F) is also available on prescription.

For patients who cannot tolerate toothpaste, or who cannot rinse out, dipping the toothbrush in fluoride mouthwash (0.2% sodium fluoride = 1,000 ppm F) will ensure that there is some form of topical fluoride regularly in the mouth. Provided the toothbrush is shaken well before it is put into the mouth there should be no excess ingestion of fluoride. For children under six years of age a daily 0.05% sodium fluoride mouth rinse (250 ppm F) can be used instead.

There are low-foaming toothpastes available and some contain fluoride in combination with chlorhexidine, which can be helpful for patients who have difficulty managing their oral hygiene.

For xerostomic patients (post-radiotherapy cancer, Sjögren's syndrome) high-concentration fluoride toothpaste as above or home application in trays of fluoride gels with a 0.4% stannous fluoride gel (1,000 ppm F) or a 1.23% sodium fluoride APF gel (12,300 ppm

F) can be advised. Rinsing with a daily (0.05% sodium fluoride) or a weekly/fortnightly rinse (0.2% sodium fluoride) is an alternative, provided the patient can rinse and spit out effectively.

Stannous fluoride (0.4%) as a gel is also incorporated into a saliva substitute which is particularly helpful for xerostomic patients who are more vulnerable to caries, especially root caries.

There is little evidence to support the use of fluoride foams but their advantage is that much less of them is required in a tray, so the potential toxicity is less and as they are less viscous they are more easily suctioned away than fluoride gels.

More recently, preparations based on a protein/calcium/phosphate combination and including 900ppm F are showing promise in helping patients with xerostomia and dental erosion, but there are currently no clinical trials to support their clinical use.

Fluoride delivered from the reservoir of a glass bead cemented to the buccal surface of molar teeth is another means of ensuring regular amounts of fluoride reach the teeth. This method of topical fluoride delivery has not yet been tried in people with impairments.

Fissure sealants

Some patients are un-cooperative for dental care and resist attempts to place fissure sealants, often because they cannot tolerate the isolation and high-volume aspiration required for the technique. Until such time as co-operation improves a **glass ionomer cement** can be applied to the fissures with no need for surface preparation. Some glass ionomers release more fluoride than others and are dual-setting, which is helpful in patients where co-operation is limited. Rapid placement followed immediately by coverage with green occlusal indicator wax helps to keep the cement dry while it sets and avoids the need to keep the area dry for a prolonged period. As well as mechanically blocking the fissures the cement acts as a fluoride reservoir to help prevent caries.

Prevention with chlorhexidine

Many carers are used to applying chlorhexidine gluconate gel (1.0%), less so using the mouthwash (0.2%), to control gingivitis. The preparation is also available as a spray, which may make its use easier in people with disabilities. Soaking dentures overnight in a solution of chlorhexidine can be helpful in cases of candidiasis.

One way to tell whether the gel or mouthwash is being used is to look for staining of the teeth, which is a side effect of the chlorhexidine. Foaming agents in ordinary toothpastes inactivate chlorhexidine and the two should not be used together. Advice to the patient or carer is to use ordinary toothpaste in the morning for fluoride protection and chlorhexidine in the evening, and it is preferable to use two separate toothbrushes. Alternatively, newer products are now available that contain both chlorhexidine and fluoride that are compatible with each other. This is much easier for patients and carers who only have one product to use, for example Kin toothpastes and gels.

Topical chlorhexidine varnish can be applied to the gingival crevices of patients with intractable periodontal problems, as well as using chlorhexidine-containing gel, mouthwash or spray at home.

Recommended tasks

(1) Carry out a risk assessment on the procedure to move a wheelchair patient from the car park to the surgery.
(2) A carer has read an article about the dangers of fluoride in the water; how will you provide reassurance that toothpaste is not only safe to use but also beneficial to their child?

Cross-infection control

In order to safeguard the health and safety of all patients and care workers it is essential that good working practices are adopted at all times. This involves careful clinical procedures for all patients regardless of whether a risk of infection has been identified. These work practices should also be implemented within a domiciliary setting. These include the use of standard precautions for all patients, such as:

- preparation of the clinical area – decontaminate the area with an appropriate solution as per your localised policy, in line with National Infection Control Standards prior to start of surgery
- use of *zoning* to reduce cross-contamination of instruments and equipment
- effective handwashing technique appropriate to the type of procedure being carried out
- use of personal protective equipment (PPE), including appropriate clothing to minimise transfer of micro-organisms between patients and staff (including uniforms, gloves, glasses and masks)
- use of single-use items where possible
- safe disposal of clinical waste, including sharps and cytotoxic waste, into the appropriate healthcare waste stream
- pre-sterilisation cleaning of instruments and equipment according to Control of Substances Hazardous to Health (COSHH) and infection control guidelines
- appropriate sterilisation and aseptic storage of all instruments and equipment (further information is available in the British Dental Association advice sheet A12 entitled Infection Control in Dentistry – December 2009).

Treatment of blood spillages

Sodium hypochlorite solution (10,000ppm) is available in granule/crystal form. It is also available in single-use spill packs, ideal for community use or domiciliary visits. Allow to crystallise over spillage, wipe up with disposable wipes and place in clinical waste bag (as per the manufacturer's instructions). Ensure staff are wearing appropriate PPE wear while doing so.

Patients with known blood-borne viruses

Standard precautions as detailed above should be used with all patients, but staff should be aware of the greater risk associated with treating this group of patients. There should also be a documented policy within the dental surgery regarding the appropriate follow up of a percutaneous injury (e.g. needle stick injury) from a patient with a known blood-borne virus.

Patients with CJD or related disorders

(See also section on Prion diseases)

While the transmission of Creutzfeldt–Jakob disease (CJD) via dentistry is considered to be low risk, the Department of Health (2007) advises that all endodontic files and reamers be treated as single-use, as a precaution to reduce any risk of vCJD transmission. In addition to standard precautions in general use within dentistry, treatment of patients with CJD and related disorders should be undertaken following the guidelines given below.

- Patients should be treated at the end of a clinical session.
- Unnecessary equipment should be removed from the clinical area.
- Operators should wear disposable personal protective equipment including disposable clinical gowns.
- Single-use instruments should be used where possible.
- Aerosol production should be kept to a minimum and only used if deemed necessary to give emergency pain relief.
- **Do not use** a centralised suction system. A portable designated unit with disposable reservoir and tubing should be used – these should be incinerated following use.
- On completion of treatment, instruments that cannot be discarded should be *quarantined* as detailed below.
- A *runner nurse* is essential throughout the procedure.
- Items for disposal should be placed in appropriate sharps bins sealed and labelled as CJD waste, and arrangements should be made for immediate collection.

Processing of instruments used for CJD patients

A number of studies have been carried out in relation to the effective decontamination and sterilisation of instruments following use on patients who are at risk or are carriers of CJD. These suggest that the most effective method would be that of the standard achieved within a Central Sterile Services Unit, to include use of ultrasonic cleaners and automated washer disinfectors as opposed to manual cleaning. It would be expected that each trust would have a local policy for treatment of such patients.

For the most up-to-date recommendations of how to process instruments following the treatment of such patients please see CJD-related publications on the Department of Health website (www.doh.gov.uk).

If this protocol cannot be followed within the normal working environment, patients should be referred to a local hospital with an effective working policy for treating patients with CJD.

Medical emergencies

All staff providing care for any patient must be alert to the potential for a medical emergency. This is particularly the case for people with impairments, for whom the risk is higher. The dental team needs to be alert to the needs of patients whose systemic disease is not well controlled, e.g. an impending convulsion or diabetic collapse. It is a requirement that all staff have the necessary skills to provide basic life support and that such routines are practised regularly within the surgery. Where dental treatment under sedation is provided, all staff administering and monitoring such procedures must have the appropriate training and experience to satisfy the UK Department of Health and General Dental Council guidelines (see Chapter 4).

Recommended tasks

(1) A mother is experiencing difficulties cleaning her child's mouth, gaining access to the mouth and getting the brush in for sufficient time. What advice would you give? What alternatives would you suggest she might try?

(2) Describe the ideal layout of equipment and instruments to prepare your surgery to make *zoning* effective and efficient for you, the dentist and the patient.

(3) A patient collapses in the surgery; list the sequence of events you need to perform to manage the collapse. Practise this with other staff by springing a surprise 'collapse' on them when they are not expecting it.

Learning disability

Definitions

Learning difficulties, mental retardation and intellectual impairment are all terms applied to people who have significant limitations in performing normal day-to-day activities because of reduced intellectual functioning. The most appropriate term, learning disability, relates to someone who has significant problems associated with education and socialising. This may be because of inherited or acquired disorders. The cause usually does not bear any relation to the subsequent deficiencies in performing the normal activities of peers, such as self-care and other activities of daily living, like school, work and leisure. The majority of people affected have only mild impairment. Associated medical problems are conditions such as seizures and heart defects.

The specific conditions most commonly seen in dental practice are Down syndrome, Fragile X syndrome, autism spectrum disorder (ASD) and attention deficit hyperactivity disorders (ADHD). Learning disability is sometimes called mental handicap, mental subnormality, retardation or mental deficiency. It is a general category characterised by low intelligence, failure of adaptation and early age of onset. Low general intelligence is the main characteristic. People affected are slow in their general mental development and they may have difficulties in attention, perception, memory and thinking. They may be stronger in some skills than others, for example music and computing, but generally they are of low intellectual attainment. People with a profound learning impairment will be dependent on others for help with personal skills as well as daily living. The dental team will be largely reliant on carers to assist the patient with oral hygiene measures. This can be helped by input from CDS/PDS services to help deliver oral health maintenance programmes specific to the needs of the client group and carers. These can be implemented by an Oral Health Education (OHE) qualified dental nurse in residential homes, adult centres and schools as appropriate. An Oral Care Plan, to be integrated with the general Care Plan, is helpful in focusing carers on oral hygiene and dietary needs.

Down syndrome

Down syndrome occurs in about 1 in 1,100 live births of the population. It is a genetic condition with three different effects on chromosome 21. Males and females are equally affected. Features of dental significance are as follows.

General

- Learning disability – ability to remember oral hygiene routines.
- Increased prevalence of hepatitis B, especially in males in residential care.
- Increased risk of coeliac disease (3.6%) – may be related to enamel defects seen in some people with Down syndrome.
- Increased likelihood of gastro-oesophageal reflux disease (GORD) – asymptomatic, gastric cancer in males.
- Increased prevalence of thyroid disease.
- Leukaemia (acute lymphoblastic leukaemia (ALL) and acute myeloid leukaemia (AML)).
- Alzheimer's disease (short-term memory and daily routines, e.g. oral care) in older people.
- Congenital heart defects – new guidelines (NICE; www.nice.org.uk/Guidance/CG64) mean that a smaller group of patients will now require antibiotic prophylaxis before dental treatment.

- Instability of cervical joints – care in handling especially when unconscious (GA).
- Problems of obesity also impose a GA risk.
- Cataracts in older patients – affects visual learning.
- Epilepsy – 2% of children and 10% of adults.

Oral and dental considerations

- Reduced caries prevalence – may be due to delayed eruption, smaller/fewer teeth or differences in saliva.
- Increased risk of periodontal disease due to altered immune system, reduced manual dexterity, reduced muscle tone leading to less natural cleansing/drooling and open-mouth posture resulting in dry mouth/poor oral clearance.
- Increased prevalence of tooth wear – erosion from GORD and bruxism. Some patients are treated with botulin toxin ('Botox') to relieve grinding.

Fragile X syndrome

This is the next most common syndrome, with learning difficulties, after Down syndrome. It is a neurodevelopmental disorder due to a mutation on the X chromosome. It is therefore seen in males, who may present with long, coarse faces or large ears, which may be low set. It is often undiagnosed but should be suspected in males living in residential care with a learning disability of unknown origin. It is of dental significance because prolapse of the heart's mitral valve (MVP) occurs in up to 80% of affected people and this may require antibiotic prophylaxis before dental treatment. About 20% will have seizures; usually partial motor, which are responsive to anticonvulsants.

Autism spectrum disorder (ASD)

This is a psychiatric disorder of childhood which may have a genetic cause. The prevalence is 2–5 per 10,000 with a male/female ratio of 4–5:1. Communications and social skills are impaired and affected children rely on repetitive routines, restricted in scope. Associated conditions are Fragile X (2–8%), epilepsy (30%), tuberous sclerosis (1–3%) and learning disability (75%). Treatment relies on intensive behaviour modelling and stimulant drugs.

Features of dental relevance are:

- sweetened medicines and prolonged retention of food in the mouth (*pouching*), which may contribute to increased caries prevalence
- phenytoin to control behaviour may produce gingival overgrowth
- bruxism
- poor attention span/distraction – high lateral vision
- reliance on familiar routines, minimal visual stimulation/distraction, rehearsal of visits, short visits, non-verbal communication.

Patients with Asperger syndrome, which is a variant of ASD, mostly have a very high IQ but poor social and communication skills. Other features are an inability to form relationships, an apparent lack of empathy, one-sided conversations, clumsiness and total, intense absorption in a particular area, for example, bus routes.

Attention Deficit Hyperactivity Disorder (ADHD)

ADHD affects 3–5% of school-age children and for 60% the disorder persists into adult life. As with many other impairments, boys are affected more than girls in a ratio of 3:1, although the rates even out in adulthood. Approximately 18–35% will have an additional psychiatric disorder. The features are hyperactivity, impulsiveness and inattentiveness for the age of the child. A child is usually assessed using a set of diagnostic criteria (e.g. *Diagnostic and Statistical Manual of Mental Disorders* – DSM IV) from which the child has to score positively for six of the nine symptoms in order for a diagnosis to be made. The disorder tends to diminish with age but in about half of those affected, signs and symptoms persist into adolescence. Adults are more likely to be of lower socioeconomic status, to have left school early, have difficulty keeping a job, possess more driving violations, have used illegal substances and smoke cigarettes. Affected adults are also more likely to report signs and symptoms of psychological maladjustment and to have relationship problems.

Treatment is usually with central nervous system (CNS) stimulants and tricyclic antidepressants (TCAs). Care must be used in the choice of vasoconstrictor if the patient is taking TCAs because epinephrine and TCAs may interact. Methylphenidate (Ritalin), a CNS stimulant, slows the metabolism of TCAs and warfarin.

Genetic diseases and syndromes

There are a number of conditions that produce intellectual impairment, either of unknown cause or with a strong genetic or familial link.

Many of these conditions have a genetic or environmental cause or a combination of the two. In some cases these result in a syndrome – where there is a recognisable, reproducible pattern of malformations as, for example, in Down syndrome. This is distinct from an anomalad or sequence where there is a pattern of anomalies arising from one structural defect, for example Pierre-Robin anomalad or sequence (see Cleft lip and palate, below).

Genetic problems may be single-gene defects which can be autosomal dominant (e.g. osteogenesis imperfecta; see acquired and congenital disorders of bone) or autosomal recessive (e.g. cystic fibrosis; see below), or X-linked recessive (e.g. the ectodermal dysplasias; see below). Chromosomal abnormalities centre around an alteration in the number of chromosomes, e.g. Down syndrome and trisomy 21.

Some conditions are multifactorial and have both a genetic and an environmental cause, as seen in spina bifida and cleft lip and palate, although some types, such as cleft palate with lip pitting (Van der Woude syndrome) are strongly genetic in aetiology.

Recommended tasks

(1) Consider the communication problems faced by people with learning disabilities. How might you help such a person to feel at ease in the surgery?
(2) How would you prepare for a dental appointment for a patient whose referral letter documented they had autism?

Physical impairment

Cerebral palsy

Cerebral palsy (CP) is a non-progressive neuromuscular disorder causing varying degrees of physical impairment. There are six movement forms, namely:

- spastic-hypertonic (70%)
- athetoid (16–20%)
- ataxic
- rigid
- hypotonic (reduced muscle tone)
- mixed.

It is acquired pre-, peri- or postnatally. The degree of impairment will be dependent on the extent of cerebral damage – one limb (monoplegic); all limbs (quadriplegic). Use of nitrous oxide sedation or oral benzodiazepines may reduce muscle hypertonicity as will well-positioned supports. Some patients are prescribed intramuscular botulinum toxin to improve limb function.

There may be associated epilepsy, learning disability, sensory and emotional disorders, speech and communication defects, and dysphagia (difficulty in swallowing). Care needs to be used with aspirators to avoid choking. Children with cerebral palsy may not grow well and are given food supplements (high in NMEs) and/or fed by nasogastric tube for a time or fed directly into the stomach (perendoscopy endoscopic gastrostomy ['PEG'] tube). Some medicines, for example clarithromycin, block these tubes and alternatives need to be prescribed. Some children with CP experience symptoms of gastro-oesophageal reflux despite surgery to correct this or even after a PEG has been fitted. This type of reflux can be painful as the stomach contents are very acidic and cause severe 'heartburn'. The distress this produces in a patient who cannot communicate pain is sometimes thought to be due to an oro-dental cause. If stomach acids are regurgitated into the mouth frequently, this can be a cause of significant dental erosion in patients with CP.

Oral and dental considerations

- Increased dental caries: caused by sweetened medicines, poor oral clearance, xerostomia (dry mouth).

- Periodontal disease: tube-fed or PEG nutrition increases prevalence of calculus.
- Drug-induced gingival overgrowth, e.g. phenytoin, although not routinely used nowadays.
- Chronological enamel hypoplasia: related to the timing of the insult that causes the CP – pre-, peri- or postnatal.
- Attrition due to bruxism, which may be treated with botulinum toxin injections.
- Erosion: CP patients with surgical correction for drooling, e.g. duct repositioning/ligation, salivary gland removal, may have parotitis (inflammation of parotid gland), rampant caries, especially of lower incisors, and a recurrence of hypersalivation.
- Untreated malocclusions.
- Self-inflicted trauma may be a consequence of a malocclusion and requires splint therapy, orthodontic treatment or occasionally dental extractions.
- People with impaired speech need time to make themselves understood. The use of Makaton (sign and symbol language) will help some patients.

If patients use a wheelchair, they can be helped to transfer to the dental chair with the use of a hoist, a banana board or a dental unit adapted to take their dental chair. Alternatively, there are surgery unit modifications available to allow the patient's wheelchair to be accommodated in a retroclined manner beside the dental unit. Supportive cushions (**Tumle cushions** are available from www.dental-directory.co.uk) for dental treatment may enable less impaired patients to be seated comfortably in the dental chair. Treatment can be delivered away from the surgery with the use of portable equipment.

Oral and dental considerations

- Poor oro-motor control means that high-volume chairside aspiration needs to be constant. This is essential whether centralised suction or a portable unit is used and should be remembered when preparing for domiciliary visits. A long-reach Yanker-type suction tip should be used, to ensure access to a clear airway.

- Staff must be aware of the potential for, and trained in the management of, seizures while the patient is under treatment.

- The use of sedation is indicated if uncontrolled movements prevent safe treatment and/or if required for anxiety management. This can be delivered by a variety of routes: oral (or via the gastrostomy site); rectal with suppositories; intra-nasal (midazolam with lidocaine); inhalational (nitrous oxide/oxygen) or intravenous (a benzodiazepine usually, although reversal with flumazenil is contraindicated if seizures are controlled by benzodiazepines). The route and drug should be decided in consultation with the patient's physician or general practitioner if there is no physician.

Spina bifida

Spina bifida arises from non-fusion of one or more posterior vertebral arches, with or without protrusion of some or all of the contents of the spinal canal. It may be accompanied by hydrocephalus in up to 95% of cases. In 50–60% of affected children the defect is inherited and environmental agents may be responsible in the remainder. In the UK the incidence is 2.5 per 1,000 births and, unlike other malformations, is commoner in females. A quarter of children also have epilepsy and about a third of people have some degree of intellectual impairment.

People with spina bifida will, unless the defect is slight, require a wheelchair to move around. Depending on where the lesion is, the person may also be incontinent. Urinary tract infections (UTIs) are frequent and thus regular courses of antibiotics are common-place. Hydrocephalus, unless arrested, is treated by the insertion of a **shunt** (Spitz-Holter valve) to drain fluid from the ventricles into either the superior vena cava, or the perito-neal cavity. If the former is done, antibiotic prophylaxis may be needed for invasive dental care, since a bacteraemia of oral origin, which may block the shunt, would cause a rise in intracranial pressure leading to seizures. If the shunt is a ventriculo-peritoneal one, no such prophylaxis is required. Constant antibiotics for UTIs may mean a modifica-tion to the usual prescription for such a patient. The material of some shunts sensitises those affected to latex products and this question in the medical history is especially important in these patients.

People who are confined to a wheelchair for much of the time will need similar wheel-chair transfers or dental chair modifications as for CP. The oral and dental care of people with spina bifida is otherwise no different from other patients.

Acquired and congenital disorders of bone

Osteogenesis imperfecta

Osteogenesis imperfecta is a group of inherited connective tissue defects of collagen, seen as increased bone fragility and lax joints. It is important to consider osteogenesis imper-fecta in cases of reported non-accidental injury (NAI). Other signs and symptoms are chronic bone pain, hearing loss, mitral/aortic valve defects, bruising, chronic constipa-tion (immobility), mid-thorax kyphosis (crush fracture of vertebrae) and pectus excava-tum (chest deep front to back).

Oral and dental considerations

- Pelvis is unstable making sitting in a chair difficult.
- Cardiac defects may need antibiotic prophylaxis.
- Dentinogenesis imperfecta in 50% of cases with grey/brown discoloration of dentine, which is more obvious in earlier erupting teeth and in the primary dentition.
- Rapid, early tooth wear and sensitivity means full coronal coverage is required which also maintains the occlusal vertical dimension. Teeth are usually sensitive to cold air from aspirator tips.
- Extractions may produce fractures of the mandible and should only be planned in consultation with the physician.
- General anaesthesia is to be avoided because of the potential for a rise in intra-thoracic temperature during anaesthesia, so prevention is really important in these patients.

Similar inherited dentine defects are seen in Ehlers-Danlos syndrome, vitamin D-resistant rickets, vitamin D-dependent rickets and hypophosphatasia.

Osteomalacia

This is a disturbance of bone mineralisation (rickets in growing bone). It is associated with a deficiency of **vitamin D** where the dietary source is inadequate or due to lack of sunlight (seen in immigrant women who remain well covered and tend not to go outside thus reducing the exposure to this source of vitamin D by the action of sun on the skin), in renal disease or from anticonvulsant therapy. The effects seen are bone fracture and deformity in children, and primarily in the long bones in adults. Tooth eruption is only affected in severe disease. The condition is treated by correcting the cause and supplementing vitamin D/calcium intake.

Osteoporosis

This is the physiological loss of bone, accelerated by ageing, oestrogen decline and immobility. It becomes pathological as a consequence of lifestyle (smoking, excess alcohol and certain drugs, e.g. heparin) and some endocrine conditions. Its prevention relies on regular exercise, adequate diet, avoidance of excess alcohol and smoking cessation. Hormonal replacement therapy, despite the side effects, helps in older (>70 years), postmenopausal women. The dental team has a responsibility to counsel patients on lifestyle factors.

There may be associated bony changes seen on jaw films and intra-oral radiographs, for example loss of bone height not directly related to periodontal disease. Patients who have osteoporosis may be prescribed bisphosphonate drugs to prevent bone loss. These drugs reduce bone turnover and as a consequence, reduce the blood supply to the bone. As a result, any trauma to bone, be it from infections, for example from an abscessed tooth, or tooth extraction means that healing is delayed or may never occur and the patient is left with bone exposed in their mouth that may need to be surgically resected.

Arthritis

Arthritis is a common, degenerative, disabling condition. The two commonest types are osteoarthritis and rheumatoid arthritis.

Osteoarthritis
This is more usually associated with ageing, although trauma to joints may be contributory, for example from bleeding into the joints in people with haemophilia.

Patients report pain from joints and eventually there is limitation in movement, which is disabling if the joints of the lower limbs, in particular, are involved.

Patients are helped by keeping mobile, physiotherapy and non-steroidal anti-inflammatory drugs (NSAIDs) which counter the low-grade inflammation that is usually present.

Oral and dental considerations

■ Patients will need modifications to seating in the dental chair in order to be comfortable. Neck support is particularly important when the spine is involved.

■ The dental team can help with modifications to toothbrushes and give advice on custom-made brushes for cleaning dentures effectively.

■ Drug interactions are important to consider; patients with arthritis may be vulnerable to anaemia, infections and delayed healing as a consequence of the use of anti-inflammatory drugs and corticosteroids.

Rheumatoid arthritis

This is a less common condition than osteoarthritis, probably genetic or autoimmune in origin, affecting the synovial joints at the extremities, hands, knees and feet. The onset is slow, with early morning stiffness of the inflamed joints, although moving after a period of inactivity brings on pain. Eventually there is total joint destruction, distortion of ligaments and even ankylosis (bone-to-bone union with no ligament in between) to produce significant deformity and disability. About 10–15% of patients become dependent on a wheelchair to move around.

Treatment consists of advice to rest the painful joint with splint support if this is helpful. Drug therapy relies on NSAIDs and corticosteroids. Injections of gold may be useful and surgery is also an option.

Oral and dental considerations are similar to those for osteoarthritis, although special attention needs to be paid to the temporomandibular joints (TMJ) if these are affected: supportive care, with heat, exercise and NSAIDs is the first line of treatment, with surgery and subsequent prosthodontic care a necessity for some patients.

This condition is particularly disabling when it occurs in the growing child (juvenile idiopathic arthritis), and the dental team will need to plan long term for the degree of impairment experienced by these children.

Sjögren's syndrome is more commonly associated with rheumatoid arthritis. The effects of this condition on salivary glands means that the dental team need to ensure that salivary gland stimulation (pilocarpine in selected cases) or saliva substitutes are used in a timely fashion to avoid the devastation to the dentition that follows when xerostomia becomes established.

Newer, high-fluoride toothpastes (2,500ppm F and 5,000ppm F) available on prescription only are particularly advantageous in this high-risk group of patients.

Inherited disorders of muscle

Muscular dystrophies

These are genetic disorders involving voluntary muscle with progressive weakness and wasting. The muscle fibres are replaced by fatty and fibrous tissue. There are a number of types: Duchenne (males only), Becker and those based on muscle groups affected.

Duchenne type is an X-linked disorder due to a mutation of the dystrophin gene. Two-thirds of the mothers of isolated cases are carriers, 50% of female siblings will be carriers and 50% of boys will be affected. Death in the second decade of life is usually because of involvement of respiratory muscles. The other observed features are scoliosis (curvature of the spine; **kyphosis** is anterior curvature, **lordosis** is posterior curvature), muscle contractures, loss of walking (7–13 years) and reduced IQ. Orally, the swallowing reflex is affected and oral clearance is poor.

Oral and dental considerations

- Efficient aspiration is essential during treatment and oral cleanliness may be an additional challenge.
- General anaesthesia is contraindicated because it requires intensive care admission, possibly for weeks, post-operatively.
- It is necessary to reduce the dosage of local anaesthesia because of poor tolerance.
- Malocclusions may be present because of the altered balance between the soft tissues.
- Flaccid soft tissues, an open-mouth posture and muscle weakness mean oral hygiene is likely to be poor.

Becker type is less severe and survival is longer. Facioscapulohumeral muscular dystrophy affects masticatory muscles more than the other facial muscles, leading to weakness of the circumoral muscles.

Cleft lip and palate

This is one of the commonest congenital malformations and the cause is multifactorial. Approximately 1 in 700 live births are affected and 1 in 20 children born to a parent with a cleft will be affected. The cause is unclear but is due to varying degrees of genetic, environmental and combined influences. Babies with lip pits tend to have a strong familial link with **clefting**.

Clefts are subdivided, based on anatomical limits, as follows.

- Primary palate – lip and alveolus
  The primary palate is that portion of the palate in front of the incisive foramen. These clefts may be uni- or bilateral and involve just a notch in the vermilion border of the lip or all the way back to the limit of the primary palate. As well as clefting, the nose is deviated to the non-cleft side in unilateral clefts with the base (ala) of the nares flattened to give the typical cleft appearance.

- Cleft of the lip and palate
  These may be complete (communicates directly with the nasal cavity), incomplete and, as with the primary palate, both uni- or bilateral. The secondary palate is involved. In a unilateral cleft, the minor segment of the alveolus tends to move palatally, to collapse inwards, emphasising the width of the cleft and posing more problems in aligning the segments for both the plastic surgeon and the orthodontist.

- Cleft palate only
  In this type of cleft, only the secondary palate is involved, although only the soft palate may have a cleft, and even that only as a submucous cleft, where the muscle is not joined, but the overlying mucosa is intact. This will affect speech.

Approximately 20% of babies born with a cleft have a syndrome or other underlying conditions. Dental anomalies that may be seen in children with clefts are:

- missing teeth and/or extra teeth, especially in the line of the cleft, usually in the region of the maxillary lateral incisor
- teeth of an abnormal size and shape
- enamel hypoplasia (enamel defects): not uncommon in the permanent incisors and may have more to do with early surgical trauma during palatal repair than to inherited defects of enamel
- ectopic (not in the normal place) eruption of first permanent molar teeth in the early mixed dentition stage (6–8 years), which may impact into and resorb the distal surface of the second primary molar and necessitate its removal.

Babies born with a cleft that involves the palate may have feeding difficulties, and early contact with a parent support group as well as knowledgeable maternity ward staff can do much to help the new mother. Feeding is aided by using a bottle designed to assist the flow of milk by squeezing, rather than relying on the child producing a vacuum with the teat pressed against the palate, to encourage a flow of milk. Gently squeezing the special baby bottles (Rosti bottles) encourages a good flow of milk and avoids the baby using up precious energy in sucking hopelessly. Mothers can still feed using expressed breast milk if they wish to do so.
  Aims and objectives of treatment and care are as follows.

- Early lip repair to foster good aesthetics to help parental bonding with the child.
- Palatal repair so that speech development is enhanced.
- Maintenance of an intact dentition.
- Good ENT supervision to avoid concurrent problems with middle ear infections and deafness.
- Speech and language therapy as indicated.

Timetable of care
A multiprofessional approach to the care of children with clefts is vital to optimise the outcome. A team will look after each child and monitor their progress from birth until such time as growth is complete – at about 18 years of age.
  Children with clefts should receive early preventive dental advice since sound teeth are vital to the successful alignment of arches. Lip repair is usually carried out between six weeks and three months, depending on the centre's protocol and the baby's health and weight. Palate repair usually takes place at around six months. In some countries repair is delayed until much later because of the potential of surgery to restrict growth. However, early surgery (before 10 months of age) is favoured to encourage good speech with an intact musculature in the oropharyngeal region.

Babies with clefts of the palate are more prone to middle ear infections because of the compromised muscles surrounding the inner auditory meatus. Early referral to an ENT surgeon will enable prompt treatment with grommets or T-tubes to avoid these sequelae. However, children and adults with repaired clefts may have some hearing impairment.

Further surgery at around 4–5 years of age may correct any nasal deformity and improve appearance before schooling starts. Speech assessment, with speech therapy at school, continues alongside dental and surgical care.

At around 8–9 years of age in children with cleft palates, orthodontic care may be initiated to expand the maxillary arch in readiness for a bone graft from the iliac crest of the hip to the cleft area to encourage the permanent canine to erupt into good alignment. Teeth will not erupt if there is no bone. Most orthodontic treatment starts after 8–9 years of age with alignment of the upper arch using fixed appliances. The relative underdevelopment of the maxilla in cleft patients means that they often have an Angle's class III malocclusion and on occasions this is so severe that maxillary teeth can only be aligned inside the lower arch. Such patients may be offered orthognathic surgery when their growth is completed, to allow a more class I relationship between the dental bases and thus improve facial profile.

Restorative care alongside good preventive care can do much to restore hypoplastic or missing teeth once the main orthodontic and surgical phases of treatment are complete.

Ectopic eruption of first permanent molars is seen more frequently in children with cleft palates. With early intervention it may be possible to retain affected primary molars and allow the ectopic permanent molar to erupt into a good position.

Ectodermal dysplasias

The ectodermal dysplasias are a group of about 150 inherited disorders that involve all the structures that develop from ectoderm, i.e. teeth, skin, hair, nails and sweat glands. The commonest forms are **anhidrotic X-linked** (occurring in males only) ectodermal dysplasia and **incontinentia pigmenti**, which affects only females.

Patients with ectodermal dysplasias have:

- frontal bossing
- fine sparse hair
- absent eyebrows and lashes
- low-set ears
- dry skin
- maxillary hypoplasia
- missing teeth: hypodontia, few missing teeth; oligodontia, six or more missing teeth; anodontia, no teeth
- teeth of abnormal shape, especially conical.

Some females may have mild symptoms. In the anhidrotic form, the complete absence of sweat glands makes temperature control problematic and dangerous over-heating can occur. Hypodontia is a feature of a large number of the syndromes.

Treatment must be multiprofessional with close liaison between the paediatric dentist, orthodontist, oral surgeon and restorative dentist to offer the best care to children and adolescents.

Preventive care is vital to retain what few teeth some of these patients have. Infra-occluded teeth need to be conservatively managed, especially if they do not have a permanent successor. Misshapen and small teeth can be modified with composite materials either as interim or permanent solutions, at least until more definitive restorative care is instituted after orthodontic treatment.

Provision of dentures for children without teeth before they start school is important if there is demand for such prostheses. The child's need for teeth and to look the same as their peers should not be underestimated. Sensitive dental care can do much to contribute to the child's fragile self-esteem and confidence.

There is much scope for interdisciplinary care for patients where there are buried teeth that can be encouraged to erupt with the aid of surgical exposure with or without orthodontic traction. Magnets may be used to encourage buried teeth to erupt with one pole of the magnet cemented to the occlusal surface of the buried tooth (after surgical exposure) and the opposing pole secured in the fitting surface of a removable appliance. This technique can also be used in, for example, cleidocranial dysplasia where there are often multiple buried teeth.

Once orthodontic alignment is complete and the necessary retention phase established, restorative management of the optimised spaces can be undertaken with adhesive or fixed bridgework, partial dentures, over-dentures and implants. Implants are deferred until growth is complete, at around 16–18 years of age. However, in the edentulous jaw of the child with anodontia, there is no reason why implants cannot be placed since there is no alveolar bone present and thus ankylosis and the burying of the implant structure will not occur.

Incontinentia pigmenti is a similar condition seen mostly in girls and in addition to the dental defects noted above, there are also skin defects.

Sensory impairments

Visual impairment

Visual impairments vary from total blindness to sight limitations of size, colour, distance and shape. The causes may be congenital or acquired. Common causes are outlined in Table 3.1. Occasionally, both hearing and vision are involved as in syndromes such as rubella syndrome and in the elderly patient.

Oral and dental considerations

■ The oral health of children with visual impairment is no different from the normal population and with good home care this can be maintained.

■ Consideration should be given to the design and format of written material available for use by patients who may be visually impaired, for example instructions for the

Table 3.1 The common congenital and acquired causes of visual impairment.

Congenital	Genetic/acquired
Infections	Infections
rubella	meningitis
Developmental	Prematurity
cataracts	
micropthalmus	
Malformations	Degenerative diseases
Ehlers–Danlos syndrome	Hunter's syndrome
Crouzon's syndrome	Prader–Willi syndrome
Pierre–Robin anomalad	
	Tumours
	retinoblastoma
	Glaucoma
	Drugs

wearing of orthodontic appliances and diet history sheets. Highly stylised type should be avoided and a mix of upper and lower case should be used. Letter size should be at least 3.2mm (one-eighth inch) high and be on uncoated (non-glare) paper. The best contrast for ease of reading is black type on white or off-white paper.

■ It is important to ascertain what help a person with a visual impairment requires. Some patients value their independence and resent being helped into the surgery. Many patients with visual impairment will have an increased sensitivity to bright lights and perhaps touch. Careful positioning of the operating light is therefore important and the sensation of touch should be used to enhance the patient's perception of what is being done; for example, being allowed to feel the instruments and dental materials.

■ It is not unusual for people to shout at those with a visual impairment. These people are usually not deaf and should therefore be addressed in a normal voice. It is important to the patient, and not only those with visual impairments, that conversation is addressed to them and not to the person with them.

■ Because vision is impaired and the sense of touch may be heightened, it can be startling for a patient suddenly to feel a cold mirror in the mouth without advanced warning. A *tell then feel then do* approach is even more important for those who may be unnerved by sudden strange contact. With these considerations in mind, there are no areas of dental treatment that are considered unsuitable for a person with a visual impairment, provided that they or their carer can maintain oral hygiene at home. Insertion of dentures or orthodontic appliances may initially be difficult and techniques such as flossing take time to master. It is important to allow time in the surgery to ensure the patient is comfortable with these before allowing them home to practise alone.

■ All important written documentation should be made available in Braille or audio form for those patients who have complete visual impairment, for example pre- and postoperative instructions for conscious sedation, or post-extraction instructions. As these must be given in both verbal and written form, consideration must be given to this under the Disability Discrimination Act (www.disability.gov.uk).

Moon texting, a system of reading and writing in which tactile symbols based on lines and curves are used to represent letters, numbers and pictures, is also an effective method of documenting written paperwork for adults who have lost their sight later in life. Advice can also be obtained from the Royal National Institute for the Blind with respect to adequate signage and documentation for this patient group (www.rnib.org.uk). Some community dental services have compiled an audiotape detailing the services and facilities available in order to help visually impaired people access dental care. The local *Talking Pages* newspaper may be willing to publicise this resource.

Deafness and hearing impairment

Loss of hearing is an impairment often acquired with age. However, many are born with either partial or total loss of hearing and this can occur in isolation or in combination with other impairments, for example rubella syndrome (auditory, visual, intellectual and cardiac defects). People with Williams' syndrome have an increased sensitivity to high-pitched sounds (**hyperaceusis**) and do not tolerate the noise, for example of aspirators or dental drills.

People born with clefts of the hard palate may acquire a hearing deficit as a consequence of chronic middle ear infections. This occurs because of poor muscle control of the internal auditory meatus because the muscles in this area do not function well. A hearing impairment may also be acquired with age and many elderly people cannot communicate because of deafness and may therefore need an aid to enhance sound.

Oral and dental care considerations

■ Patients who have a hearing impairment may be anxious, or even appear hostile, because they feel they are not going to understand what is being asked of them.

■ Patients may not hear what has been said but pretend they have done so to avoid embarrassment. In this situation visual aids assume an even greater importance.

■ It is essential for optimal hearing that all extraneous background noise is removed when communicating with the hearing-impaired person. Piped music in the surgery and noise from the reception area, as well as internal noises like aspirators and scavenging systems should be turned off or the volume lowered.

Cochlear implants are provided to patients who have lost all hearing in both ears and currently there are about 2,400 children in the UK who have received such devices. Additionally, 300 children a year are provided with these implants. A cochlear implant consists of a radio receiver implanted in the ear and a decoder with a magnet which is placed approximately on the mastoid process, above and behind the pinna.

Removable external microphone/radio transmitters can be damaged by equipment that interferes with electronic devices. As with patients with cardiac pacemakers, electronic scalers, electrosurgical equipment, some pulp testers and apex locators should not be used with these patients. There are few data to indicate what the oral health of people with hearing impairments is like. In the past, institutional care has allowed a fairly uniform standard of oral hygiene and dietary control. Greater integration into mainstream schools has meant that children with hearing impairments now do much the same as their peers. Like many other impaired children, hearing impaired patients are initially wary of battery operated toothbrushes because of the sensation they produce intra-orally. Although these brushes have not been shown to be better in terms of plaque removal than a well-manipulated manual brush, in children particularly, the novelty may be a motivating factor to use this type of brush.

Many deaf or hearing-impaired people will wear aids to enable them to pick up more sounds and older people may have skills not only in lip reading but also in signing. However, there is now a trend towards discouraging the use of signing and to positively encourage a child to acquire some speech, utilising any residual vocal potential. For those children who can lip-read it is necessary to sit well in front of the child, with good lighting to the operator's face. Masks are therefore to be put to one side and bearded operators should ensure that facial hair does not obscure clear visualisation of lip movement. The services of a British Sign Language interpreter can be purchased if there are no staff qualified in this mode of communication. These can be contacted via the Royal National Institute for Deaf People (www.rnid.org.uk).

People wearing hearing devices may be disturbed by the high-pitched noise produced by dental handpieces and ultrasonic scalers. This may make them less co-operative and less amenable to treatment. Similarly, the conduction of vibrations from the handpiece and burs via bone is more disturbing for the hearing-impaired person. After initial communications are complete it may be advisable to suggest that the hearing device is removed or turned off and only re-inserted on completion of the dental treatment in time for final instructions. In any event, very young children often have difficulty keeping the aids in place simply because of the size of the immature pinnae. This is especially so when lying supine in the dental chair.

Recommended tasks

(1) A patient who relies on a wheelchair and who needs inhalation sedation cannot easily be moved from their chair. Think of ways of optimising the patient's comfort and safety while at the same time ensuring that the dental team is able to provide the dental treatment effectively.

(2) A patient who has spina bifida has a latex allergy but needs dental treatment. How will this be organised and delivered? What alternatives can be considered?

(3) An older patient with rheumatoid arthritis and significant hand deformity has complete dentures. What problems will be faced when wearing and caring for these dentures?

Cardiovascular system

Disorders of blood

Blood is made up of plasma, red cells (erythrocytes), white cells (leucocytes or granulocytes) and platelets (thrombocytes). Plasma contains proteins and other components responsible for the functions of blood.

Specific defects related to cell numbers are:

- erythrocytes – anaemia (too few); polycythaemia (too many)
- leucocytes – leucopenia (too few white cells); leucocytosis (too many white cells)
- platelets – thrombocytopenia (too few red cells); thrombocythaemia (too many red cells).

Anaemias

These are due either to a failure of the body to make sufficient red cells, e.g. bone marrow aplasia (aplastic anaemia) or bone marrow hyperplasia (iron deficiency anaemia). Alternatively, anaemias are known by the effect on the size and shape of the red cells: normochromic and normocytic (normal), hypochromic and microcytic (pale and small), normochromic and macrocytic (colour normal and large cells).

There are many causes of normocytic anaemias, such as acute blood loss, diseases like rheumatoid arthritis, tuberculosis, problems related to the bone marrow, e.g. leukaemias, and premature breakdown of the red cells, e.g. sickle cell trait/disease.

Patients appear pale, complain of tiredness and have no energy. They are breathless on exertion, have dizzy spells, may complain of ringing in the ears, have a rapid pulse and may have heart problems (angina). Memory may be affected. Treatment relies on identifying the cause of the anaemia and managing it while treating with blood replacement.

Microcytic anaemias occur as a result of faulty haemoglobin production, usually because of iron deficiency. Haemoglobin is responsible for the carriage of oxygen around the body. Patients are tired, breathless and report palpitations, dizziness and poor memory. They appear pale and have a rapid pulse. The spleen is enlarged due to the breakdown of faulty red cells. The oral tissues appear pale once the haemoglobin drops below 8g/dl. The main risk for dental care is for patients requiring GA, because the oxygen-carrying capacity of the blood is reduced.

Macrocytic anaemias occur due to a deficiency of vitamin B_{12} and folate, which are needed to make white cells and platelets. In these patients, there is no secretion of intrinsic factor in the stomach wall to combine with the extrinsic factor (vitamin B_{12}) and so deficiency follows. This can be treated by injections of vitamin B_{12}.

Folic acid deficiency also occurs because of malabsorption, seen for example in coeliac disease or in chronic alcoholism. Drugs can also interfere with absorption, such as in epileptic patients taking phenytoin or in cancer patients receiving methotrexate. This is why a careful medical history is so important as well as a high index of suspicion when the patient's reported history does not match the signs, e.g. alcoholism. Patients with this type of anaemia have all the signs and symptoms of anaemia generally.

Haemolytic anaemias

These are seen where there is premature destruction of the red cells in congenital conditions such as sickle cell trait/disease and thalassaemia, where the haemoglobin is defective. Acquired defects are seen in, for example, infections like malaria. Affected patients have all the signs and symptoms of general anaemia but will also appear jaundiced due to the bilirubin in the blood as a result of the increased breakdown of the red cells. Patients who have sickle cell disease are vulnerable to low oxygen (hypoxia) or dehydration, for example under GA, when the cells *sickle*, clump together and block blood vessels. This is painful and potentially serious, particularly in the brain.

Blood dyscrasias

It is important to decide from the patient's history if this is inherited or acquired. Tooth extraction may be the first challenge that someone with a mild inherited bleeding disorder may experience.

These disorders can be divided as follows.

Coagulation disorders

- Intrinsic
    - congenital (e.g. haemophilias)
    - acquired (e.g. heparin therapy)
- Extrinsic
    - acquired (e.g. liver disease, warfarin therapy and malabsorption).

Platelet disorders

Thrombocytopenia (reduction in numbers) may be due to:

- decreased formation (bone marrow problems)
- increased breakdown (immune thrombocytopenia purpura, ITP)
- platelet function defects
- congenital (e.g. von Willebrand's disease)
- acquired (e.g. aspirin therapy).

Vessel wall defects

- Congenital (e.g. Ehlers-Danlos syndrome)
- Acquired (e.g. Schönlein-Henoch purpura; scurvy)
- Fibrinolytic disorders (e.g. streptokinase therapy).

These defects are tested using different laboratory procedures. Another important test is the bleeding time (normal 9 minutes).

Haemophilia A
This is an X-linked recessive condition and therefore only seen in males. It is graded according to severity:

■ severe: <1% of normal factor VIII levels
■ moderate: 1–5% factor VIII
■ mild: >5–25% factor VIII.

For surgical procedures, factor VIII needs to be raised to 25–50% of normal with factor VIII concentrate infusion by the haemophilia team. This is followed up with epsilon-aminocaproic acid (EACA), an antifibrinolytic agent that prevents the clot from breaking up, taken four times a day for about one week to stabilise the clot. For less invasive procedures such as restorative dentistry, the factor VIII level needs to be raised to 15–20% of normal.

Milder cases (factor levels of greater than 10%) can often be managed without factor VIII replacement but with the use of desmopressin (DDAVP, 1-deamino-8-arginine-vasopressin), which encourages the temporary increase of factor VIII, together with one of the antifibrinolytic agents, EACA or tranexamic acid and the use of intra-ligamentary anaesthesia, since this technique avoids the risk of subsequent bleeding.

Factor replacement carries a small risk of infection with blood-borne viruses. Some patients will have antibodies to the factor after repeated use, and it is costly, so should be avoided where possible. Patients who have antibodies (15% of haemophiliacs) may be treated with the use of factor IX.

Haemophilia B (factor IX deficiency, Christmas disease)
This is managed at a haemophilia centre with infusion of factor IX or fresh frozen plasma (FFP), prior to the dental procedure. Again this is not without consequences since sometimes factors within the replacement may cause intravascular clotting and emboli.

Haemophilia C (factor XI deficiency)
People with haemophilia C should also be managed at a haemophilia centre, where they will receive factor replacement via an infusion of FFP prior to the dental procedure. As with other patients with a factor deficiency, they should be monitored at the centre after the dental treatment. The dental nurse will need to liaise closely with the centre about the timing of appointments.

Von Willebrand's disease
This is an autosomal dominant inherited condition so is seen in both males and females. It is a disorder of platelet function as well as factor XIII deficiency. Prior to dental procedures the haemophilia centre will cover patients with DDAVP (type 1 von Willebrand's) or cryoprecipitate (type II von Willebrand's disease).

Thrombocytopenia

This is a disorder that may be inherited, acquired or with no known cause (idiopathic). It is defined as a platelet count of less than 100,000/microlitre. It is vital that there is communication between the dental team and the patient's physician, since the thrombocytopenia may be temporary and the dental procedure could possibly be postponed until platelet levels are increased. If treatment cannot be postponed or if the thrombocytopenia is likely to be permanent, then a platelet transfusion will be required. The following drugs cause thrombocytopenia.

- **Aspirin**, taken for chronic pain (e.g. arthritis, juvenile idiopathic arthritis) and for prevention of a stroke (or cerebrovascular accident, CVA) and coronary artery occlusion. The dangers of stopping the aspirin outweigh the risk of postoperative haemorrhage, which can be managed by local measures (packing/suturing). Aspirin should not be prescribed for children and adolescents under 16 years of age because of the danger of developing Reye's syndrome – a rare but dangerous condition with liver and brain effects, which is often fatal.

- **Warfarin**, which is a vitamin K antagonist, is taken by patients with heart disease, those with prosthetic valves and after a stroke (CVA). The patient's INR (international normalised ratio) should be checked so that it is at a value of 4 or less prior to dental surgery. Discussion with the patient's physician should take place about the proposed treatment.

White cell defects

Raised white cell counts (leucocytosis)

Neutrophil leucocytosis is usually due to bacterial infection or seen after a myocardial infarct (MI) or acute trauma, whereas a lymphocytosis is seen in viral infections and lymphatic leukaemias and lymphomas. Treatment is aimed at addressing the cause.

Reduced white cell counts (neutropenia)

This is seen in relation to viral infections as well as during treatment for cancer. Patients are more vulnerable to infections, often by organisms present normally in the mouth. Patients need to be barrier-nursed and infections treated aggressively.

Neoplastic disease

The most common of these are the lymphomas and leukaemias. **Lymphomas** are malignant overgrowth of lymphoid cells, lymph glands, spleen and liver, divided into Hodgkin's and non-Hodgkin's lymphomas.

Hodgkin's disease/lymphoma is usually seen in young men and the first sign may be enlarged lymph nodes in the neck. Patients may also have the signs of anaemia, thrombocytopenia and neutropenia. Patients are treated with radiotherapy and chemotherapy and some patients, depending on the area irradiated and the cytotoxic drugs used, will have all the oral signs and symptoms related to these treatments – mucositis (ulceration, redness and sore oral tissues), discrete oral ulceration, xerostomia. Patients requiring oral surgery involving bone have the potential to develop osteoradionecrosis after radiation because of the compromised blood supply to the bone. The five-year survival rate is about 60%.

Non-Hodgkin's lymphomas are more common and have many subtypes. Their prevalence increases with age. The clinical features are similar to Hodgkin's disease. Treatment depends on the type and involves different chemotherapy regimes. The outlook is poor but many with low-grade disease survive for many years.

Leukaemias are a group of diseases, some of which may be due to chromosome defects (chronic myeloid). Radiation can also be a cause. The group of diseases is characterised by extra numbers of normal, precursor cells in the bone marrow. They are classified into acute and chronic and according to the cell type affected: myeloid or lymphoblastic/lymphatic. Patients have anaemia because of the crowding out of the bone marrow with the precursors of abnormal white blood cells.

The types of leukamias are:

- acute lymphoblastic leukaemia – usually children; 95% five-year survival rate
- acute myeloid – normally adults, may develop from chronic form
- chronic lymphatic – usually in middle age
- chronic myeloid – commonly in old age.

The general signs and symptoms are:

- anaemia because of reduced production of red blood cells
- bleeding tendency because of reduced platelet production
- susceptibility to infections because of reduced normal granulocyte production
- infections – many are treated with radiotherapy and chemotherapy and some with bone marrow transplantation.

The oral signs and symptoms are:

- anaemia – pale gums
- gingival hypertrophy due to an inability to respond to infection
- ulceration due to altered immunity and some cytotoxic drugs
- infections – viral (e.g. herpes) and especially fungal (candida)
- bleeding tendency – gingival oozing, prolonged bleeding after surgery, purple/blue patches on soft tissues
- xerostomia – and caries as a consequence
- dysphagia (difficulty swallowing) because of lack of saliva
- cervical lymphadenopathy.

Longer-term effects in the growing child are:

- alteration in growth if radiotherapy to bony growth centres
- loss of lamina dura, visible on radiograph

- stunted roots
- teeth fail to develop or are very small.

Cardiovascular disease

Cardiovascular disease can be broadly subdivided into the following categories.

- Congenital heart defects (CHD)
  - □ genetic – Down syndrome (septal defects); osteogenesis imperfecta (aortic and valve defects); Marfan syndrome (aorta, septal and valve defects)
  - □ environmental – rubella (patent ductus arteriosus; septal defects and pulmonary valve/artery defects).

- Ischaemic heart disease
  - □ angina pectoris
  - □ myocardial infarction.

- Hypertension.

Oral and dental issues in CHD

- General:
  - □ antibiotic prophylaxis
  - □ anaesthesia
  - □ bleeding.

- Oral (cyanotic disease):
  - □ delayed eruption
  - □ enamel hypoplasia.

Anaesthesia considerations in CHD

- General anaesthesia:
  - □ risk of arrhythmias
  - □ myocardial disease
  - □ conditions treated with digoxin/β-blockers.

- Relative analgesia (nitrous oxide inhalation sedation):
  - □ may be positively helpful with management because of superior levels of oxygen delivered during inhalation sedation (at the very least 30%, compared with 21% in room air).

- Local analgesia – avoid epinephrine in patients with:
  - □ myocardial disease
  - □ arrhythmias
  - □ Tetralogy of Fallot.

CHD and bleeding

Patients may have:

- warfarin after replacement valve surgery
- aspirin for shunts
- streptokinase for cardiac catheterisation
- defective platelet function (cyanotic heart disease)
- increased fibrinolytic activity (cyanotic heart disease).

The medical history *must* be checked at each visit. From the evidence available it seems sensible *not* to stop aspirin therapy prior to oral surgical procedures, but local measures, such as packing and suturing of the socket after extractions may be necessary because of an extended bleeding time.

CHD and dental procedures

Development of infective endocarditis

Infective endocarditis results from organisms settling on a pre-existing lesion, e.g. faulty valve. The lesion consists of an accumulation of fibrin, platelets and blood products, and develops as a consequence of disruption of the endothelial lining due to abnormal development (e.g. CHD), disease or turbulent blood flow. The endothelium is later colonised by organisms which get incorporated into the vegetative lesion.

In the UK, the National Institute for Health and Clinical Effectiveness (NICE) now recommends that antibiotic prophylaxis is not given prior to dental treatment in patients who previously were thought, because of the type of heart defect, to be at risk of developing infective endocarditis. Neither is the use of chlorhexidine mouthwash prior to dental treatment recommended.

The evidence linking infective endocarditis and dental procedures is weak. NICE concluded that the risk of anaphylaxis from antibiotic use was greater than the risk of developing infective endocarditis. It must be remembered that antibiotic cover is not always 100% effective and a balance must be struck between the risk of anaphylaxis, microorganism resistance and infective endocarditis. Many patients will produce a significant bacteraemia each time they eat or brush their teeth.

Prosthetic joints

There was a fourfold increase in joint replacements in the USA during the 1990s. Approximately 72,000 hip procedures were recorded in the National Joint Registry in 2007 and the estimated number of hip replacements will increase by 40% over the next 30 years because of demographic change alone. In the UK, in the 1950s and 1960s, there was a 15–25% prevalence rate of postoperative infections associated with prosthetic joint surgery. Infection of such prostheses can occur early or late. Early infection may be related to a peri-operative source of the infection. Late onset prosthetic joint infection (LPJI) may be related in some cases to an oral source. This is potentially serious as LPJI carries a high mortality of 18–50%. However, in the USA at least, routine antibiotic cover for these patients would cost $480,000 to prevent one case of LPJI. The risk of anaphylaxis is greater than LPJI.

Antibiotic cover is required for in-dwelling catheters, neurosurgical shunts and other implants only if:

- the catheter is near the right side of the heart
- the patient has a newly placed cardiac stent (within two weeks)
- the patient is on systemic medications (given because the patient is immunocompromised)
- the patient is on haemodialysis (not continuous ambulatory peritoneal dialysis, CAPD)
- there is hydrocephaly – if ventriculo-atrial shunt (not ventriculo-peritoneal shunt) – which has an infection rate of 5–30% and a mortality rate of 40%.

The protocol for prevention of infection in operative sites in the mouth is as follows.

- Use antibiotic cover for high contamination, for example periodontal surgery for immunocompromised people, patients at risk of infective endocarditis or with prosthetic joints.
- Use antibiotic cover for medical history predisposing to periodontal disease (for example poorly controlled diabetes).
- Pre-operative swabbing of the operative site with chlorhexidine (0.2% solution or 1% gel) is warranted.

Anaphylaxis

This is an emergency arising from a patient's exposure to an allergen (e.g. drugs such as penicillin, latex, wasp or bee stings, eggs, peanuts). The reaction occurs within minutes of contact with the allergen producing vasodilatation resulting in hypotension (often a dramatic fall in blood pressure) and shock. Laryngeal oedema results in stridor (high-pitched whistling sound because of respiratory obstruction) and there is an asthma-like wheeze. Treatment consists of calling for emergency help, maintaining the airway, raising the legs to increase blood pressure, administering oxygen and 0.5mg of 1:1000 epinephrine at 10-minute intervals and intravenous hydrocortisone 100mg until resuscitation help arrives. The dental nurse's role is to work as part of the team having rehearsed for such emergencies, but principally to call for an ambulance, ensure that the necessary oxygen and drugs are at hand and assist in accordance with appropriate training.

Angina pectoris

This is a temporary chest pain when there are increased demands on the heart and arises as a result of local ischaemia (lack of blood flow) when the coronary arteries are narrowed by atherosclerosis. There may eventually be a myocardial infarct where an area of heart muscle is deprived of its blood supply and dies ('heart attack').

It is important to know the history of the disease, frequency of attacks, known precipitating factors such as the stress of a dental visit or climbing stairs. The patient should have nitroglycerin tablets or spray (produces vasodilatation) available to place under their tongue in case of an attack. Appointments should be kept short. If the patient is very stressed the dentist may consider advising the patient to take a nitroglycerin tablet or use their spray before an appointment or to use some form of sedation (oral or inhalation) for its anxiolytic effect.

The use of epinephrine as a vasoconstrictor is contraindicated by some authorities, but on balance an ineffective LA without this vasoconstrictor may cause more pain and anxiety and may precipitate an attack.

Other signs of heart disease are shortness of breath, cyanosis, puffy, swollen ankles (oedema), prominent neck veins, palpitations and pain in the lower limbs on exertion (vessels blocked by atherosclerotic plaques).

Myocardial infarction, 'heart attack'

Myocardial infarction (MI) occurs when a plug of platelets and fibrin block off a coronary vessel producing an area of infarction (loss of blood supply) to the heart muscle. The piece of heart muscle supplied effectively dies. The signs are the same as for angina, but more severe, and not helped by resting or the usual drugs. Patients may require angioplasty – where a small balloon is inflated inside the coronary vessel to push the atherosclerotic plaque blocking the vessel through the wall of the vessel to allow blood to flow again normally. Alternatively, a coronary artery bypass graft (CABG) may be performed where the section of blocked vessel is replaced with a piece of vein from the leg.

The dental team must consult with the patient's physician as to the extent of heart muscle damage and precautions about future dental care such as the use of drugs. If the MI is recent (within six months) it is advisable to delay elective procedures, especially under GA, since a repeat MI is more likely in this interval. There are no direct dental effects apart from gingival overgrowth as a consequence of the use of calcium channel blockers. However, in children, dental development is delayed, along with a general delay in growth.

Patients who have had an MI may be on anticoagulants, e.g. warfarin or aspirin. The INR should be of the order of 4 or lower for any dental procedures likely to cause bleeding, such as extractions or periodontal surgery. The risk of stopping the anticoagulants, possibly resulting in a stroke, outweighs the benefit for haemostasis after the dental procedure. Bleeding can usually be controlled by local measures, e.g. pressure, packing and sutures. Aspirin affects platelet activity for 7–10 days.

Hypertension

This is defined as a systemic arterial pressure that is consistently raised above average. The average for young adults is 140 (systolic)/90 (diastolic) mmHg. The result of persistently raised blood pressure can be a stroke (CVA) or heart or renal failure. In older people these values may rise much higher. In most cases the cause is unknown, in others it is related to lifestyle (stress, smoking, obesity, drugs or a combination). Hypertension can occur with other diseases that raise the blood pressure, for example through hormone effects in renal or endocrine diseases.

Patients with hypertension will be taking a number of drugs, such as β-adrenergic blockers, angiotensin-converting enzyme (ACE) inhibitors, diuretics, calcium antagonists and α-adrenergic blockers.

Anticoagulants

These are used in a number of conditions such as:

- prevention of thrombo-embolism which leads to MI or CVA (stroke)
- prevention of systemic embolism in patients with prosthetic heart valves or atrial fibrillation
- prevention of recurrent infection and death in patients with valvular heart disease.

Drugs used for anticoagulation are:

- aspirin – alters platelet function for the whole life cycle (7–10 days).
- NSAIDs – interfere with platelet activation, but the effect is reversible.
- warfarin – interferes with the coagulation cascade.
- heparin – inhibits formation of thrombin (needed for fibrin production and platelet activation).

General management of anticoagulated patients is usually started in hospital with intravenous heparin and then maintained at home with oral warfarin. If oral surgery is required for patients with atrial fibrillation, pulmonary embolus or deep venous thrombosis (DVT), they should be treated in a hospital.

Management of anticoagulated patient for invasive surgery

(1) INR levels should be checked pre-surgery (day of surgery), usually in the range of 2–3.5.
(2) LA with epinephrine should be used; no NSAIDs or Cox-2 inhibitors for pain relief.
(3) Any sockets should be sutured and these should be removed one week later.
(4) Haemostatic agent (Surgicel/Instat/Beriplast) should be used.
(5) The patient should be advised to use tranexamic acid mouthwash 5% (prevents the clot breaking up) as a mouthwash, four times daily for two days.
(6) All patients must have verbal and written postoperative instructions and pressure packs (gauze) for home use.
(7) Give the carer/patient a 24-hour contact number, not that of an answering machine.

Cancer of the head and neck region

Head and neck cancer represents a mixed group of malignancies affecting a number of sites in the nasopharyngeal tract. Most are sensitive to a treatment regime of surgery followed by radiotherapy and, increasingly, in combination with chemotherapy. These are usually squamous cell carcinomas.

Many of the patients who present with head and neck cancer do so by virtue of their lifestyle; patients are predominantly from lower socioeconomic groups, are likely to be poor dental attenders, neglect their oral health, and smoke and drink to excess. The disease is therefore potentially preventable.

Oral and dental considerations

- Head and neck cancer patients often require extensive dental care prior to curative surgery and/or radiotherapy if their oral health is not to be further compromised after cancer treatment. These patients are more prone to extensive and rapid dental caries. It is important to the successful outcome of rehabilitative care, which may include implant therapy, that patients retain as many of their standing teeth as possible because this not only improves the stability of dentures but has been shown significantly to improve the quality of life for cancer patients.

- It is vital that dental extractions are undertaken *before* radiotherapy in order to avoid the serious sequelae of osteoradionecrosis, which is a risk if the pre-treatment extraction of teeth has not been undertaken. Radiotherapy to the muscles of mastication produces stricture, which prevents full mouth opening. This side effect can seriously limit access to the oral cavity for dental treatment, which is sufficient reason alone to carry out dental care prior to radiotherapy.

- Some patients will require obturators to be made because surgery may remove part of the jaws. Patients who require radiotherapy to the head and neck region will require the fabrication of a stent to shield dental tissues from the therapeutic beam. For post-radiotherapy patients, intra-oral appliances that act as a reservoir for topical fluoride therapy are advisable and the dentist should have these ready for the patient post-surgery.

Mucositis, seen without exception in head and neck irradiation but also with chemotherapy, is the commonest and most distressing side effect of treatment. It impacts seriously on a patient's quality of life in terms of pain, inability to eat, swallow and talk. Patients need to be monitored carefully because mucositis in combination with neutropenia can lead to septicaemia and be potentially life threatening. It can be so severe as to necessitate the interruption of cancer treatment. Prevention of mucositis, which is also a sequel of high-dose chemotherapy, is important and should be undertaken in conjunction with the inter-professional team managing the patient's care. Although benzydamine hydrochloride (Difflam) is effective in reducing the symptoms of mucositis in most cases, other agents, with the exception of ice chips, are not.

Patients with head and neck cancer who undergo radiotherapy will experience profound lack of saliva (xerostomia) in most cases. The management of this relies on aggressive caries prevention, regular dental care and saliva stimulants/substitutes where needed by patients.

Palliative care

The five-year survival rate of head and neck cancer is 40%, although this is dependent on the stage. Palliative care is defined as the active, total care of patients whose condition or disease is not responsive to curative treatment. The aim of such care is the relief of symptoms, including pain, and the active support of patient and family members, physically and psychologically, in order to ensure the best quality of life for all. There is an important role for dental input to a palliative care team since oral signs and symptoms of disease can be the most distressing.

Recommended tasks

(1) The wife of a patient recently diagnosed with heart disease rings prior to his appointment worried about the effects of dental treatment. Outline the way in which you would reassure her.
(2) Patients with cancer of the head and neck have a number of lifestyle features in common. Detail the health promotion advice you would design for the waiting room as an aid to prevention.
(3) At the next meeting of the trust or your practice you are asked to update dental nurses, as part of continuing professional development, on the revised protocol for the management of people at high risk of endocarditis. Design the slides/drawings you would use to illustrate your talk.
(4) A patient with a known bleeding disorder requires an extraction. Describe to your trainee dental nurse the procedures to be adopted, the people to contact and the instructions the patient/carer will need.

Respiratory disorders

Acute upper respiratory infections

These are commonly associated with the common cold and make the delivery of dental care more trying for the patient as well as increasing the exposure of the operator to infection. When a patent nasal airway is mandatory in, for example, inhalation sedation or GA, elective treatment needs to be deferred.

Asthma

This is defined as repeated, reversible attacks of wheeze on breathing out, shortness of breath and a cough as a result of narrowing of the airway. Inflammation (oedema) and infection (mucus plugs) may follow. It is a syndrome caused by allergy (dust mites, foods, drugs), pollution, infections, stress, exercise and non-compliance with drugs, and is seen in atopic individuals (eczema, hay fever).

Management of asthma consists of:

■ avoidance of allergens and known precipitating factors
■ the use of inhaled bronchodilators and steroids.

To avoid the potential for an acute attack:

■ sit the patient up
■ check the airway for any obstructions
■ advise the patient to use their bronchodilator inhaler.

The patient should be admitted urgently to hospital if the attack continues despite these measures. On admission, the patient may be given oxygen, nebulised bronchodilators, systemic steroids, antimicrobial drugs (if infection is the cause) and ventilation if the attack progresses to **status asthmaticus** (sudden and sustained aggravation of asthma).

The use of epinephrine, aspirin and NSAIDs in asthmatic patients should be avoided. Local anaesthetic agents such as articaine should be used with caution. There is the potential for candida infection in the palate from the use of inhalers. Asthmatic patients may be more susceptible to dental erosion as a consequence of gastro-oesophageal reflux because of coughing. Patients on steroids may have a steroid crisis. Respiratory depressants, especially sedatives and tranquillisers, should be avoided.

Chronic obstructive airway disease

This is also called chronic bronchitis or emphysema. It presents as bronchospasm and destruction/distension of the alveoli and is commonly seen in smokers.

Patients may be taking steroids and so may need supplemental steroids for invasive, stressful dental care because the endogenous supply of steroid will be suppressed. They may also be predisposed to oral candida infection as well. Patients taking theophylline should not be given erythromycin and some other antimicrobials because they result in toxic levels of theophylline.

Sedatives, tranquillisers, hypnotics and narcotics should be avoided. High-flow oxygen may take away the respiratory drive and as such may be a relative contraindication to use of nitrous oxide sedation during which levels of oxygen are higher than in inspired room air. Consultation with the patient's physician will clarify whether this is a real problem.

Scoliosis

Patients who have a lateral curvature of the spine (kyphosis, anterior curvature; lordosis, posterior curvature) may have associated cardiac and respiratory disorders.

Oral and dental considerations

- General anaesthetics may be contraindicated in a person who has severe scoliosis because of the poor ventilation of portions of the respiratory tree.
- Patient comfort is paramount – seating with good support (Tumle cushions) is very important.
- Patients may wear a brace – the Milwaukee brace encases the thorax and abdomen and has a chin cap extension; such orthopaedic splinting may produce a malocclusion.
- Chairside aspiration must be high vacuum to protect the airway in a patient in whom respiratory infection would be complex to manage.

Cystic fibrosis

This is not strictly a respiratory disorder but it predominantly affects the respiratory tree. It is the most common inherited condition in humans with 1 in 25 of the population as carriers. The disorder is of mucus-secreting exocrine glands, therefore effects are seen principally in the respiratory and gastrointestinal tracts. Patients will be taking a number of drugs, some of which may have affected the teeth during development. Problems with the pancreas mean that diabetes is seen in these patients. Orally/dentally patients may present with:

- discoloured teeth (from underlying disease and/or antibiotic therapy)
- enamel hypoplasia
- caries resistance (because of high pH of saliva)
- increased prevalence of calculus
- salivary gland enlargement.

Water lines in dental clinics should be carefully sterilised to avoid contamination with *Pseudomonas aeruginosa*, which is very resistant to treatment once it colonises the lungs. Patients may be uncomfortable if treated supine and will need daily physiotherapy. Some patients will require parenteral nutritional supplements as well as prophylactic antibiotics.

Tuberculosis

This used to be the most common infective disease, but better living conditions and widespread availability of treatment with antibiotics reduced its prevalence. However, drug resistance and human immunodeficiency virus (HIV) infection has brought about a recurrence of this infection. Patients with active tuberculosis (TB) lose weight, complain of feeling tired, have night sweats and are breathless. They have a chronic cough with blood in the sputum (haemoptysis).

Transmission of TB is usually by droplets but occasionally from infected, non-pasteurised milk. Healing may take place and the only sign in later life is calcified nodes on a lung x-ray. Progression of TB may occur through blood spread to involve other organs or re-activation of a previous infection, seen in the lungs as cavitation.

Patients with active disease (positive sputum) or who are still coughing should not receive dental care, except for dental emergencies. Most patients will have negative sputum cultures after three to four weeks of treatment and are then not infective. Non-compliance with drug therapy, which takes months, is the usual cause of a prolonged infective period.

Endocrine disorders

Integration of the functions of the specialised organs and tissues of the body is undertaken by two mechanisms:

- electrical impulses carried in the peripheral and central nervous system
- hormones produced in the endocrine glands.

The glands that carry out this function are the:

- pituitary
- hypothalamus
- parathyroids
- thyroid
- adrenals
- ovaries
- testes and placenta
- islets of Langerhans in the pancreas.

Loss of function of one of these produces symptoms that can be relieved if the hormone function is substituted by replacement therapy.

Pituitary gland

The pituitary gland, situated at the base of the brain, regulates the activity of many of the other endocrine glands by the production of stimulating hormones. It lies in close proximity to a number of important nerves, the cranial nerves in particular, so that alteration in its size, for example by a neoplasm, puts pressure on these and can cause visual disturbances. The pituitary exerts its influence mainly by stimulating other glands, but it does have a primary function in control of growth through the production of growth hormone. Over-production during the growing period results in gigantism, while under-production produces a dwarf. In the adult, over-production results in gigantism at the extremities – acromegaly. The patient may complain that dentures no longer fit. Accompanying signs and symptoms are sweating, heart disease and diabetes.

The other relevant hormone secreted by the pituitary is antidiuretic hormone (ADH) which regulates the uptake of water via the kidney and helps control fluid balance. Failure to do this produces diabetes insipidus and the affected patient loses litres of urine per day and drinks excessively. This is managed by DDAVP (see p. 109).

Aspects of oral and dental significance

In **hyperpituitarism**:

■ precocious dental development
■ osteoporosis
■ thickening of facial and cranial base bony structures
■ hypercementosis.

In **hypopituitarism**:

■ delayed dental development
■ alteration in the facial skeleton and cranial base dimensions
■ anterior open bite
■ link with adrenal and thyroid function may precipitate a hypopituitary coma in response to stress.

Thyroid gland

This gland is situated at the base of the neck with a lobe either side of the trachea. Its activity is controlled by thyroid-stimulating hormone (TSH) from the pituitary gland. This is regulated by the amount of thyroid hormone in the blood, which feeds back to the pituitary so preventing over- or under-production. The thyroid hormone plays a central part in regulating the metabolic rate.

Goitre

The thyroid gland can be prominent in cases of goitre. The hormone thyroxine is made up in part of iodine; if there is insufficient iodine in the diet there is under-production of thyroxine. The pituitary gland then receives less circulating thyroxine and so produces more TSH, causing the gland to eventually enlarge. This is corrected by adding iodine to table salt in areas where such a deficiency would otherwise occur.

More commonly, such effects are seen nowadays in young women and may be related to oestrogen because they are commonly seen at times of hormonal upheaval such as the onset of menstruation or pregnancy. Other goitres are due to an adenoma. Thyroiditis may also occur due to viral infections or autoimmune disease – Hashimoto's thyroiditis. Malignant tumours can occur and are treated by thyroidectomy or injection of radioactive iodine.

Hypofunction

Congenital hypothyroidism, called cretinism, is rare in the UK because of screening at birth. In adults it may occur due to autoimmune disease, surgical removal or a defect in the pituitary control. Patients complain of feeling cold and weight gain. They seem lethargic, slow and look puffy, particularly around the eyes. The effects on the heart are slowing of the rate (bradycardia), and an increase in blood cholesterol eventually results in ischaemic heart disease. Such patients are treated by thyroxine and care must be used in administering LA containing epinephrine. These patients respond poorly to stress and infection.

Hyperfunction

Hyperfunction is usually due to an autoimmune disorder – Graves' disease. This is seen mainly in young women. The effects of auto-antibodies also produce the characteristic eye effect – proptosis (forward positioning of eyeball, i.e. protuberant) – as a result of the reduction in intra-ocular volume. The signs and symptoms are the opposite of those seen in hypothyroidism, namely weight loss, increased heart rate (tachycardia), agitation and tremor, and intolerance to heat. Stress, trauma or acute infection can bring on a thyroid storm (thyrotoxic crisis) if the condition is not stable.

Parathyroid glands

The function of these glands is of relevance to dentistry because they are involved in the control of calcium and phosphate levels. The four glands are situated at the back of the thyroid glands. Their activity is not controlled by the pituitary, like other glands, but by the levels of calcium in the blood.

Parathyroid hormone (PTH) promotes:

- increased absorption of calcium from the intestines
- increased retention of calcium, by action in the renal tubules
- osteoclastic activity in bone, releasing calcium into the blood
- increased excretion of phosphates by the kidney.

Hyperparathyroidism

PTH excess is usually as a consequence of a tumour. This produces demineralisation of bone and large cyst-like areas appear on a radiograph. Fractures may occur. Because high levels of calcium and phosphate are being excreted through the kidneys, calculi (renal stones) may develop.

Hypoparathyroidism

Lack of PTH means that calcium is not readily mobilised from bone and blood levels fall. In the growing child this happens rapidly as calcium is taken up into developing bone. As well as bone, calcium is involved in other cells in the body; it plays a very important role in keeping cell membranes intact. In the absence of calcium, cell membranes become more permeable, and in muscles, depolarisation occurs spontaneously and the fibres twitch and go into spasm. This is called **tetany**. Tetany produces tingling and cramps, spasm of the hands and seizures. Tetany is also seen in alkalosis. Hysterical patients may hyperventilate, losing excess carbon dioxide (CO_2), producing alkalosis and tetany. Reassurance and re-breathing expired air (breathing in and out of a paper bag) will help to re-establish normal CO_2 levels.

Oral and dental effects

- Anterior open bite and class II skeletal base relationships.
- Delayed dental development, spaced dentitions.
- Enamel hypoplasia.

Adrenal glands

The two glands are situated on top of the kidneys. The outer portion of each gland (cortex) produces steroid hormones and the inner part (medulla) produces epinephrine and norepinephrine.

Adrenal cortex

Adrenocorticotrophic hormone (ACTH) secreted by the pituitary stimulates the adrenal cortex to produce steroid hormones, which are responsible for glucose metabolism. The most common of these are cortisone and hydrocortisone, and they act in the opposite way to insulin, i.e. by increasing blood glucose. These hormones also play a part in suppressing the immune system. The other steroid hormones produced are responsible for sodium and potassium metabolism (aldosterone) and for secondary sexual characteristics (testosterone and oestrogen), although most testosterone and oestrogen is produced by the testes and ovaries respectively.

Hypofunction (Addison's disease)

Hyposecretion is as a result of autoimmune destruction of the gland, steroid therapy, surgical removal or problems with the pituitary gland. Patients will complain of tiredness, weakness, may appear confused and, in the longer term, will have weight loss. Sodium and potassium handling is altered so patients will complain of thirst all the time. A patient may have a heart attack because of these raised levels of potassium or because of arrhythmias.

Oral and dental considerations

■ Patients may feel faint on sitting up from the dental chair.
■ Patients respond poorly to the stress of infections or dental procedures.
■ There may be pigmentation of the gums (due to stimulation of melanocytes).

It is vital to consult the patient's physician to determine what additional steroids should be given to cover any dental procedures and where these procedures should be carried out.

Hyperfunction (Cushing's syndrome)

Hyperfunction arises as a consequence of overproduction of ACTH from, for example, a pituitary or adrenal tumour or because of chronic high-dose steroids such as those used for immunosuppression after transplantation.

Patients have classic rounded (**moon**) faces and an increase in body fat accompanied by muscle wasting, especially of the arms and legs. Women show an increase in facial hair. Sodium and therefore water is retained. Such a clinical presentation could be confused with obese alcoholics.

Oral and dental considerations

■ Patients who have been on courses of steroids are in danger of a steroid crisis if exposed to stressful situations because they are unable to produce sufficient of their own as a consequence of wasting of the adrenal gland. Patients for whom this applies must be covered adequately for stressful dental procedures. It is sensible to discuss the proposed dental treatment with the patient's doctor/physician, who may feel it advisable to prescribe an antibiotic because of the immunosuppression and the likely consequences of postoperative infection. Treatment under sedation can be useful to allay anxiety. The normal daily output of hydrocortisone is 20mg, therefore patients taking low doses for short time periods are unlikely to need supplementation.

■ Patients who are on larger doses or for longer periods should, in consultation with their physician, double the daily dose on the morning of dental treatment, up to the normal physiologic output of adrenal glands (20mg/day). Higher doses (>40mg/day) of prednisolone would not normally require a supplemental dose for routine care but will for surgery with or without GA (see below).

■ The steroid dose for mild to moderately stressful procedures should be doubled on the day of surgery. For more stressful procedures in patients at high risk, prednisolone 60mg should be given on the day of surgery and reduced rapidly over the following three days to the patient's usual dose.

Protocol for managing patients who have stopped taking steroids in the recent past:

- <3 months: treat as if on steroids
- >3 months: no peri-operative steroids.

Patients on high dose immunosuppression are advised to take their usual doses during the peri-operative period (e.g. 60mg prednisolone daily needs 250mg hydrocortisone infusion during the peri-operative period).

Adrenal medulla

Epinephrine and norepinephrine are produced in the adrenal medulla. Epinephrine is the hormone responsible for the **fight or flight** response mechanism that is triggered in stressful situations. It increases heart rate, alertness and levels of glucose and fat in the blood, etc.

The most likely, but unusual, disorder of the medulla is hypertension as a consequence of a tumour (phaeochromocytoma).

Pancreas – islets of Langerhans

Diabetes mellitus

This is the most common endocrine disorder of childhood, and may have a genetic, viral or autoimmune cause. The islets of Langerhans cells within the pancreas secrete **insulin**, which is responsive to levels of glucose in the blood. As well as regulating the concentration of glucose in the blood it also increases the rate of synthesis of fat, glycogen and proteins.

Four types of diabetes mellitus have been described. **Type 1** or insulin-dependent diabetes mellitus (IDDM), formerly called juvenile onset, accounts for about 10% of all diabetic patients. It affects two people for every thousand of the population. These patients produce little or no insulin and have a greater tendency to develop ketoacidosis (excess ketone bodies – formed when fatty acids are broken down in the liver as an energy source – in people unable to metabolise glucose). Early in the disease, some patients may not need insulin.

Patients who are controlled by diet alone can be managed as normal patients. Those who are being treated with oral hypoglycaemic drugs (to stimulate residual insulin secretion) should not take their normal drugs on the day of any planned surgery but should restart their drugs the following day. Where diabetic control is poor, these patients should be hospitalised for stabilisation before dental surgery.

Antibiotics are not indicated for diabetic patients as there is little evidence to support their use except that response to infection is poor and may complicate diabetic management.

Type II or non-insulin-dependent (formerly called adult onset) is the most common form and accounts for 90% of all diabetes. This is the non-ketosis-prone form of diabetes where there are decreased amounts of insulin or insulin with decreased activity. A third of type II patients are treated by weight loss, a third by diet and antidiabetic drugs, and the remainder need insulin.

These patients should be admitted to hospital for management of their diabetes during dental surgery.

Type III diabetes is induced by drugs, hormones and genetic syndromes as well as diseases of the pancreas such as Cushing's syndrome, acromegaly and cystic fibrosis. **Type IV** is related to pregnancy.

In all types, treatment is aimed at keeping the blood glucose levels constant. Pancreatic transplants may, in the future, be a viable alternative.

There are a number of long-term complications seen in diabetic patients.

- Visual impairment. Cataracts are a feature of long-standing diabetes.
- Infections are commonplace and probably related to altered neutrophil functions and an increase of glucose in the urine and other body secretions.
- Because of their diabetes, these patients may have premature cardiovascular disease.
- Renal disease is seen early on in the condition and is related to the cardiovascular disease; together with chronic urinary tract infections (UTIs) it leads to renal failure.
- Patients have motor nerve neuropathy leading to diabetic neuropathy, and in combination with the cardiovascular changes and susceptibility to infection, patients will present with, for example, an ulcerated leg that fails to heal.

Specific oral/dental features are:

- decreased salivary flow (fluid changes)
- candida infection (prone to infection)
- dental caries (if control is poor)
- erosion (gastrointestinal tract disturbances)
- periodontal problems (microvascular changes)
- slow wound healing.

Diabetic acidosis results from dehydration as water is excreted with the glucose. There is raised blood glucose from fat (producing acids) and protein breakdown as a result of lack of insulin. Patients are treated with dietary control and appropriate medication depending on their need for insulin. Prior to dental treatment, the dental team needs to know the drugs used and how they are taken (e.g. oral, injected), the frequency and the level of control. In relation to this, the number of hospital admissions and the reasons (e.g. loss of control, infections) are relevant.

Hyperglycaemia (excess glucose in the blood)

If untreated this will lead to diabetic coma and death. It is caused by poor control and can be seen in association with dental infection. The patient will have signs as above, i.e. thirst, dry skin, passing of large quantities of urine, weakness, air hunger (gasping for breath), rapid pulse, low blood pressure, stomach cramps, hunger and nausea before becoming unconscious over a period of days. This develops slowly so the patient is unlikely to present for dental care. However, if it is suspected, glucose should be given by mouth to distinguish from hypoglycaemia if the patient is still conscious, or intravenous glucagon if not. Medical attention should be sought.

Hypoglycaemia (shortage of glucose in the blood)

This is seen where there is an imbalance between the insulin taken, the diet and the energy expended. This develops more rapidly than hyperglycaemia. A patient attending a dental appointment may avoid eating and precipitate a hypoglycaemic attack. Stress adds to the likelihood of such an event. The patient will be pale, sweaty, anxious and may appear confused, even aggressive. They may complain of headaches, nausea and palpitations. Most patients will recognise the warning signs and will carry a supply of glucose with them – usually as sugar lumps or confectionery. The collapsed patient needs Basic Life Support (BLS) and urgent medical attention.

Oral and dental considerations

- Close co-operation with the patient's physician is paramount.
- Diabetic patients who are well controlled should have appointments early in the day when diabetic control is likely to be better.

Recommended tasks

(1) A regular dental patient who is diabetic appears unwell. What are the features that help you decide whether they may be hypo- or hyperglycaemic?

(2) What are the essential features of all the endocrine conditions that are of direct relevance to the safe delivery of dental care?

(3) A new nurse comes to the practice/clinic. Take them through the protocol to be followed when referring patients for dental care under GA, including the pre-operative instructions to the patient/carer.

Gastrointestinal and related disorders

Gastrointestinal tract disorders

There are a number of conditions seen in special care dentistry that come within the remit of predominantly gastrointestinal disorders.

Congenital disorders

Peutz-Jeghers syndrome is characterised by duodenal polyps which may result in part of the bowel telescoping in on itself, resulting in gangrene of the affected section of bowel if not treated. Occasionally, these polyps undergo malignant transformation. There are associated pigmented macules/polyps around the mouth.

Gardner's syndrome – an inherited condition in which there are multiple osteomas, epidermoid cysts and multiple polyps in the colon, which usually undergo malignant change in about the fourth decade of life. Multiple supernumerary teeth are associated with this condition. A dental screening film that detects osteomas/supernumeraries may be the first clue to the disease in someone with chronic diarrhoea or ulcerative colitis.

Acquired gastrointestinal disorders

Coeliac disease (gluten sensitivity) has a familial tendency and is seen in geographical clusters such as the west of Ireland. It is a condition that has a higher prevalence in people with Down syndrome. Coeliac disease arises as a consequence of intolerance to gluten (contained in many cereals) with a reaction between T lymphocytes in the gut wall and gluten. Eventually the villi in the wall of the intestine flatten off and malabsorption follows. A gluten-free diet allows healing, which takes up to three months, with the duodenal portion of the gut the last to heal. Dentally, chronological enamel hypoplasia is seen.

Ulcerative colitis involves the large bowel only, with changes confined to the mucosal lining of the bowel. Patients complain of diarrhoea and weight loss; anaemia is common as a consequence of rectal bleeding. Management is with systemic corticosteroids and oral 5-aminosalicylic acid (5-ASA) drugs. Surgery may be indicated if malignancy supervenes. Orally, there may be ulcers recorded in up to 20% of patients with the disease.

Crohn's disease is a granulomatous disease that occurs in both the small and large bowel, but in discrete areas. Gradual thickening and sclerosis of the bowel wall results in malabsorption, but there may also be perforation and intestinal obstruction. The disease follows a course of remission and relapse. Patients complain of weight loss, diarrhoea, pain and have signs of anaemia. Management is by dietary means. Corticosteroids and even immunosuppression with, for example, ciclosporin or azathioprine may be necessary for periods of time.

Orally, there may be a cobblestone appearance of the buccal mucosa (seen in orofacial granulomatosis as well) and aphthous ulcers. The latter may be the first indication of the presence of Crohn's disease. These can be painful and can make dental treatment difficult because of the discomfort. Care is needed in the placement of the aspirator tip and other manipulation of the oral tissues. Depending on how long-standing the disease is, there may be enamel hypoplasia.

Long-term immunosuppression with steroids can lead to candida and other infections and ciclosporin can lead to gingival hypertrophy.

Gastro-oesophageal disease (GORD/GERD) is a condition in which gastric contents are regurgitated back up into the oesophagus, possibly also with pepsin or bile. In some instances the stomach contents may reach the mouth. If the condition is chronic, there is ulceration of the oesophagus because it is not designed to withstand the low pH of gastric acid. In some patients, there may be aspiration of gastric contents exacerbating a chronic lung condition like asthma. The two conditions may in fact be linked and which comes first is sometimes unclear.

GORD is more common in situations where intra-abdominal pressure is raised. This can be from obesity, late pregnancy, lying supine, large meals with alcohol, hiatus hernia, diabetes and renal disease, and is also related to lifestyle factors, e.g. tobacco, some foods and drugs. It is a common condition in patients where muscle tone is altered, for example in cerebral palsy.

Untreated, patients may progress from oesophageal ulceration to stricture as a consequence of repeated ulceration, and finally to squamous metaplasia (early cancer change in the squamous lining cells of the oesophagus). **Barrett's oesophagus** is the term applied to the latter. Where there is bleeding from ulcerated areas, iron deficiency anaemia will be seen. If the reflux is severe enough to reach the oral cavity, dental erosion is evident on the palatal surfaces of upper teeth and on the occlusal, and sometimes buccal, surfaces of lower teeth.

Management consists of accurate diagnosis, which may involve intra-oesophageal pH monitoring and then treatment consisting of lifestyle changes, management with antacids, layering agents (e.g. Gaviscon), H_2 receptor agonists (Cimetidine/Ranitidine), proton-pump inhibitors (Omeprazole) to reduce acid production and drugs to increase lower oesophageal sphincter tone (Cisapride) and thus facilitate better stomach emptying. Strictures (constriction of the oesophagus from repeated scarring from acid attacks) can be freed by dilatation, and surgery is indicated for hiatus hernias.

Liver disease

The liver performs the following functions in the body:

- regulation of metabolites (carbohydrates, proteins and fats)
- production of bile, including the conversion of bilirubin from the breakdown of haemoglobin so that it can be excreted in bile salts into the duodenum
- detoxification of absorbed toxic materials including drugs, many of which pass through the liver
- synthesis of clotting factors under the influence of vitamin K.

Jaundice

This occurs as a result of accumulation of bilirubin in the circulating blood. It may be obstructive or haemolytic.

- **Obstructive jaundice**: bile cannot flow from the liver either because of a blockage in the bile ducts or disease of the liver itself. Bile is necessary for fat digestion and so fat appears in the stools. Fat soluble vitamin K (necessary for the production of clotting factors) absorption is also affected so eventually clotting will be affected.

- **Haemolytic jaundice**: premature breakdown of haemoglobin produces excess circulating bilirubin that the liver cannot handle. One of the inborn errors of metabolism, glucose-6-dehydrogenase deficiency, classically has haemolytic anaemia as a symptom and learning disability can also be a feature. Certain drugs induce anaemia in these patients. Prilocaine (Citanest®) LA should be avoided in patients with this condition.

Acute and chronic liver disease produce elevated serum bilirubin levels.

Acute hepatitis

Acute hepatitis occurs as a result of:

- increasingly, alcoholism
- infection – viral hepatitis is the most common liver disease worldwide
- drugs, e.g. acute paracetamol poisoning.

These conditions may become chronic and if severe may be an indication for transplantation.

Hepatitis A (infectious hepatitis)

This is commonly spread as a result of poor hygiene, e.g. inadequate handwashing after toileting, contaminated water and food. Patients experience fever, nausea, vomiting, anorexia and appear jaundiced. Patients have lifetime immunity after recovering from infection. People travelling to areas where hepatitis is endemic are usually advised to have immunoglobulin A immediately prior to travel.

Hepatitis B (serum hepatitis)

Hepatitis B is transmitted primarily by intimate contact with body fluids. The incubation period is two to six months, which is much longer than with hepatitis A. Intravenous drug abusers, immigrants from developing countries, Down syndrome males in residential care and other institutionalised populations such as prisoners, and those in receipt of blood products, e.g. patients with haemophilia, have a higher risk of contracting hepatitis B. Some patients progress to chronic liver disease and hepatic cancer and 2% become carriers.

All staff working with potentially infected patients should have an antibody titre in excess of 100mIU/ml to hepatitis B.

Hepatitis C (non-A, non-B) and hepatitis D

These are mostly contracted from blood transfusion products. In addition to the symptoms described above, patients complain of pain in the area of the liver.

Vaccination for hepatitis B also confers protection against hepatitis D.

Chronic liver disease (cirrhosis)

In addition to the signs and symptoms of jaundice, patients with chronic liver disease have a tendency to bleed. This arises because the portal vein becomes occluded and hypertension follows. In addition, anastomoses (connections) between the portal and other systemic veins develop varices (dilated veins), usually at the lower end of the oesophagus, which if ruptured by the increased blood pressure, result in dramatic bleeds. A lowered concentration of plasma proteins and retention of sodium and thus water, together with portal hypertension, result in large accumulations of fluid in the peritoneum (ascites). Patients may have grossly distended abdomens.

Patients who present with liver failure need careful consideration prior to dental treatment. They may be jaundiced, have impaired clotting functions and an inability to detoxify many routine drugs, e.g. LA, antibiotics, analgesics, sedatives and tranquillisers.

Adequate sterilisation protocols must be observed for all patients, irrespective of their medical history. All potentially contaminated instruments should be treated as follows.

(1) All instruments should be removed from the dental surgery to a designated area for processing. Ideally they should be placed directly into a washer disinfector. This should then be followed by sterilisation in a vacuum autoclave according to the manufacturers' specifications.
(2) If this is not possible, the following process should be used. While wearing heavy-duty gloves, wash first under running water, place in an ultrasonic bath with appropriate solution for 10 minutes, rinse, dry and inspect for residual debris. This should be removed by hand.
(3) Where sterilisation of instruments is not possible, disposables *must* be used.
(4) Chemical sterilisation is no longer an accepted practice.
(5) All handpieces and triple air-syringes should be flushed through with water for two minutes at the beginning of the day and for 20 seconds between patients to reduce the chance of microbial contamination.
(6) Where possible, sterile bottled water systems should be used for dental units and these should be drained daily and purged to clear all air/water lines.

The following events may occur post-transplantation:

- graft rejection, but this is usually managed with drugs
- bleeding from oesophageal varices as well as the liver itself
- opportunistic infections – immuno-compromised patient; hepatitis B, C, D; hairy leukoplakia; and Kaposi's sarcoma
- anxiety and depression following on from immediate post-transplant sense of well-being.

Other blood-borne viruses (HIV)

HIV infects T lymphocytes to produce severe disease and eventually death. Patients develop a number of infections as a consequence of immunosuppression, particularly pneumonias, tuberculosis, encephalitis, other neurological problems and tumours (particularly the rare **Kaposi's sarcoma**). HIV infection ultimately progresses to a collection of signs and symptoms termed the acquired human immunodeficiency syndrome (**AIDS**).

The virus is transmitted in body fluids and infection has been most prevalent in those groups in the population who are at risk by virtue of:

- lifestyle (intravenous drug abusers, homosexuals)
- accidental exposure (patients with haemophilia, transfusion recipients in countries where blood products are not screened, possibly in transplanted donor organs, babies breast-fed by infected mothers, needlestick injuries).

Patients may present with general signs and symptoms:

- chronic (long-standing) viral infections, e.g. herpes simplex and zoster, cytomegalovirus
- bacterial, e.g. pneumonias, drug-resistant tuberculosis
- fungal, e.g. candida
- neurological defects from infections, e.g. encephalitis, peripheral neuropathy
- tumours, e.g. Kaposi's sarcoma, non-Hodgkin's lymphoma.

Oral effects

- Candida infection occurs early on in the disease; its progression to involve the oesophagus may result in difficulty in swallowing.
- Ulcerative gingivitis and periodontitis.
- Hairy leukoplakia, seen in patients who are immunosuppressed and not just patients infected with HIV. This is due to infection with Epstein-Barr virus and affects the lateral border of the tongue after secretion of the virus from adjacent salivary glands.
- Kaposi's sarcoma exists together with herpes virus infection and as well as predominantly affecting the skin, this raised, purple-coloured lesion is seen commonly intra-orally in patients with HIV (although occasionally seen in renal transplant patients as a consequence of immunosuppression).

Treatment is managed by a multiprofessional team and consists of management of infections and neoplasia, antiretroviral therapy, and appropriate counselling and support.

Dental management

- Respecting patient confidentiality at all times is paramount and all healthcare workers must be mindful of this while at the same time conscious of their duty to protect other staff and patients.

- Since most patients will be unaware of their disease state, all dental patients should be managed with adherence to the highest standards of infection control. Staff should have appropriate PPE, including facemasks, preferably incorporating transparent face shields as protection from aerosol contamination. Cuts and wounds should be covered before effective handwashing and gloving. It is desirable that all staff should be vaccinated for hepatitis B, although it is acknowledged that not everyone will seroconvert and have satisfactory antibody titres. Such staff should be offered appropriate counselling and be made aware of the policy to be followed should they obtain a percutaneous injury during their work practices.

- Needles should never be resheathed directly by hand and mechanisms must be in place to manage used needles, both for resheathing and disposal into a sharps receptacle. Disposables should be sealed in strong bags that cannot easily be punctured, according to the local waste disposal policy.

- Specimens from patients should be double-sealed in strong plastic bags and the receiving laboratory notified. Similarly, impressions must be disinfected in an appropriate sodium hypochlorite solution and sealed before transfer to the laboratory, which should be notified accordingly.

- Instruments that can be sterilised should be processed appropriately following best practice recommendations within the dental surgery or sent to a Central Sterile Supply Department. Instruments that cannot be heat sterilised must be replaced with disposables prior to starting treatment. Surfaces that potentially may be contaminated should be covered with material that can be removed and disposed of between patients. Surfaces should be swabbed with an appropriate solution as per local infection control policy.

Spleen

This organ is responsible for the production of some antibodies (IgM) and for the removal of worn-out red blood cells and other waste products. Although theoretically the spleen is not an essential organ, dental patients who have had their spleen removed are usually covered by prophylactic antibiotics, especially if there is other, underlying disease. Children may be more at risk than adults.

Renal disease

Patients with renal disease are more likely to be seen in primary dental care, with better survival both for those undergoing dialysis and for patients who have renal transplants. The kidneys are responsible for maintaining homoeostasis – the nephrons in the kidneys filter over 7 litres of blood an hour, and if all this went unfiltered the body would lose all its water and salt content in half a day. Solutes such as sodium, potassium, glucose, amino acids, by-products of metabolic processes and some drugs are filtered out. Depending on the body's needs, some are retained by reabsorption into the blood and the remainder are excreted in the urine.

Patients may have either acute or chronic renal disease. **Acute renal failure** must be treated immediately, otherwise there is irreversible damage to the kidney's filtration system and cardiac changes occur. Treatment is by dialysis; usually haemodialysis three times a week for 4–5 hours each time.

Chronic renal disease occurs with a gradual reduction in the number of functioning nephrons and evidence of this may only become apparent when the number is reduced by 75%. Because the kidney is concerned with blood pressure control, as well as red cell production and calcium balance via its role in vitamin D absorption, the effects are noted elsewhere in the body. End-stage renal failure usually follows and is treated by dialysis; this may be by haemodialysis or peritoneal dialysis, depending on a number of factors.

Peritoneal dialysis involves an exchange of fluids through a catheter in the peritoneum so that toxins are removed over a few hours. This avoids travel to a centre for haemodialysis and is cheaper. If there are recurrent infections at the site of the catheter, and especially peritonitis, the patient needs to be placed on haemodialysis. Continuous ambulatory peritoneal dialysis (CAPD) enables patients to have a reasonably normal lifestyle with dialysis going on via the peritoneum. Home-based peritoneal dialysis is used especially for younger patients to prevent interference with schooling, and can be undertaken overnight.

The ideal is a renal transplant but patients are reliant on a suitable donor and in some areas there may be an upper age limit.

The signs and symptoms seen in the oral soft tissues are:

- dry mouth – decreased salivary flow rate
- metallic taste after dialysis – due to uraemia
- enlarged tongue – due to uraemia
- reduced response to infection (bacterial, viral or fungal)
- no correlation between levels of plaque and calculus with the degree of gingivitis. Increased calculus deposits are as a result of raised pH of saliva.

Bony intra-oral signs include:

- loss of lamina dura
- changes in radiodensity on x-rays
- radiolucent lesions in the jaws
- calcification in soft tissues
- malocclusions.

The teeth may show:

- intrinsic staining (due to the disease or antibiotics or both)
- enamel hypoplasia
- reduced caries prevalence (raised salivary pH from urea breakdown products in saliva)
- delayed eruption.

Dental considerations in patients on renal dialysis

- These patients will be on heparin for dialysis to prevent any blockage of the arterio-venous shunt in their arm. This will complicate bleeding as the half-life of heparin is about 4–6 hours. Any surgical procedures should therefore be deferred until the day after dialysis, when toxins in the blood are also reduced.

- Physicians usually prefer patients with shunts to receive antibiotic prophylaxis although there is no evidence to justify its use in these circumstances. The kidney's capacity to handle some antibiotics is altered and should be avoided long term. For example, potassium-containing penicillins, tetracyclines and cephalosporins are all toxic to the kidney; erythromycin is a safer alternative.

- Normal infection control procedures should be instituted. Because of dialysis, the prevalence of blood-borne viruses, hepatitis B, C and D, and HIV are potentially greater. Dialysis also predisposes patients to bony changes (renal osteodystrophy) and secondary hyperparathyroidism (see parathyroid glands), which is seen as cystic-like lesions in the jaw bones on routine dental orthopantomograms.

Patients with renal disease have:

- anaemia, unless well controlled. This is secondary to the uraemia, a lack of erythro-poietin production by the kidney, blood loss during dialysis and the shortened life span of the red blood cells. It is treated by iron supplements. This is a consideration for patients contemplating GA
- biochemical abnormalities
- hepatitis risk from dialysis
- renal bone disease
- raised blood pressure (hypertension)
- need for antibiotics to protect the arterio-venous anastomoses.

Renal transplant patients

Patients with end-stage renal failure may be successful in obtaining a cadaveric donor organ or allograft from a matched donor, usually a close relative. Once normal renal function is restored after transplantation, the patient can be treated as if the kidney is normal. However, they will be taking a number of drugs, namely:

- immunosuppressants to prevent rejection of the graft
- antibiotics for prophylaxis against UTI
- antihypertensives for blood pressure control
- calcium channel blockers for blood pressure control.

These can have side effects such as gingival overgrowth. The patient's care should take into account management of these drug-related effects as well as underlying diseases, e.g. diabetes, that may have predisposed the patient to renal failure. As well as care with antibiotics, other drugs that are excreted via the kidney should be used only after consultation with the patient's physician, e.g. NSAIDs and paracetamol for prolonged use. Aspirin seems to be less toxic to the kidney. Not all transplants are successful and the patient may still require dialysis, so antibiotic prophylaxis to protect arterio-venous shunts, anaemia and heparinisation needs to be considered prior to dental treatment. Dentists need to be aware of the potential for neoplastic change within the drug-induced gingival overgrowth.

Other organ transplants

Heart-lung transplants are becoming a viable consideration in patients with cystic fibrosis. Heart and kidney transplants are more commonplace and liver transplants are becoming more routine.

Bone marrow transplantation is advocated for:

- lymphomas
- relapsed leukaemias
- aplastic anaemia
- severe combined immunodeficiency (SCID).

Oral and dental considerations

- Patients undergo total body irradiation and methotrexate prophylaxis for graft versus host disease prior to transplantation and will be severely immunocompromised for some weeks thereafter, so any dental care should be carried out prior to total body irradiation and only once the immunosuppressed state is nearing normality. Antibiotic cover is essential.

- Patients may require systemic antivirals prophylactically and will require antibiotics for any invasive dental care.

- Oral hygiene is severely compromised during the peri-transplant time; mouth soreness from mucositis (reddening, soreness and ulceration of the oral mucosa) makes insistence on toothbrushing impossible. Extremely soft toothbrushes (Ultrasuave) may be tolerated. A 0.2% chlorhexidine solution diluted 50:50 to make it less astringent will help keep the mouth clean and prevent any oral source of secondary bacterial infection. The 1% gel version can be applied locally to especially sore areas using a clean finger or cotton wool bud.

- Benzydamine hydrochloride (Difflam) – as a spray in children under 12 years of age – may relieve the pain of mucositis unless it is really severe.

- Preventive measures may be needed against oral candida.

- Oral sponges that contain lemon and glycerine can be very erosive and are not advocated because of the danger of enamel erosion.

- Preventive measures for caries can be by topical applications of neutral sodium fluoride products (stannous fluoride is astringent to oral tissues).

- Saliva stimulants/substitutes may be necessary for patients in whom salivary gland function has been diminished or lost entirely by the radiotherapy.

- Ice chips have been shown in trials to give the most effective relief from mucositis induced by chemotherapy. Chlorhexidine has minimal if any effect in this clinical situation.

Recommended tasks

(1) A patient with a blood-borne viral infection fails to attend his appointment. When you ring him he says he did not attend because he feels he may be stigmatised by staff. Outline how you will reassure him by telephone about the way he will be looked after to minimise this feeling.

(2) Consider how you will explain to the mother of a child with renal disease why the child's teeth are stained and pitted and their gums are overgrown.

(3) What aspects of dental care need to be carefully managed to reduce the risks of sequelae for the patient with liver disease?

Neurological and psychiatric disorders

Epilepsy

This is a symptom rather than a disease, divided into generalised and partial. The causes of seizures are numerous and may not be determined in some cases (25%). Epilepsy may be genetic or acquired.

- Genetic – if one parent is affected there is a 4% risk, if both parents then a 10–14% risk. Associated genetic conditions with increasing prevalence of seizure disorders are: Sturge-Weber, Down, Fragile X syndromes, and von Recklinghausen's neurofibromatosis.

- Acquired – brain damage, cerebrovascular accidents (strokes), brain tumours, alcohol intoxication.

Clinical presentation

Tonic-clonic seizures (used to be called grand mal)

Patients occasionally will sense an aura a few seconds before a seizure. There may be facial flushing, dilated pupils and rolling eyes, drooling, and increased blood pressure and pulse. During the attack there will be twitching of the extremities which may last minutes. After the seizure, the patient will appear dazed and slow to recover, complaining of a headache. There may be incontinence of both urine and faeces.

*Absences (*used to be called petit mal*)*
These are seen more commonly in younger people. These attacks last for a few seconds only and resemble an *absence*, but may occur tens of times a day. The patient appears vacant and staring.

Most people are considered to have active seizures if they have had an attack within the previous two years. Attacks are usually managed with drugs and in the majority of patients only one drug is needed. The drugs commonly used are carbamazepine, sodium valproate, clonazepam, lamotrigine, ethosuximide. Where these cannot control the seizures, other drugs in combination are needed: vigabatrin, lamotrigine, gabapentin, topiramate, all with a slightly different range of effects and side effects. Phenytoin, with all the problems of gingival overgrowth, is no longer the first choice of drug.

Common problems with the current drugs are:

- weight gain
- sedation
- interactions with other drugs (e.g. aspirin, NSAIDs, antifungals and phenytoin; erythromycin with carbamazepine and sodium valproate)
- side effects such as oral ulceration with ethosuximide, benzodiazepines and midazolam/flumazenil (reversal agent); gingival hypertrophy; birth defects; and in severely affected individuals, seizures despite a combination of therapies.

Oral and dental considerations

- The seizure history should be checked at each visit and the possibility of drug interactions with any change in drugs considered.

- For routine dental procedures, local anaesthetics are safe to use in normal doses. Some common sedative agents, e.g. midazolam, are used to control seizures either orally or as intramuscular injections; diazepam can be given rectally as a suppository. Nitrous oxide is not a cerebral irritant and is therefore safe. Dental care under GA should be provided in a hospital setting (but note that sodium valproate affects platelets and there is therefore potential for bleeding after surgery).The reversal agent used for IV sedation, flumazenil, should not be used with patients who are taking benzodiazepines for control of other conditions.

- Aggressive preventive care is vital because of the potential effects of sugar-based medicines, xerostomia, gingival hypertrophy and the likelihood of dental trauma in patients with poorly controlled seizures.

The majority of patients become free of seizures but at least half need to maintain their drug regime. Death due to seizures primarily occurs because of:

- accidents, maybe as a consequence of a seizure
- effects of the drugs used for control
- asphyxiation/bronchopneumonia due to aspiration

- heart-related effects
- status epilepticus (persistent seizure – life-threatening).

Acquired and degenerative

Multiple sclerosis

Multiple sclerosis (MS) is a disease that affects the central nervous system (CNS). It is a chronic autoimmune, demyelinating (loss of myelin sheath around nerve fibres) disease affecting young adults (20–40 years), usually females. It is characterised by periods of remission and relapse. The areas of demyelination affect the spinal cord and areas of the brain. There are four types of MS.

- Benign – mild attacks with complete recovery (with little or no disability after 15 years).
- Relapsing/remitting (25%) – with increasing disability after each relapse.
- Secondary progressive (40%) – relapsing/remitting initially, progressing after 15–20 years to no remission periods.
- Primary progressive (15%) steadily worsening with little/no remission.

The symptoms are dependent on the area of the CNS affected and the extent of demyelination. Patients report transitory weakness, sensory disturbance affecting a limb and cognitive effects, seen as personality changes and mood swings. There are co-ordination defects and tremor, visual disturbances, dysphagia, slurred speech and hearing defects, and problems with breathing, bladder and bowel control. Chronic pain can be the most disabling effect and impacts seriously on the patient's quality of life.

There are a number of signs of MS relevant to the dental team.

- **Trigeminal neuralgia**: the dentist may be consulted because this is one of the early signs, characterised by an intense pain involving one or more branches of the trigeminal nerve. It is managed with carbamazepine, phenytoin or sodium valproate, or if a trigger can be found, by cryotherapy or injection of LA.
- Trigeminal sensory neuropathy and facial palsy.
- Lateral gaze defect.
- Abnormal peri-oral hypersensitivity or anaesthesia. Altered sensations in this area mean that the dental team should be cautious about offering treatment in situations where the report of dental pain is vague and reliable signs and symptoms are absent.

Oral and dental considerations

- In addition to the signs and symptoms detailed above, treatment is mainly symptomatic and essentially based on physiotherapy and drug therapy. The drugs used can produce dental sequelae.

- Oral baclofen, tizanidine, dantrolene, gabapentin and diazepam all reduce muscle spasticity.
- Drugs for bladder dysfunction may produce a dry mouth.
- Cannabis assists in spasticity and bladder control but has significant oral side effects, such as gingivitis, white patches, candidiasis (also from steroids), epithelial dysplasia/carcinoma and xerostomia. The drug may also interfere with LA and intravenous sedative agents.
- Other drugs, such as antidepressants, anticholinergics (for incontinence), antihistamines (for dizziness) and antispasmodics, produce a dry mouth and predispose patients to dental caries.
- Cytotoxics and β-interferon, which delay the disease progression as well as the degree of disability, can result in oral ulceration and blood dyscrasias.
- Infections aggravate the disease and so dental infections must be eradicated. Disease prevention is crucial. Patients may need special help with mouth cleaning, especially with advanced tremors. Other factors that worsen the signs and symptoms are anaesthetics and surgery, as well as other stressful events, which should therefore be avoided where possible.
- Despite reports in the lay press there has been no sound scientific evidence to link mercury from amalgam fillings with MS.

Motor neurone disease

This is a progressive condition of older people with no known cause, involving degenerative changes in the cells of the brain and nerve-conducting pathways. Patients have weakness of the head and neck muscles, as well as eating, swallowing and speech difficulties. The tongue may be reduced in size, cannot be stuck out and quivers.

Oral and dental considerations

- Patients may have difficulty in managing oral secretions and, in particular, swallowing.
- Good aspiration is essential.
- Consideration of the length of the appointment because of the muscle weakness.
- Patients may be transported in a wheelchair.

Myasthenia gravis

Myasthenia gravis (MG) is an autoimmune disease of muscles, which experience extreme but painless fatigue that is relieved by rest and made worse by infection or stress. It is a rare cause of arthrogryposis multiplex congenita (joint contractures and other deformities), when antibodies from the mother cross the placenta. MG can occur from one year of age, after childbirth and after the use of muscle relaxants used in GA.

Patients report drooping of the eyelids and double vision, as well as difficulty in swallowing, speaking or chewing (bulbar palsy), drooling, neck or limb weakness. Respiratory weakness can be life-threatening.

Patients receive treatment to relieve their symptoms and may be taking azathioprine and prednisolone, both of which are immunosuppressants. They may also be taking anticholinesterase drugs. For muscles to function, acetylcholine is released at the junction between a stimulating nerve and the muscle fibre. The enzyme cholinesterase destroys the acetylcholine, thus preventing the nerve transmission that stimulates the muscle to work, hence the use of anticholinesterase drugs.

Patients may also be taking atropine to help with drooling, which will result in a dry mouth. Patients who have had this form of therapy for a long time may be so used to the dry mouth that they do not report symptoms from it.

Patients who have taken excess anticholinesterase drugs may have a cholinergic crisis, the signs of which are excess saliva production, tears, increased sweating, vomiting and contraction of the pupils.

Parkinson's disease

This is a neurological disorder of unknown cause. It is a progressive, degenerative disease mainly affecting those over the age of 50 years. A loss of the chemical neurotransmitter dopamine leads to increased adrenergic activity, similar to the effects of some of the drugs used to treat MS. Treatment is aimed therefore at replacing dopamine.

The signs and symptoms of the condition are:

- slow, staccato-like movement
- shuffling, with a rigid body and lack of facial expression – mask-like appearance
- rigidity and flexure of the upper body
- postural instability – unsteady on their feet
- tremor of the arms and head even at rest
- speech difficulties
- drooling due to swallowing difficulties, rather than excess saliva production.

Oral and dental considerations

- The body posture signs and symptoms listed above make sitting in the dental chair and opening the mouth more difficult, and the tremor, if present, can compromise the safe delivery of treatment. Mouldable head supports are an advantage in such patients, as is the use of mouth props.

- Many of these patients have difficulty with the control of their airway and extreme care must be taken by the dental team in ensuring that oral secretions and water, such as that from the high-speed handpiece and ultrasonic scaler, are aspirated away rapidly. Keeping the patient upright in the dental chair is therefore helpful, as is the use of rubber dam, if this can be tolerated.

- More can be accomplished if dental appointments are within a couple of hours of taking the antiparkinsonian drugs.

■ Splint therapy can be helpful in patients who experience pain secondary to the muscle tremor and where rigidity is a feature of the disease.

Some drugs react with other medication such as levodopa (which is converted into dopamine in the brain) but reacts with benzodiazepines and epinephrine in dental LA. Some drugs may produce excess saliva while others produce the opposite effect. Patients are advised to use frequent sips of water or sugar-free gum or sweets to stimulate saliva. **Artificial saliva** may be required. This needs to take into account religious and cultural preferences; for example, Saliva Orthana contains pig gastric mucin. Others (e.g. Biotene) interact with the normal foaming agents found in toothpastes and are inactivated. Not all contain fluoride (only Saliva Orthana and Luborant spray and Biotene toothpaste). The pH of some is low and their use is not advised for patients who are dentate. Tooth Mousse, a topical, water-based, sugar-free cream containing casein phosphopeptide–amorphous calcium phosphate and fluoride, is useful for patients who have a dry mouth and are at risk of caries.

Where excess salivation, or poor control of saliva exists, botulinum toxin ('Botox') injected bilaterally into the parotid glands has been tried with some success and no noted side effects.

Home care may be compromised by the ability of the patient to carry out oral hygiene procedures and a partner or carer may need to help with this task as well as with removing and inserting dentures. Personalised instruction may be given to the carer to aid the patient, such as a mouth care programme to suit the specific needs of that patient.

Alzheimer's disease

This is just one of the causes of dementia that produces a decline in intellectual capacity. Alzheimer's disease is due to an as yet unknown wasting of nerve fibres in the brain. It accounts for half of all cases of dementia in older people (5% of people over 65 years; 20% of those over 80 years of age). Cases are sporadic but may be inherited. Older Down syndrome patients have many of the signs consistent with Alzheimer's disease, such as loss of cognitive function and the inability to carry out their usual daily routines, for example toothbrushing. Early brain trauma may be an aetiological factor and aluminium deposits have also been implicated. Caffeine is proposed as being protective.

The signs and symptoms of Alzheimer's disease are as follows.

■ Patients have a loss of short-term memory initially but are able to recall events decades previously. As a consequence of the memory loss, patients become frustrated, agitated and may appear disoriented. The latter leads them to behave bizarrely in strange surroundings, for example a new dental surgery.
■ Personality changes.
■ Purposeful wandering secondary to memory loss. For example, the patient may get up at 3am, shave, dress and then wander off outside.

- Confusion. Patients with higher levels of functioning are at greater risk of suicide attempts.
- Deterioration in personal hygiene which may be related to dyspraxia (a disorder of the organisation and planning of physical movement) and the inability to recognise everyday items such as a toothbrush and toothpaste.
- Loss of language skills.
- Immobility and generalised wasting of the whole body. Poor nutrition because of swallowing difficulties may be resolved by the use of a surgical procedure (PEG) in which a permanent entry is made into the stomach for feeding.
- Incontinence.

These patients will have been investigated for the other possible causes of their symptoms, especially thyroid disease, vitamin B_{12}, folate deficiencies and benign cerebral tumours.

Oral and dental considerations

- Patients may be taking a variety of drugs. Cholinesterase inhibitors are the most likely, but some others are potentially useful: hormone replacement therapy (HRT); anti-inflammatory drugs; high-dose vitamin E; and Ginkgo biloba. There are no clinical trials yet to support alternative therapies.

- Side effects of drugs include xerostomia. The dental team needs to plan dental care taking this into account. In dentate patients the risk of dental caries is increased. In edentulous patients, lack of saliva makes denture wearing difficult.

- Dental treatment will become increasingly difficult to deliver as the condition of the patient worsens with advancing disease. It is sensible to plan treatment with this in mind and to retain teeth that are viable long term but to remove teeth of poor prognosis, which the patient will not be able to maintain, e.g. teeth with furcation involvement, as long as this does not compromise denture design.

- Older patients tolerate drugs less well. They have reduced levels of albumin in the blood to which many drugs bind so that free, circulating drug levels are higher. In addition, liver mass and circulation is reduced and so drug breakdown and excretion via this route is reduced; there may, therefore, be toxic levels of drugs circulating. Similar effects are noted with drugs excreted via the kidneys.

- There is the potential for interactions with prescribed medications.

- In elderly patients, many drugs produce peak blood levels twice as high and have a half-life twice as long as those seen in younger patients.

As a general approach to dental care, many of the patients with dementia revert almost to a second childhood and so approaching dental care with this in mind is helpful. A careful, simple step-by-step explanation of what is to be done, as well as giving the patient time to get used to the idea, is advisable. This way, irrational behaviour and distress on the part of the patient can be avoided.

Acquired brain injury

This occurs either as a result of trauma such as from road traffic accidents or indirectly as a result of surgery for tumours and other cranial pathology. Similar results are also observed in young children in cases of non-accidental injury.

The signs and symptoms are similar to those observed in patients who have had a stroke (CVA). They are:

- unilateral weakness (hemiplegia), paralysis and/or paraesthesias
- communication difficulties involving vision, hearing and speech
- altered behaviour with psychiatric and emotional disorders.

While there is slow recovery, not all function may be fully restored and on the evidence in the literature, most patients will retain behavioural and sensorimotor (especially speech) difficulties even a year after the event.

Oral and dental considerations

- An awareness by the dental team that the patient may have concurrent, underlying disease, for example cardiovascular disease, the management of which will also affect how dental care is delivered.
- There may have been significant oral and dental changes as a result of the cause of the brain injury, for example jaw fractures and avulsed teeth consequent to a road traffic accident.
- Patients will be undergoing intensive rehabilitation, including physiotherapy and occupational therapy. Work with a speech and language therapist may also help with drooling.
- Tolerance of operative procedures may be reduced and short appointments are indicated, at least initially.
- Pain, for example from fractured and exposed teeth, should be dealt with promptly. It is not the role of the primary care dentist to manage jaw fractures, although they may have been missed by a casualty officer if not accompanied by signs and symptoms. Old, healed fractures are sometimes seen on an orthopantomogram (OPT).
- Patients who have had surgery for tumours or other pathology may be taking a number of drugs, many of which will have a bearing on what the dental team may be doing, for example the patient who has panhypopituitarism consequent to removal of the pituitary due to an adenoma. Such patients may need additional steroids prior to dental surgery.
- Difficulty in swallowing may mean that patients cannot clear oral secretions or cope with large volumes of fluids so that high-volume suction is mandatory.
- Allowing the patient to stay upright is helpful.

- Some patients may be in a wheelchair during the early stages of their recovery and allowances have to be made for providing care with the patient in their own chair if no mechanism such as a hoist or modified dental chair exists to allow them to be treated in a dental chair.
- On occasions, it may be preferable to provide care in a domiciliary setting or even on a hospital ward. The availability of a custom-made domiciliary kit, including a dental motor, suction, curing light and air supply, greatly enhances the range of dental care that can be offered.
- Patients may acclimatise poorly to new prostheses and consideration should be given to duplication of existing dentures where at all possible.

Spinal cord injury

Patients with spinal cord injuries have usually sustained these in accidents and until the time of the accident may have experienced routine dental and home oral care.

The level of impairment suffered post injury will depend on the level at which the lesion occurs. Damage to the lower end of the spinal cord results in paralysis of the lower limbs, so-called **hemiplegia** or **diplegia**. Patients may also have no control of bladder and bowel functions. These patients will be in a wheelchair and so treatment is limited by the facilities offered by the primary dental care provider. Dental staff need to be trained in safe handling and moving of such patients either with the aid of a hoist to move them from their chair to the dental chair, or transfer of the patient's wheelchair into the dental unit itself. Patients who have no lower limb sensation need to be moved regularly to avoid pressure sores. When they have no bladder sensation, regular voiding is important to avoid over-distension which can cause a dramatic rise in blood pressure. Blood pressure monitoring of such patients is therefore desirable.

Patients with spinal cord injury at a higher level have **quadriplegia**, with all four limbs affected. As well as the precautions noted above, the swallowing and gag reflexes are affected. Dental care with the use of a rubber dam and good aspiration to hand, as well as a calm atmosphere to diminish the patient's anxiety, are important. The dentist may be asked to make mouthsticks to facilitate the use of equipment such as a computer keyboard by the patient who is unable to use their upper limbs.

As with all patients, careful history taking will reveal details of those patients who are taking anticlotting drugs such as warfarin or aspirin. The INR value for the former and the bleeding time for the latter may need to be identified before invasive dental care is offered.

Cerebrovascular accident (CVA; stroke)

CVA is caused by one of the following.

- Bleeding into the brain from a congenital defect such as a ruptured aneurysm or occasionally because of the use of anticoagulants, e.g. warfarin used in patients who have had heart surgery and/or who have high blood pressure. This accounts for about 20% of all strokes. A common site for such bleeds is a congenital weakness of the circle of Willis at the base of the brain. Bleeding from here results in a subarachnoid haemorrhage with sudden onset of severe headache, neck stiffness and loss of consciousness. If not recognised and comprehensively managed, death is highly likely.

■ Blockage of a small or large blood vessel with a blood clot (**thrombus**). This type of stroke is more commonly seen in patients who have high blood pressure (hypertension). There may, in hindsight, often have been a warning with transient ischaemic attacks (TIAs) leading to a full-blown stroke. These have little effect after the first 24 hours, but such patients will normally be on low-dose aspirin (75–300mg/day) for prophylaxis. Falls in elderly people may be as a consequence of such *mini-strokes*.

■ An embolus in the brain, coming from the area of the carotid bifurcation in the neck, as well as in patients in atrial fibrillation, especially in patients with a history of valve disease. It arises when atheromatous plaques rupture. This is of more sudden onset and recovery is slower. Patients who have had a stroke as a result of atrial fibrillation may well be taking anticoagulants, e.g. warfarin.

Signs and symptoms of a CVA will depend on where the occlusion (blockage) occurs, but will present as weakness or paralysis, which may involve the facial muscles. In right-handed people the left side of the brain is dominant but in left-handers either side may be dominant. There may be difficulty in eating and swallowing. If you suspect that the person is having a stroke, get them to hold their hands out in front, to smile and to say their name. If they are unable to do these things, call an ambulance and let them know you think the person has had a stroke.

The patient will complain of a headache, nausea and even vomiting, and double incontinence, as well as experiencing numbness or paralysis of a limb or side of the body. There may be vision and speech disturbances (**dysarthria**) as well as disorders of language (**dysphasia**), both written and spoken. The latter is particularly frustrating for patient and relative alike, struggling to find the right word, and is a deficit that originates in a higher brain centre than purely speech disturbances.

Recovery is seen in approximately two-thirds of patients, with death occurring in the remainder. Of those who recover, half will be at risk of subsequent strokes and the remainder will be dependent on others for their daily care. Such repeated strokes account for a significant burden of dementia.

In recovery, patients are nursed in hospital with frequent observation to prevent infection, commonly chest infections, pneumonia and bed sores. Patients are fed by nasogastric tube if unconscious or directly into the stomach by a PEG procedure, since swallowing may be poor and the danger of aspiration into the lungs with resultant infection is a constant danger. Simultaneously, the various therapists will aid the patient's recovery by physiotherapy to encourage early mobility, speech therapy to overcome dysarthria and occupational therapy to equip the patient to cope with a degree of independent living, once recovery is well advanced. Liaison with the therapist can be mutually beneficial in allowing the exchange of ideas and techniques that may benefit the patient's rehabilitation orally and dentally.

All the oral and dental considerations outlined in the care of people with acquired brain injury apply here. Oral hygiene in the early days after a stroke needs to be managed by ward staff or the principal carer. Mouth sponges that are frequently used on wards contain lemon and glycerine and while they moisten the dehydrated oral cavity well, in the dentate patient their continued use puts enamel and dentine at risk of erosion. In patients who can tolerate oral feeding, weakened orofacial musculature means that there may be *pouching* of food in the buccal mucosa and carers/nursing staff need to be aware of this and know how to clear the mouth of old food debris. The use of a toothbrush that also permits aspiration (suction toothbrush) is useful in mouth cleaning for the unconscious or semi-conscious patient. The lips should be moistened with Vaseline before and after mouth cleaning to aid patient comfort.

During aftercare patients may be medicated with aspirin or warfarin and dental care planning needs to take this into account, as well as any antihypertensive drugs that may now be prescribed for the patient.

Huntingdon's chorea

This is an inherited degenerative disease of the central nervous system identified as a defect in chromosome 4. The clinical features of the condition are psychiatric disorders (psychoses, depression, aggression and loss of impulse control), motor disturbances and dementia. Cognitive disturbances involve particularly memory and concentration. There is **hyperkinesia** (abnormal increase in motor function and activity), which results in staggering, and **hyperlordosis** (increased curvatures seen normally in the lumbar and cervical regions of the spine), and in the orofacial region the tongue is affected. The drugs used to treat the psychiatric disorders may actually make the hyperkinesia worse. There are serious effects on speech and swallowing and bruxism may be a feature.

Oral and dental considerations

- The hyperkinesia makes the safe delivery of care virtually impossible unless there is a degree of control.

- Hyperkinesia of the orofacial muscles may result in trauma and fractures, resulting in broken teeth which may be easily inhaled.

- Denture wearing may be compromised because of the uncontrolled movements and the lack of saliva (xerostomia). The use of implants should therefore be considered in these patients.

- Communication may be hampered by the speech defects.

- Anticholinergic drugs produce xerostomia and this can have a disastrous effect on the teeth and soft tissues, particularly when coupled with the poor oral hygiene seen as a result of the general disinterest that forms part of the natural course of the disease.

- Dental care needs to be planned early in the disease so that long-term decisions can be made in consultation with the neurologist managing the patient's general care.

- Planning needs to be radical. Teeth of poor prognosis, including those with advanced loss of support and/or furcation involvement, should be extracted. Topical fluoride therapy using high-dose forms such as varnishes (2300ppm F) and prescribed toothpastes at fluoride concentrations of 2800–5000ppm F that are used for other high caries risk patients should be considered.

- Anaesthesia is complex in patients with Huntingdon's chorea; premedication with smaller than normal doses of oral midazolam, titrated to that individual patient's needs, is safe, but any agent affecting the central nervous system has to be used with caution. Aspiration is a real risk in these patients and control of saliva is poor in the recovery phase. High-speed aspiration is essential. This, combined with the poor muscle control, weakness and malnutrition in some cases make safe delivery of dental care under GA hazardous. However, a stable oral state contributes to the social and psychological integration of the patient.

- Good communication between the physician and the carer is essential; nobody will know the patient as well as their regular, long-term carer.

Prion diseases

These diseases have come into prominence recently as a group of fatal neurodegenerative disorders caused by the accumulation of an abnormal protein in the central nervous system. Those most familiar to the dental team are sporadic **Creutzfeldt–Jakob disease** (CJD) and **new variant CJD**.

In these conditions, the brain and spinal cord undergo a spongy degeneration in a slowly progressing disease that has an incubation period of up to 20 years.

Sporadic CJD affects older people and is preceded by symptoms of headache, tiredness and weight loss. There is rapid mental deterioration accompanied by ataxia and blindness, progressing to mutism (inability to speak). An iatrogenic (caused by the clinician/dental team) form, spread by improperly sterilised instruments, grafts and growth hormone should be eradicated with greater awareness and knowledge of the potential for this to occur.

Variant CJD has been linked to **bovine spongiform encephalopathy (BSE)** in cattle and is found in a much younger age group than sporadic CJD. Affected individuals, who may or may not have eaten infected beef (some sufferers have claimed to be vegetarian), have behavioural and psychiatric disease over a number of months, accompanied physically by involuntary movements, progressing to mutism and dementia.

Sporadic CJD is seen in relatively elderly people and some of the signs and symptoms may be confused with other acquired neurodegenerative diseases seen more commonly in this age group. Variant CJD affects a young age group who, given the rapid progression of the disease and the likelihood that the collection of symptoms lead rapidly to a diagnosis, are unlikely to present for routine dental care. However, such patients may require palliative care and this must be provided in the same way as for other patients, taking into account the infection control measures required to prevent the spread of the disease.

There is no current evidence for the transmission of prion diseases from oral tissue, although it is known that gingival tissue from infected individuals contains more prion protein material than pulpal tissue. Bone graft material from outside the UK is not thought to carry a risk. Patients who have received growth hormone after 1985 are not thought to be at risk since they have been given a commercial, non-human pituitary-derived growth hormone instead. In the UK, potential transplant tissue from patients who have had brain or spinal cord operations before August 1992 will not be accepted for grafting.

Further details of appropriate infection control measures are described in the section on Cross-infection control (p. 89).

Psychiatric disorders

Neurosis

Depression
This may be part of the individual's make-up or appear as a consequence of traumatic life events. It may accompany other underlying medical problems, for example the demented patient with high cognitive function or the person with a learning disability, and can lead to attempted suicide. More temporary depression may be seen as part of postnatal events.

Patients who are depressed appear outwardly sad and may even be tearful. They will be chronically tired if their sleep pattern is disturbed, often waking in the early hours of the morning and unable to sleep thereafter. Some patients may lose weight, with no apparent interest in food, while others overeat. Memory is poor and the individual is distracted and cannot concentrate on any task reliably.

Oral and dental considerations

- Electro-convulsive therapy (ECT) is sometimes used to treat very severe depression and the patient's dentition needs to be sound before this treatment. During ECT the electrodes are applied just above the ears in the temporal area. Drugs used to sedate the patient or produce anaesthesia (if the patient is to be paralysed) will reduce the reflexes that protect the airway, so loose teeth must be removed, as should dentures, at the time of the treatment. Patients having ECT will normally be provided with a mouthguard to protect teeth from clenching trauma during the treatment.

- Patients are usually treated with selective serotonin reuptake inhibitors (SSRIs) which may react with other drugs such as warfarin, increasing its effect. Some SSRIs react with asthma medication making it more available. In poorly controlled epileptic patients, seizures may become more frequent. Some patients experience bruxism while taking SSRIs. Other drugs that may still be used in patients with depression are the monoamine oxidase inhibitors (MAOIs) and the tricyclic antidepressants (TCAs). There is controversy surrounding their use and interactions with epinephrine used in dental LAs. Epinephrine-containing LA should not be used in patients taking MAOIs because of the potential to increase blood pressure. In a vulnerable patient this could cause a myocardial infarct or a stroke, or even death.

- Because of the interaction with epinephrine in LA solution, it is wise to use self-aspirating syringes when using epinephrine-containing LA in patients taking TCAs, to prevent accidental intra-vascular injections, and to limit the total dose used.

- Orally, these patients may have neglected themselves. Oral hygiene is generally not a priority and in the chronically depressed patient there may be all the signs of a very neglected dentition. Such patients may have orofacial pain, which is ill defined, and drug therapy may produce xerostomia with all the consequences of rapid caries progression.

- Supportive dental therapy is important, with the aid of a carer to oversee oral hygiene and preventive care. Patients may not remember the need to brush, use floss and fluoride mouthwash on their own. Chairside preventive care is therefore more important and regular short appointments are useful with high-dose topical fluorides (2300ppm F varnishes) and/or high dose (2800/5000ppm F) toothpastes prescribed. Patients may benefit from the use of chlorhexidine varnishes as these are known to reduce the concentration of oral flora in the gingival crevice for up to six months. In psychiatric units, it is advisable to have an oral hygiene regime written into the patient's daily nursing care plan. This will help maintain any work carried out by the dental team and in addition, the interest shown in the patient by the dental team together with their efforts to maintain the dentition may help to boost the patient's low self-esteem.

Manic depression (bipolar disorder)

There is a related depressive disorder, manic depression, in which patients alternate between exhilaration and profound depression. It is also referred to as bipolar disorder. During a manic phase patients may engage overenthusiastically in oral hygiene practices causing tooth wear (abrasion). Illegal substance use may also result in erosion and attrition of enamel and dentine. During bouts of depression such patients have no interest in their oral health and all the effects noted above for chronic depression are seen.

Treatment of the manic symptoms is usually with lithium and the antipsychotic (neuroleptic) drugs used in the treatment of schizophrenia (see Psychoses, p. 153). The depressive phase is managed with short-term antidepressants.

Orally, patients taking these drugs notice side effects: lithium produces xerostomia and sometimes hypersalivation. Where xerostomia is predominant, use of saliva substitutes (see p. 143) can enable the patient to tolerate the drug therapy.

Circulating blood levels of lithium may also be raised by the use of NSAIDs and these should only be used in short courses for dental pain. The antipsychotics interfere with the cardiovascular system, reducing the number of circulating cells (red and white blood cells and platelets) and causing a fall in blood pressure (hypotension). As a class of drugs they also interact with sedation agents such as midazolam and nitrous oxide producing respiratory depression. Interactions with some of the antipsychotics, such as the TCAs and epinephrine in LA, are potentially a problem but the use of self-aspirating syringes and a limit on the amount of LA used (three cartridges in adults) should be safe.

Anxiety states

These are seen as exaggerated responses to stressful situations and are not an uncommon reaction in relation to dentistry. Irrational fear is defined as a **phobia**. Stress results in release of endogenous epinephrine and the long-term, chronic effects of this are to produce hypertension (raised blood pressure) and gastrointestinal effects such as reflux disease. Patients who cannot cope in stressful situations may become hysterical and hyperventilate. The blowing off of carbon dioxide can lead to tetany and collapse (see section on Parathyroid glands, p. 123). Getting the patient to re-breathe from a paper bag can redress this rapidly. Treatment of anxiety disorders rests with empathy on the part of a counsellor and medication if indicated, as for depressive states.

Dentally, patients will be helped by an empathetic approach to their problem, alongside a course of desensitisation to help them overcome their anxiety/fear. Sedation is a useful adjunct in this acclimatisation process.

Post-traumatic stress disorder

Post-traumatic stress disorder is defined as 'following exposure to a traumatic event that is outside the range of usual human experience, a person re-experiences the event'. This phenomenon can be experienced after significant events like natural disasters, accidents or rape. Patients react by reliving the experience either consciously or through nightmares. Individuals affected may wall themselves off from the rest of the world, thus making inter-personal relations with family and colleagues difficult. Medically these patients may also have outward signs of stress. Examples are heart disease and gastrointestinal disorders that are related to stress, such as ulcerative colitis. Such people are more vulnerable to alcohol and substance abuse.

The oral and dental features seen in such patients mirror those seen in other patients with psychiatric conditions: neglected dentition, malnutrition, poor or absent oral hygiene, TMJ disorders and tooth wear in those using illegal substances or the chronic alcoholic patient.

Establishing an empathetic, supportive relationship with the dental team is the first goal in enabling the patient to rehabilitate, dentally at least. Aiding the patient to restore their mouth and improve appearance can help in raising their feeling of self-worth. As with all these psychologically damaged patients, aggressive prevention is vital since the combined effects of neglect, malnutrition and maybe substance abuse need to be vigorously countered while trying to re-establish good habits.

Personality disorders

These are serious defects of personality leading to antisocial behaviour as a consequence of psychotic states. Such patients are removed from the reality of everyday life and need usually to be detained in a secure unit, at least temporarily. The move to establish community living for many residents of such residential units has led to isolated cases of re-offending and, on occasions, death of innocent individuals.

Psychoses

These are divided into functional, such as **schizophrenia**, and organic, such as **dementia**. Dementia is broadly covered under Alzheimer's disease (see p. 143), which is a form of dementia.

Schizophrenia

This is a psychiatric disorder in which the thought disturbances and personality disorganisation reduce the individual's capacity to integrate and communicate with others. Patients are alternately compliant and stubborn, emotionally labile and suffer from delusions. Paranoid schizophrenics regard most things with great wariness, including dental situations.

The patient's experience of these bizarre delusions results in one of the early signs of the disorder, thinking that they hear voices. The individual may become increasingly withdrawn as a consequence, with an inability to communicate with others. Treatment is usually supportive and with antipsychotic drugs, which interact with other medicaments and produce their own side effects.

Antipsychotic drugs produce cardiovascular and neurological effects. The cardiovascular effects manifest as an increased heart rate and an inability to respond rapidly to changes in position so that, for example, raising the dental chair too quickly may make the patient feel faint (orthostatic hypotension).

The effect on the blood is to reduce the number of cells (red and white) and platelets. The most notable neurological effect is **tardive dyskinesia**. In and around the mouth this is manifest as writhing movements of the facial muscles, lip-smacking and chewing. Generally the patient will be restless and keeping still in the dental chair while on this medication will be a challenge. This class of drugs also causes xerostomia, with profound effects on the teeth in terms of rapid progression of dental caries.

Many of these drugs also interact with the vasoconstrictor epinephrine in LA. The choice and dose of anaesthetic is therefore important. Interaction with drugs that depress the central nervous system also leads to severe respiratory depression so sedative agents need to be used with caution and only after consultation with the patient's physician.

Oral and dental considerations include assessment of the overall condition of the patient and this is best accomplished with the patient's physician, who will also be able to indicate the patient's competence to give informed consent for dental procedures.

Consultation with an anaesthetist prior to GA for such patients is important to consider the potential effects of interactions between prescribed drugs for the schizophrenia and central nervous system depressants and other drugs used during GA, as well as the ECG (electrocardiogram) effects noted with these medications.

As with other patients who have psychiatric disorders, these patients may have similar signs of dental neglect such as broken-down dentition, few if any restorations, missing teeth and advanced periodontal disease. There may be drug-related effects such as mucositis (sore mouth), xerostomia (dry mouth), parotitis (parotid gland inflammation) and tooth wear consequent on tardive dyskinesia and illegal substance use. Denture teeth may be broken off as a consequence of tardive dyskinesia and the design of dentures must take this risk into account.

Eating disorders

The main eating disorders **anorexia nervosa** and **bulimia nervosa** are multifactorial syndromes that more commonly affect young females but are seen increasingly in boys. Obesity in adolescents has increased by 75% in the past three decades. **Pica**, the eating of non-nutritive substances, is seen more commonly in people with severe learning disabilities.

Anorexia nervosa and bulimia nervosa are triggered by dietary restriction, usually as a result of a disordered body image. Media and peer pressure on the requirement to be thin contributes to this, although some adolescents may have underlying psychiatric disease. Cultural transition, seen now with the migration of people from one country to another, either voluntarily or as asylum seekers and refugees, makes for pressures on young people, compounded by demographic constraints that favour eating disorders. Negative self-esteem may be a trigger. Altering their weight in this way may be the only area in which the adolescent feels they can exert any control in their life.

Depressive disorders during adolescence are now known to be risk factors for eating disorder onset, recurrent weight fluctuations after previous eating disorders, dietary restriction and purging behaviour. Disruptive and personality disorders also contribute to specific weight problems. Patients who do better are those in whom there are no other underlying illnesses, a relatively short history to the illness, minimal family psychiatric disease and in anorexia nervosa, a higher minimal weight.

The clinical features seen are an obsession about their weight and a secretiveness about the condition. In anorexia nervosa, patients will wear clothing that is often inappropriate for the season or outside temperature in order to disguise their thinness. While the bulimic patient may have almost normal body weight or be overweight, they will control their weight by alternate bingeing and purging. The patient with anorexia will avoid anything that may add weight and take delight in losing pounds. There is some cross-over with bulimia, in that patients may present as vomiting anorectics.

The physiological effects are seen in electrolyte disturbances from the use of laxatives as well as impaired nutrition, cardiac dysrhythmias and even sudden cardiac death. In anorectics, there may be partial hypoplasia of the bone marrow, but the circulating levels of white blood cells do not always reflect the extent of the damage to the bone marrow. These effects are usually reversible with good nutrition.

Treatment of these conditions relies on psychotherapy, family therapy and re-nutrition. Drugs may be less helpful, although anti-depressants may be used for relapse prevention. Newer peptides involved in appetite and body weight control may be helpful to this group in the future.

Oral and dental considerations

- Patients may be fanatical about oral hygiene to the extent that there is evidence of abrasion and significant gingival recession.
- Bizarre eating patterns seen in bulimia may predispose to biochemical imbalances, the consequences of which may be seen in the soft tissues, for example hypervitaminosis A and yellow discoloration of the skin and oral mucous membrane from excess dietary intake of foodstuffs containing this nutrient (e.g. carrots).
- Bizarre dietary practices may also result in dental erosion, which is seen in vomiting anorectic and bulimic patients.
- Careful observation of the hands may reveal calluses on the fronts of the fingers (**Russell's sign**), which have been produced by inserting the hands, against the teeth, into the throat to induce vomiting.

The dental team needs to approach such patients with consideration and empathy. Probing questions about their dietary habits may alienate the patients, who may not return for dental visits. It is not the province of the dentist to undertake the psychiatric care needed but if, from the oral signs and symptoms, a member of the dental team suspects that the patient may have an eating disorder, discussion with the patient's general practitioner in the first instance is warranted. Discussion with the patient's parent, where the patient is still a minor in the eyes of the law, is difficult. The duty to respect the confidentiality of the patient is essential, but the dentist's duty of care to the patient may need the support of the parent. This should be broached with the patient in the first instance.

Rapid tooth wear, seen in vomiting patients, is one of the few situations where there is an indication to restore, even though the cause may not have been controlled. To wait until this happens will leave some patients with a dentition level with the gingival margin. Full-coverage crowns, perhaps only stainless steel crowns in the first instance, may be advisable until definitive treatment can commence. Restoring less abraded or eroded tooth surfaces with glass ionomer cements can relieve symptoms of sensitivity, as can topical fluoride applications both at the chairside and at home. Treatment delivered in a non-judgemental way is vital for the establishment of good rapport between patient and the dental team.

Drug and substance abuse

Illegal drugs

It may be difficult to obtain an accurate history of this from the patient and only a high index of suspicion may lead to this diagnosis. However, a patient's right to confidentiality must be respected at all times provided it does not entail harm to others.

The history may reveal enough to confirm the use of illegal drugs, but not always. In patients who are intravenous drug users the likelihood of them having hepatitis B, C or D infection and possibly HIV infection is high. All the precautions listed in the section on management of patients with blood-borne viruses hold true here. In practical terms, universal precautions mean that, because many patients are unaware of their level of infectivity, all patients are treated as if they are potentially infective, thus maximising the protection not only of the dental team but of other patients as well.

Patients with these viruses may have reduced liver function and so blood clotting may be affected. With patients requiring surgery, these factors should be checked pre-operatively. Some of these patients will have cardiac defects and should be identified pre-operatively, even for routine dental care, as antibiotic prophylaxis may be required, for example with patients who have murmurs or a history of infective endocarditis. Such patients may have psychiatric conditions and it is important to determine if that is the case, as well as any medication they may be taking for this. Illegal drugs as well as prescribed drugs may interact with those prescribed by the dentist and the patient must be made aware of the potential for this to happen, for example cocaine and epinephrine.

Oral and dental considerations

- Is the patient competent to consent to dental care?
- Patients tend often to have recently neglected dentition and periodontal states depending on how long standing their drug abuse habit has been.
- There may be rampant caries not only because of the drugs used but also due to the accompanying xerostomia.
- Patients on Ecstasy may have dental erosion because of the extreme dehydration brought about by the drug and consumption of carbonated drinks as a consequence.
- Some drugs are used in the buccal pouch and may have a direct erosive effect on the adjacent teeth.
- Grinding (attrition) may also be a dental feature.

Alcohol abuse

Again, obtaining an accurate history is virtually impossible, as most alcoholic persons are good at disguising their habit. If a member of the dental team suspects that the patient is an alcoholic, one of the accepted screening questionnaires can be helpful. A history of delirium tremens or of gastrointestinal bleeds gives an indication of the severity of the condition.

Patients with established addiction may have altered liver function and as this impacts on invasive dental care, because of an increased bleeding tendency, liver function tests as well as coagulation factors should be assayed. Antibiotics may be indicated peri- and postoperatively to prevent infection arising from low protein (albumin) levels. Long-standing alcoholic persons often have neglected dentitions because of non-interest in their oral state. There may be soft tissue effects as a consequence of malnutrition and dental disease, mainly tooth wear due to vomiting. Such patients may also be smokers and this, combined with alcoholism and malnutrition, exposes the patient to an increased risk of oral cancer.

Patients should be seen earlier rather than later in the day. If the patient is assessed as being drunk by any of the staff, treatment should be deferred since the patient may become aggressive or abusive and injure themselves and staff. An incoherent patient is not in a position to give valid consent.

Clinically, patients may appear sedated and may refuse an LA; their protective reflexes are likely to be impaired and so their airway is at risk.

Prisoners

In prisoners, two specific impairments of relevance to dental care may be seen: an increased prevalence of psychiatric disorders and hepatitis B and HIV infections.

Two-thirds of women prisoners have some form of mental disorder. Statistics indicate that 40% of women have been in receipt of help for mental or emotional problems before imprisonment, which is double the rate for male prisoners. Fifty per cent of women in prison take psychotropic drugs but only 17% of them will have been prescribed these drugs before starting to serve their sentences.

Data from cross-sectional studies in Irish prisons (no UK data is available) show that 6% have antibodies to hepatitis B core antigen, 22% have antibodies to hepatitis C virus, while 2% have antibodies to HIV. The rates were lower for the 33% of offenders who had not been in prison before. The range for those admitting to intravenous drug abuse was from 7% for those entering prison for the first time to 40% for reoffenders. Tattooing in prison is an independent risk factor for hepatitis C infection in prisoners who claim never to have used injected drugs.

Oral and dental considerations

- As with all patients, strict adherence to infection control procedures must be observed.
- Vigilance needs to be maintained for disease-related clinical signs in patients in whom the infection rate with HIV in particular is known to be high.
- The oral and dental status of prisoners is likely to be poorer than that of the free population.
- Oral and dental effects of illegal substance abuse, such as tooth wear and soft-tissue neoplastic change as described in the relevant sections, are a consideration in this population.

Recommended tasks

(1) You see a number of patients for dental care who use a wheelchair. Outline the case you would make to your manager to accomplish safe handling of such patients in the dental surgery.

(2) A patient with unstable epilepsy is due to attend for dental care. What precautions would you need to take in case of a seizure while under treatment?

(3) There has been much written recently in the newspapers and some magazines about the detrimental effects of mercury; a patient with MS wants all her amalgam fillings removed. Describe how you would counter the arguments for this.

(4) Describe how you would prepare the surgery for an adolescent patient who has muscular dystrophy and who requires inhalation sedation for dental treatment.

(5) Detail the layout you would design for a leaflet to help patients with Alzheimer's disease and their carers cope with oral and denture hygiene.

(6) The dental team is planning a survey of homeless people based on a drop-in centre; what are the preparations you will need to make for the survey day?

(7) You suspect that a patient has an eating disorder. What observations would you make to help the dentist in writing a report for the patient's general practitioner?

(8) You see a number of patients with psychiatric disease in the clinic. What are the features of their disease that conflict with the smooth running of the clinic, and how might these be best managed?

References and further reading

British Dental Association (2003) A12 Advice Sheet – Infection Control in Dentistry.

Department of Health (2008) Commissioning Systems Management HTM 01-05 Decontamination in Primary Care Dental Services. London: Department of Health.

Department of Health (2007) Gateway reference 8100. London: Department of Health.

Griffiths J and Boyle S (2005) *Holistic Oral Care (2e)*. London: FDI World Dental Press.

Lockhart PB, Meechan JG and Nunn JH (2004) *Dental Care of the Medically Complex Patient* (5e). Oxford: Elsevier.

Nunn JH and Klingberg G (2009) Dental care for the child and adolescent with disabilities. In: Koch G, Poulsen S and Dahllof G (eds) *Pediatric Dentistry. A Clinical Approach*. Oxford: Blackwell-Munksgaard.

Walker JT, Dickinson J, Sutton JM, Marsh PD and Raven ND (2008) Implications for Creutzfeldt-Jakob Disease (CJD) in dentistry: a review of current knowledge. *Journal of Dental Research* **87**: 511–519.

Walker JT, Dickinson J, Sutton JM, Raven ND and Marsh PD (2007) Cleanability of dental instruments – implications of residual protein and risks from Creutzfeldt-Jakob disease. *British Dental Journal* **203**: 395–401.

4 Sedation

Lesley Longman and Pat Heap

This chapter is not meant to be exhaustive and the reader is advised to read the syllabus from the NEBDN to ensure that any omissions can be covered by reading other texts or from a course on conscious sedation.

Management of anxiety

Dentists have a duty to provide and patients have a right to expect adequate pain and anxiety control. Pharmacological methods of pain and anxiety control include local anaesthesia and conscious sedation techniques.

Maintaining Standards (General Dental Council, 2001)

The avoidance of dental care due to fear of dentistry is a well-known barrier to oral health. Many anxious or phobic patients will accept dental treatment if managed by sympathetic staff with the assistance of psychological therapies. However, a proportion of the population will require sedation to help them accept dental treatment. It should be remembered that while fear of dentistry is commonplace, there are other reasons why patients may refuse dental care, for example the patient may have behavioural problems or lack the capacity to understand the proposed treatment. When managing patients who are reluctant to have dental treatment it is important to understand the difference between anxiety and phobia.

Phobia: An irrational fear of a particular object or situation – the fear response is excessive and disproportionate to the threat posed.

- The stimulus is comparatively small compared to the severity of reaction.
- This is a lasting, abnormal fear that is usually deep rooted in a patient's emotions and often its origin cannot be explained, although this is not always the case.
- The patient has little or no control over the phobia and logic is not a feature.
- A phobia can significantly change a patient's behaviour.
- Embarrassment and shame are often present.

Anxiety: A human emotion that causes feelings of apprehension, tension and discomfort and is associated with increased activity of the sympathetic nervous system.

■ Anxiety is a learnt response.
■ Anxiety can be beneficial (e.g. it is often anxiety that precipitates a candidate to study for examinations), but anxiety is not always a helpful state to be in.
■ An anxious patient is in a state of unease.
■ Anxiety can be measured by using self-reported questionnaires such as the Corah Scale or Modified Dental Anxiety Scale (see Figure 4.1, Section on Patient assessment).

Dental anxiety has implications for both the patient and the dental team. A variety of studies have shown that the prevalence of dental anxiety is high, affecting up to one-third of the UK population. The 1998 Adult Dental Health Survey identified that 32% of dentate patients in the UK population 'always feel anxious about going to the dentist'. This figure rises to 46% in dentate patients who only attend when they have some trouble with their teeth. It is interesting to note that 59% of dentate patients reported that they attended for regular dental check-ups. Anxiety therefore remains a barrier to dental care in a significant proportion of the population. Approximately 10% of the population avoids dental care because dental treatment provokes overwhelming feelings of anxiety that exceed the sufferer's ability to cope; such patients have dental phobia. Dental anxiety and phobia can be distinguished by the intensity of anxiety experienced and the patient's ability to cope with the anticipated anxiety of dental treatment. It is not unusual for a phobic patient to seek help for a dental problem from their doctor, rather than a dentist, in the hope of being prescribed painkillers or antibiotics. Many anxious/phobic patients will only seek a dental appointment when in severe or chronic pain, some are forced to do so by a friend or relative. Despite the efforts required by dental phobics to attend for treatment, it is not unusual for them to flee from the waiting room as their appointment time approaches. It is therefore not surprising that there is an association between high anxiety and missed or delayed dental appointments.

Patients who are anxious or phobic about dental treatment may have generalised concerns about many aspects of dentistry or they may have very specific worries, such as a fear of injections. Other patients have a fear of the unknown or feel that they may lose control. Anticipation of pain during dental treatment is a frequently reported reason for dental anxiety and fear. Anxiety may be based around one or more previous distressing experiences, such as pain, but it is not always possible to identify specific traumatic life events. Some adults who have accepted routine dental treatment in the past may develop dental anxiety for no obvious reason. Patients may become anxious because of incidents portrayed by family, friends and the media; this is known as vicarious learning. Not surprisingly, patient's beliefs (cognitions) about dental treatment vary considerably, as does their response to stress-provoking situations. Children respond quite differently from adults. Patients with psychological or psychiatric problems may

<u>CAN YOU TELL US HOW ANXIOUS YOU GET, IF AT ALL,
WITH YOUR DENTAL VISIT?</u>

PLEASE INDICATE BY INSERTING 'X' IN THE APPROPRIATE BOX

1. **If you went to your dentist for TREATMENT TOMORROW, how would you feel?**
   Not   *Slightly*   *Fairly*   *Very*   *Extremely*
   anxious ☐   *anxious* ☐   *anxious* ☐   *anxious* ☐   *anxious* ☐

2. **If you were sitting in the WAITING ROOM (waiting for treatment), how would you feel?**
   Not   *Slightly*   *Fairly*   *Very*   *Extremely*
   anxious ☐   *anxious* ☐   *anxious* ☐   *anxious* ☐   *anxious* ☐

3. **If you were about to have a TOOTH DRILLED, how would you feel?**
   Not   *Slightly*   *Fairly*   *Very*   *Extremely*
   anxious ☐   *anxious* ☐   *anxious* ☐   *anxious* ☐   *anxious* ☐

4. **If you were about to have your TEETH SCALED AND POLISHED, how would you feel?**
   Not   *Slightly*   *Fairly*   *Very*   *Extremely*
   anxious ☐   *anxious* ☐   *anxious* ☐   *anxious* ☐   *anxious* ☐

5. **If you were about to have a LOCAL ANAESTHETIC INJECTION in your gum, above
   an upper back tooth, how would you feel?**
   Not   *Slightly*   *Fairly*   *Very*   *Extremely*
   anxious ☐   *anxious* ☐   *anxious* ☐   *anxious* ☐   *anxious* ☐

Instructions for scoring (remove this section below before copying for use with patients)

The Modified Dental Anxiety Scale. Each item scored as follows:

Not anxious	=	1
Slightly anxious	=	2
Fairly anxious	=	3
Very anxious	=	4
Extremely anxious	=	5

Total score is a sum of all five items, range 5 to 25: cut-off is 19 or above which indicates
a highly dentally anxious patient, possibly dentally phobic.

Figure 4.1 The Modified Dental Anxiety Scale (Humphris *et al.* 1995, 2000). Reproduced
with permission.

respond unpredictably to stressful situations. Some patients will experience anxiety only
on the day of the appointment or when they enter the dental surgery. Other patients
will start to exhibit symptoms of stress as soon as they receive the dental appointment,
experiencing several sleepless nights prior to the visit. The spectrum of symptoms varies

Table 4.1 Signs and symptoms of anxiety.

■ Clenched fists (white knuckles), sweaty hands	■ Breathlessness
■ Pallor, sweating	■ Tachycardia (heart rate >100 bpm),
■ Tense, raised shoulders, sitting upright unsupported in the chair, ill at ease	■ Palpitations
	■ Hypertension
■ Fidgeting, nail biting, licking lips	■ Dry mouth
■ Hypervigilance (constantly looking around, suspicious, extremely alert and conscious of environment)	■ Frequent visits to the toilet
	■ Feeling nauseous, light headed or faint, vomiting, syncope, 'butterflies', stomach pains
■ Distracted, confused, unable to concentrate	
■ Very quiet or extremely talkative	■ Tremors
	■ Hyperventilation/panic attack

bpm, beats per minute.

from mild psychological symptoms to physical (somatic) signs and symptoms such as those listed in Table 4.1. Research has shown that many patients who have high levels of dental anxiety also display other fears or psychological problems and these may adversely influence treatment outcome.

Dental anxiety can have a profound detrimental impact on the quality of life of the sufferer. One study by Cohen *et al.* (2000) has shown that the impact of dental anxiety on peoples' lives can be divided into the five categories outlined below.

■ Physiological disruption, e.g. dry mouth, increased heart rate, sweating.
■ Cognitive changes, e.g. negative and even catastrophic thoughts and feelings, unhelpful beliefs and fears.
■ Behavioural changes, e.g. alteration of diet, attention to oral hygiene, avoidance of dental environment, crying, aggression.
■ Health changes, e.g. sleep disturbance, acceptance of poor oral health.
■ Disruption of social roles, e.g. reduced social interactions and adverse affects on performance at work. Family and personal relationships can also be adversely affected.

Management of dental anxiety

The management of anxious/phobic patients is dependent on the severity of the condition and the treatment that needs to be undertaken. The medical history of the patient also influences management. It is important to control anxiety in patients who have systemic disease that is aggravated or triggered by stress, for example hypertension, epilepsy or asthma. The spectrum of patient management varies from psychological or behavioural approaches to the use of pharmacological agents such as anxiolytic drugs or general anaesthesia (GA). The spectrum of management strategies for the anxious patient is outlined in Table 4.2, and ranges from behaviour management to local anaesthesia, sedation and general anaesthesia. Not everybody can be managed by sedation' GA is the

Table 4.2 Methods of reducing anxiety.

■ *Relaxation training* breathing progressive muscle relaxation	■ *Hypnosis* ■ *Systematic desensitisation* ■ *Biofeedback*
■ *Positive reinforcement*	■ *Acupuncture*
■ *Behaviour shaping*	■ *Sedation*
■ *Distraction* story-telling music	■ *General anaesthesia*
■ *Transfer of control to the patient* stop signal rehearsal sessions	
■ *Explanation and information* 'tell, show, do' sequence modelling permissible deception (being economical with the truth)	
■ *Negative reinforcement*	

These techniques must be carried out in a suitable environment. The operator should have a relaxed, positive and empathetic manner.

method of choice for the pre-co-operative child and for many patients with profound learning or physical disabilities.

It is important to appreciate that the use of an anxiolytic drug is not a replacement or substitute for behavioural management of an anxious patient. The use of effective and persuasive communication techniques is still required when managing a patient under sedation.

Behavioural techniques

Behavioural techniques are employed as a matter of routine by many dentists, and are perhaps most evident when children are being treated. Positive reinforcement is frequently used, as shown by the delivery of praise to an appropriately behaved patient. The age and emotional development of a child must always be taken into account when deciding on which techniques to use. Anxious patients should always be given a stop signal as this transfers an element of control to the patient. A commonly used signal is simply raising a hand and it can be helpful for the patient to rehearse this briefly before treatment. The dental team must always respond appropriately to such signals. The trust of a patient can take a long time to build up but can be very quickly undermined or destroyed.

Behavioural management can be time-consuming and expertise is required. Dentists who have access to a clinical psychologist are very much at an advantage. Patients with needle phobias can often be cured of their phobia by employing a systematic desensitisation programme. Desensitisation is a graded introduction to the feared experience/treatment – starting with the least frightening. The patient learns to cope with this before progressing to the next stage. Finally, the patient is exposed to the most threatening

Table 4.3 Management strategies for anxious patients according to anxiety type.

Anxiety type	Management strategy
Patients who fear specific stimuli e.g. needle phobics	Gradual exposure of patient to the feared stimulus (e.g. 'tell, show, do', systematic desensitisation). This approach will work better with a patient stop signal. Coping strategies such as relaxation techniques are also helpful
Patients with free-floating anxiety or generalised anxiety The patient finds many situations outside of dentistry stressful; often there will be no history of a precipitating event	The patient needs to develop coping strategies to reduce anxiety
Patients who have a fear of physical catastrophe e.g. choking, retching, asphyxiating or death	Rehearsal and explanation of the patient's psychosomatic reactions are helpful Systematic desensitisation, coping strategies and biofeedback can be beneficial once the patient acknowledges the mind–body link to their reactions
Patients who are distrustful of dentists These patients may be confrontational in how they express their fears, e.g. the dentist was always in a rush and never asked how I felt; or always made me feel as if the problems were my fault	Listening to the patient's fears and the transference of some control to the patient is helpful. Feedback must be sought from the patient throughout treatment. The establishment of a dialogue in an unhurried, open and non-judgemental manner will help improve the patient's confidence and trust

Adapted with permission from Naini *et al.* (1999).

situation. A long-term aim in the management of anxious/phobic patients is to modify their behaviour such that some or all future dental treatment may be accepted without the assistance of sedation.

Some clinicians find it useful to categorise anxious patients into four types (Table 4.3); this is because the patient category influences the choice of behavioural management strategy. It should be appreciated that whilst this classification can be helpful, patients may have features of anxiety that belong to more than one category and several management strategies are sometimes required for one patient.

Conscious sedation

The term sedation has different meanings in medicine and dentistry and this can also vary internationally. Throughout this book the term *conscious sedation* will be used as this has widespread acceptance among dental sedationists in the UK and has a precise definition. The definition that has been adopted by the General Dental Council (GDC), the Department of Health and other dental societies and advisory bodies such as the Dental

Sedation Teachers Group is that originally proposed in the Wylie Report in 1978 and is as follows:

> A technique in which the use of a drug or drugs produces a state of depression of the central nervous system enabling treatment to be carried out, but during which verbal contact with the patient is maintained throughout the period of sedation. The drugs and techniques used to provide conscious sedation for dental treatment should carry a margin of safety wide enough to render loss of consciousness unlikely.

It is imperative that the level of sedation is such that the patient remains conscious, retains protective reflexes and is able to understand and respond to verbal commands. In patients who are unable to respond to verbal contact even when fully conscious (e.g. patients with hearing impairment), the normal method of communicating with them must be maintained. The concept of *sedation* in which the criteria listed above are not fulfilled is regarded as **general anaesthesia** by the GDC. When the term *sedation* is used in this chapter the authors are referring to *conscious sedation*.

In the UK, the main sedative agents used in dentistry are:

- nitrous oxide (N_2O) administered by inhalation
- midazolam administered intravenously
- a benzodiazepine administered orally (e.g. midazolam).

The use of other sedative drugs and multiple agents (**polypharmacy**) is only occasionally indicated and their use requires additional training and expertise because of the increased risk of adverse events, including respiratory depression.

Indications for sedation

Local anaesthesia remains the mainstay of pain control during dental treatment. However, in some patients conscious sedation can be an effective method of facilitating dental treatment and is normally used in conjunction with local anaesthesia as appropriate. Sedation is a valuable tool in dentistry, it is not a therapy. Like local anaesthesia, it is an adjunct to patient management. There are some patients in whom sedation is contraindicated and in a small minority of patients it may prove to be unsuccessful. The indications for sedation are as follows.

Psychological/social: Patients who have dental anxiety or phobia and are unable to accept treatment which they view as traumatic or distressing; sedation often allows the acceptance of such treatments. This heading would also include patients who routinely faint on dental injections or report that local anaesthetic is ineffective and therefore their previous dental treatment has been painful. While failure of local anaesthesia is often due to poor technique or failure to anaesthetise an accessory nerve supply, some patients do become fearful and anxious that local anaesthetic is not going to work and sedation is helpful in controlling anxiety associated with these patients.

Medical: This category consists of several different types of patients.

(i) Anxious patients with medical conditions that are precipitated or aggravated by stressful procedures can often benefit from receiving sedation, indeed stressful treatment undertaken with sedation may be safer than carrying it out with local anaesthesia alone. Anxiety and pain can cause overactive sympathetic nervous activity (hypertension, tachycardia, arrhythmias). Normal physiological responses to anxiety and fear are not usually harmful; however, in a medically compromised patient they may present a risk to the patient's health. Sedation reduces physiological responses to anxiety and fear. Epilepsy, asthma, hypertension, angina and psychiatric conditions are examples of systemic diseases that may be exacerbated by stress.

(ii) Patients who have involuntary movements due to neuromuscular disease (e.g. cerebral palsy or Parkinson's disease) may wish to have dental treatment but are unable to physically co-operate. It is difficult to treat patients with movement disorders safely, and sedation can facilitate dental management in this group of patients.

(iii) Patients with cognitive impairment, such as individuals with learning disabilities or dementia. This group of patients may not necessarily be anxious prior to dental treatment but they may become distressed during treatment, usually due to poor understanding of the procedures. Dementia patients will often forget why they are in the dental chair and are then unable to co-operate with treatment and communication may be limited. Sedation can sometimes allow treatment to be undertaken in a non-threatening manner that the patient finds acceptable. Learning disabilities could quite rightly be seen as forming a category on its own rather than being viewed as a medical condition.

Dental: Patients who normally find dental treatment acceptable may need sedation for procedures that they view as stressful. Oral surgery procedures (e.g. surgical removal of teeth or implant placement) under local anaesthesia are understandably viewed as unpleasant by many patients. Children may view certain procedures as unpleasant but their perceptions are likely to change as they mature. Sometimes a clinician may recommend sedation because the planned procedure is expected to be particularly traumatic or prolonged, the views of the clinician will have to take the patient's wishes into account, and the threshold for this decision may change with the age of the patient. Patients who have a severe disruptive gag reflex may be included in this indication, although some would say this is psychological in origin and should therefore be classified in the psychological/social category.

General anaesthesia

General anaesthesia is a state of unconsciousness with complete loss of feeling and protective reflexes. In dentistry, GA is reserved for patients who cannot accept routine dental treatment, such as individuals with severe learning disabilities that prevent patient co-operation. In addition, GA is used for procedures that are not amenable to local anaesthesia alone or with sedation. GA remains the preferred method of pain and anxiety control in the pre-co-operative child in the UK. Over recent years there has been a move away from the use of GA in dentistry. GA is subject to stringent regulations and when required for dental treatment it is provided under consultant care in a hospital. The administration of general anaesthetics in primary care ceased following the implementation of *A Conscious Decision* (2000), a report by the Department of Health.

Recommended tasks

(1) Access on the Royal College of Surgeons of England website (i) the UK national clinical guidelines on the use of conscious sedation in paediatric dentistry (2002); (ii) the guidelines on non-pharmacological behavioural management (2002).

You can obtain a copy of these guidelines from the RCSEng website: www.rcseng.ac.uk/fds/clinical_guidelines.

(2) Read around the subject of dental anxiety and phobia. Journal publications such as Cohen *et al.* (2000) and Naini *et al.* (1999) will be helpful.

(3) Obtain a copy of *A Conscious Decision* from the Department of Health and learn more about why the use of GA has been restricted in dentistry. The full document or an executive summary may be obtained from the Department of Health website (www.dh.gov.uk/en/healthcare/primarycare/dent). Identify situations where general anaesthesia, rather than conscious sedation would be advisable for dental treatment.

Patient assessment

An assessment visit is essential for patients who require sedation. This not only allows the dental team to obtain a full dental and medical history but it can also help establish a relationship between the patient and the dental team. The patient's opinions and attitude towards dental treatment can be greatly influenced by the reception they receive. Poor rapport at the assessment visit can lead to problems and confusion at later appointments or the patient may fail to attend future appointments. The consultation should not appear to be rushed. The assessment visit ensures that the most appropriate form of pain and anxiety control and treatment is prescribed, and hopefully the patient will be able to make an informed decision about their dental management. However, no matter how clearly you think that the various management options and proposed treatment plan have been explained, some patients still fail to fully understand or retain the information given because their dental anxiety adversely affects their ability to concentrate and focus. Patient information leaflets are invaluable, but unfortunately they may remain unread. Therefore, details of the proposed treatment will need to be discussed again at the treatment visit.

Complaint and dental history

It is important that the patient tells you about their dental problems, their associated anxieties and fears, and their expectations of treatment – their expectations may not always be appropriate or realistic. Patients should be questioned as to what aspects of treatment they find frightening. Some patients are distressed the moment they receive an appointment and are unable to sleep or relax prior to their appointments. Patients may worry in anticipation of the whole treatment episode. Others may be frightened by discrete procedures, such as an injection. Interestingly, many patients who are terrified of intra-oral injections can tolerate extra-oral injections. It is often helpful to ask a patient if there was a specific experience that they associate with the onset of fear. A patient's dental history can yield valuable information that may influence their management. It is important to obtain information about the frequency of past dental attendance, the approximate timing of the last attendance and the reason for that visit, problems and bad experiences with dental treatment and details of previous sedation experience. Most patients are willing to volunteer this information but some will be reticent; it is not unusual for a patient to become distressed and emotional at the assessment visit. Many patients will also be embarrassed and it is important to be sensitive to their feelings. The use of self-reported psychometric anxiety questionnaires to evaluate patients objectively can be helpful. An example of a frequently used five-item questionnaire, the Modified Dental Anxiety Scale (MDAS), is shown in Figure 4.1. The Corah Dental Anxiety Scale was the predecessor of the MDAS and contained only four questions, however it did not mention fear of injections. Simplified versions of anxiety scales are available for use with children, examples include the *Children's Dental Fear Survey Schedule, Venham's Picture Scale* and the *Modified Child Dental Anxiety Scale*.

Medical history

A thorough medical history is required for all dental patients, irrespective of the need for sedation. A medical history proforma, such as the one produced by the British Dental Association, is preferred by many dentists. It is essential that the medical history is regularly reviewed and updated at future visits.

When assessing a patient's suitability for sedation the following factors are important.

Medical status: It is common practice for sedationists to classify their patients in terms of the risks that their medical history presents to treatment under sedation. The classification used by the **American Society of Anaesthesiologists (ASA)**, which estimates the medical risks for patients undergoing anaesthesia, is frequently adopted and is summarised in Table 4.4.

The ASA classification is a useful assessment tool; it is usual for patients in ASA groups I and II to be treated under sedation in the general dental practice setting, while patients in ASA groups III and IV should receive treatment in a specialist unit or hospital. Age is an important factor when considering dental treatment under sedation. In extremes of age, caution is required, even in healthy patients. Young patients have a reduced or

Table 4.4 American Society of Anesthesiologists (ASA) Physical Status Scale.

ASA status	Description
I	**Patients who are normal and healthy**. The health of the patient does not present problems to proposed dental treatment under sedation; the patient has no systemic disease
II	**Patients with mild to moderate systemic disease that is well controlled and is not limiting their lifestyle**, e.g. well-controlled diabetes, hypertension, epilepsy and asthma
III	**Patients with severe systemic disease that limits activity but is not incapacitating**, e.g. history of myocardial infarction (heart attack), poorly controlled epilepsy, diabetic patients with vascular complications, moderate to severe degrees of pulmonary insufficiency, chronic bronchitis, angina pectoris or healed myocardial infarction. Extreme obesity and extremes of age may be included, even though no discernable systemic disease is present (these patients may be physiologically stressed or challenged by certain dental procedures and consequently sedation or the dental management may need to be modified in ASA III patients. Most ASA III patients will be treated in a specialist clinic or hospital)
IV	**Patients who have incapacitating systemic disease that is a constant threat to life**, e.g. unstable angina, recent myocardial infarction, brittle (uncontrolled) diabetes, uncontrolled hypertension and end-stage renal disease. Also a patient with severe cardiorespiratory disease who is unable to walk upstairs or any short distance without becoming short of breath and fatigued. Treatment should be carried out in a hospital environment
V	**Patients with a terminal condition not expected to survive more than the next 24 hours with or without treatment**

unpredictable response and have immature personalities. The elderly may have increased sensitivity to sedatives and also have a reduced capacity to metabolise drugs, therefore sedatives have to be titrated slowly, in small increments, to reduce the risk of overdose. Sedation in pregnancy should be avoided whenever possible, and special precautions may be required in mothers who are breast-feeding. Significant cardiovascular or respiratory disease can be a contraindication to sedation, but patients with asthma and those who suffer from angina or hypertension may benefit from treatment under sedation if their condition is aggravated by anxiety. Liver and kidney disease are important considerations when sedatives are metabolised and excreted by these organs. Drug abusers and alcoholic patients may have impaired renal and hepatic function. Patients with severe psychological or psychiatric disease may be unpredictable to treat and antipsychotic medications can interact with sedative agents. Patients who are obese may be difficult to cannulate, and patients who are exceptionally thin may be malnourished.

Medications: CNS depressants (antidepressants, antipsychotics, tranquillisers) can potentiate (enhance) the action of sedatives.

Allergies: Allergies to the sedative agents used in dentistry are exceptionally rare; however, patients may have allergies to natural rubber latex. New products are now labelled if they are latex-free, but equipment used in sedation that may contain latex includes the reservoir bag and hoses on a relative analgesia machine. Nasal hoods, face masks, tourniquets, blood pressure cuffs and tubing now tend to be latex-free, but manufacturers should be contacted if any doubt exists when treating a latex-allergic patient.

Lifestyle factors: It can be helpful to know what employment the patient is in and if they have dependants to look after, such as children or a sick or elderly relative. The majority of patients prescribed sedation require an escort for the sedation appointment; in addition a carer should look after the patient postoperatively. It is not always possible for patients to arrange this and if they cannot, sedation would be contraindicated in an outpatient setting. Following intravenous (IV) sedation with midazolam a carer is required postoperatively for about 12 hours. It is also good practice to check on how the patient will be transferred home after treatment as this knowledge may influence the choice of sedative agent: private transport is advisable but may not always be possible.

Examination

Throughout the consultation the dental team should assess how comfortable, anxious, agitated or stressed the patient is (see Table 4.1).

Dental examination

A dental examination should be undertaken whenever possible. Not all patients will allow an intra-oral examination, for example those patients who have profound learning disabilities or a severe, disruptive gag reflex. Radiographs may also be problematic for this group of patients. A provisional treatment plan for the first sedation visit can usually be made from the assessment visit, but sometimes sedation is required to enable clinical and radiographic examination.

Blood pressure, heart rate and arterial oxygen saturation should be recorded at the assessment visit in adults. The clinician may wish to assess a patient's veins on the dorsum of the hand, forearm and antecubital fossa to predict the ease of cannulation.

Decision making

A diagnosis and treatment plan should be made at the assessment visit. Sometimes a clinician can only formulate a provisional diagnosis and interim treatment plan , because an incomplete intra-oral or radiographic examination was undertaken. Further information may also be required from the referring dentist or from the patient's medical practitioner. The indications for sedation have been discussed earlier in this chapter, but the choice of pain and anxiety relief will depend on:

- the severity of the patient's anxiety
- medical and drug history
- social circumstances

- the skill and expertise of sedation staff
- the level of co-operation from the patient and the patient's wishes
- the age of the patient.

The different methods of pain and anxiety control should be discussed with the patient (e.g. behavioural methods, local anaesthetic, sedation and possibly GA). A minority of patients will not be able to decide how to proceed and will require a further visit to discuss treatment options. In order for patients to give informed consent they must have the capacity to do so and be aware of the alternative treatment options, what the proposed treatment involves, the advantages, disadvantages and what the consequences will be if treatment is not undertaken. If sedation is planned, then ideally the consent process should begin at the assessment visit and the first part of the consent form should be signed. Medico-legal issues surrounding consent are discussed later in this chapter.

The assessment appointment has the following advantages.

- The patient is introduced to the dental team and rapport may be developed. Hopefully this will improve the patient's confidence and trust.
- The patient can inform the dentist about previous bad experiences and about their general and specific anxieties concerning dental treatment.
- Baseline values for blood pressure and pulse oximetry can be taken. This also serves to screen patients for undiagnosed hypertension.
- Potential problems in the management of the patient can be identified.
- The most appropriate form of pain and anxiety control can be prescribed.
- The dentist can assess the patient's suitability for sedation and if necessary refer to a:
  - □ specialist sedation unit
  - □ psychologist for behavioural therapy.
- The use of a topical dermal anaesthetic (for the site of cannulation), premedication or pre-operative oral sedation can be discussed (if appropriate). The treatment appointment will need to accommodate time for oral sedation and topical anaesthesia to become effective.
- Management options can be discussed and a treatment plan agreed.
- The consent process can be commenced and verbal and written pre-and postoperative advice and instructions given.
- The patient can have any questions answered, voice their concerns and be reassured.
- An appropriate treatment appointment, with the correct allocation of time, can be more accurately determined.

Information leaflets about sedation are essential. Pre-operative instructions should be given to the patient and should include both written and verbal instructions; Table 4.5 addresses the issues that need to be discussed. On occasion a patient may need to be given very specific instructions, for example a mother who is breast-feeding and is to have IV sedation with midazolam. It may be necessary for breast milk to be expressed

Table 4.5 Issues to address in pre- and postoperative instructions for patients having treatment under intravenous sedation.

The effects of the sedation you have been given may last for up to 12 hours after treatment

For your treatment appointment:
- wear loose-sleeved clothing so that your blood pressure may be taken
- do not wear nail varnish
- wear comfortable clothes and do not wear high-heeled shoes.
- you should be accompanied by a responsible adult escort and a responsible adult is required to look after you for the rest of day
- you should have a light meal two hours before your appointment; do not have any alcohol
- take your medications as usual

After sedation:
Do
- take any routine medication as usual
- arrange for someone else to look after your children (or any other people you look after) for the rest of the day
- rest for the remainder of the day and avoid strenuous exercise

Do not
- return to work for at least 12 hours
- drive, ride a bicycle, climb ladders, operate machinery or potentially dangerous domestic appliances for 12 hours after treatment
- make any important decisions, sign business or legal documents for the next 12 hours
- drink any alcohol

Consider if special instructions are required:
e.g. mothers who are breast-feeding

and discarded after sedation and the baby to receive a bottle feed. This is not always necessary and is dependent on the frequency of breast-feeding and the age and health of the baby. Nitrous oxide sedation may be a less problematic alternative for mothers who are breast-feeding. In addition it should be remembered that patients who have had oral or IV sedation cannot be the sole carers of children or other dependant persons up to 12 hours postoperatively.

Recommended tasks

(1) Study a medical history proforma and identify conditions that may be important when assessing a patient for dental treatment under sedation.
(2) A patient asks you to explain how sedation will make them feel. Rehearse your answer by role-play (ask a colleague or friend to pretend to be the patient so that you may practise your response).
(3) List the information obtained from the assessment visit that should be recorded in the patient's clinical notes.

(4) Search the internet for patient information on sedation. The British Dental Health Foundation would be a good place to start (www.dentalhealth.org.uk). Remember that management protocols will vary between countries as different definitions for sedation (e.g. USA) may be used.

(5) Access www.youranaesthetic.info/index.asp to obtain a copy of a patient information leaflet on *Your Child's General Anaesthetic for Dental Treatment*. Read the section on *risk and safety* of a GA. When do you think GA is indicated for patients who require dental treatment? Compare the pre- and postoperative instructions for sedation with those required for GA.

(6) Access the Royal College of Surgeons website for: Guideline for the Use of General Anaesthesia (GA) in Paediatric Dentistry (2008) (www.rcseng.ac.uk/fds/clinical_guidelines).

Applied physiology and anatomy

The cardiac, respiratory and vascular systems are all intricately related and disease processes affecting one system will invariably have consequences for other organs. One of the many roles of the dental nurse when assisting in the care of the sedated patient is to monitor the cardiovascular and respiratory systems. Therefore, the reader must understand the basic relevant anatomy and physiology before commencing a more detailed study of this topic. This includes the heart, the respiratory system and the coronary, pulmonary and systemic circulations. The reader should revise this information from an appropriate textbook such as *Levinson's Textbook for Dental Nurses* (Hollins, 2008).

Respiratory volumes

When a person is resting their breathing is usually quiet with a regular rise and fall of the chest – this represents the gentle expansion and relaxation of the thorax and lungs. At rest the inspiratory accessory muscles – the diaphragm and intercostal muscles – are not used. The rate at which a person breathes is called the **ventilation** or **respiration rate**. This is around 14–20 breaths per minute in a resting adult; in 2–10-year-olds the rate is increased to 20–30 breaths/min. At rest an adult inhales and exhales approximately 500 ml of air with each breath (ventilation); this is called the **tidal volume** (TV). Not all of this air takes part in gaseous exchange; only about 350 ml enters the alveoli where gaseous exchange is possible, the remaining 150 ml, known as the **dead space volume**, occupies the airway passages where no gaseous exchange occurs.

The volume of air breathed per minute is called the **minute volume** and is approximately 7 l/min. The value is calculated by multiplying the ventilation rate by the tidal volume, e.g. 14 breaths/min × 500 ml = 7000 ml/min. The depth and rate of respiration obviously varies and several factors will influence the minute volume, including anxiety. The average minute volume is a helpful guide for setting the flow rate of gases at the start of inhalation sedation. The reservoir bag should then be observed and appropriate adjustments to the flow rate made as appropriate. It is usually possible for a person to inhale further air above the tidal volume. The volume inhaled over and above the tidal volume is called the **inspiratory reserve volume** (IRV). At the end of a normal exhalation, a person can forcefully breath out; this is forcibly expelled air from the lungs and is called the **expiratory reserve volume**. The total volume of air that can be expired after a maximum inspiration (TV + IRV + ERV) is known as the **vital capacity** (VC), and is about 4.5 l for an adult. Only a small amount of this capacity is used in normal breathing. After maximum respiratory effort approximately 1.5 l of air, the **residual volume** (RV), remains in the lungs. The total lung capacity is around 6 l (TV + IRV + ERV + RV).

The efficiency of gaseous exchange in the lungs can be seriously impaired by several diseases, such as asthma, bronchitis and emphysema. Patients who smoke may have a reduced arterial oxygen saturation, increased bronchial secretions, a persistent cough and reduced lung function. Expiration is a relatively **passive** process; inspiration is an **active** event dependent on muscle activity. In an asthma attack breathing out is difficult because the bronchi are constricted (narrowed) and wheezing occurs. When the upper airway is partially obstructed, paradoxical or *see-saw* respiration occurs. The accessory muscles of respiration become active in respiration in an attempt to increase the volume of the thorax.

Control of respiration

The rate and depth of respiration is controlled by the **respiratory (ventilation) centre** which is situated in the brain. Breathing can be altered by chemical and nervous control. There are chemoreceptors situated in the aorta and carotid arteries and the respiratory centre. They are sensitive to a rise in the level of circulating carbon dioxide (CO_2), a drop in blood pH or reduced levels of circulating oxygen (O_2). Stretch receptors, situated in the lungs and respiratory muscles, can stimulate the vagus nerve to inhibit inspiration. Emotions can also affect breathing by influencing the higher centres of the brain.

An increased partial pressure of carbon dioxide ($PaCO_2$) (**hypercapnia**) is a more significant and sensitive stimulus for respiration than hypoxia; a low PaO_2 will cause an increase in ventilation rate but this is far less dramatic than the hypercapnic drive. The hypoxic drive is a *back-up* mechanism, but it may assume importance in patients with chronic lung disease. Medicines that are CNS depressants, including benzodiazepines, can reduce the respiratory drive and reduce chemoreceptor sensitivity.

Oxygen dissociation curve

Oxygen is essential to maintain life; when tissues become **hypoxic** (low oxygen levels) they die. For example, when a coronary artery becomes blocked with a thrombus an area of the myocardium (heart muscle) fails to receive oxygen. This results in a myocardial infarct (an area of dead tissue), also called a heart attack or a coronary. When the tissues of the brain are deprived of oxygen for more than three minutes irreversible brain damage occurs. In a sedated patient there is an increased risk of hypoxia because sedative drugs have the potential to cause respiratory depression. **Hypoxaemia** is defined as a low PaO_2 in the blood; this may be caused by pulmonary disease, cardiovascular collapse drug overdose or airway obstruction by a foreign body.

The alveoli of the lungs are surrounded with capillaries and this is where pulmonary gas exchange occurs. Oxygen and carbon dioxide diffuse across the alveolar-capillary walls by diffusion. Oxygen is carried around the body by haemoglobin, which is found in the red blood cells. Haemoglobin has a great affinity with oxygen and when combined to it is called oxyhaemoglobin. The amount of oxygen in the tissues is termed the **oxygen tension** or the **partial pressure of oxygen** (PaO_2), and is now measured in kilopascals (kPa). It used to be measured in millimetres of mercury (mmHg). The relationship between the PaO_2 and the percentage saturation of haemoglobin with oxygen is not linear – this is clear from the **oxygen dissociation curve** (Figure 4.2); the line is described as having a sigmoid or 'S' shape. The top of the graph is fairly flat and this represents what happens in the lungs; even if the partial pressure of oxygen in the alveoli falls, a high percentage saturation of haemoglobin is maintained. The steep part of the curve represents the PaO_2 levels found in the tissues. In the tissues, a small fall in PaO_2 will cause a larger percentage fall in the saturation level of haemoglobin, therefore oxygen is released in areas of low oxygen tension. Thus the sigmoid shape of the oxygen saturation curve ensures that the red blood cell haemoglobin combines with oxygen in the lungs (areas of high partial pressures of oxygen) and releases oxygen when in the tissues.

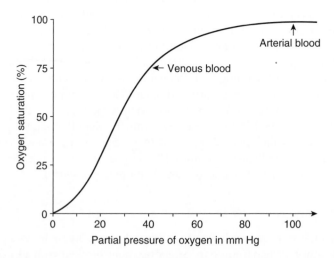

Figure 4.2 The oxygen dissociation curve showing the relationship between the partial pressure of oxygen (PaO_2) and the percentage saturation of haemoglobin with oxygen (SaO_2). The shape of the oxygen dissociation curve favours the loading of haemoglobin with oxygen in the lungs and the release of oxygen in the tissues. (Adapted from Mallett and Dougherty, 2000.)

Pulse oximetry

Pulse oximetry is a non-invasive method of electromechanically monitoring arterial oxygen saturation (SaO_2, sometimes shown as SpO_2). Pulse oximetry enables the operator to detect the early onset of hypoxia during procedures involving conscious sedation. Visual signs of **cyanosis** will only be detected by a skilled operator when the SaO_2 falls below 85%. The use of a pulse oximeter will enable the clinician to be aware of any impairment of oxygenation before cyanosis develops. Patients will normally have oxygen saturation levels of 96–100%.

Pulse oximeters have the following features.

- A probe with a light-emitting diode and a photosensor (usually a finger probe; toe and ear probes are available but they are thought to be less reliable).
- A digital display window showing the pulse rate and the percentage SaO_2 of the haemoglobin. Many units also have a graphic display where the patient's **pulse pressure** is shown in a plethysmographic waveform (this is not an ECG (electrocardiogram) tracing).
- Audible alarms for the pulse and oxygen saturation programmed to activate when critical values are reached. These levels can be reset, for example the pulse alarm settings will need to be altered for a marathon runner who has a resting pulse rate of 48.
- Battery back-up in case of power failure.

Pulse oximetry combines the principles of spectrophotometry with plethysmography. **Spectrophotometry** uses light absorption and emission to measure a change in the concentration of oxyhaemoglobin. There is a change in colour in red blood cells as they gain or lose oxygen, consequently oxygenated and deoxygenated blood transmit and absorb different amounts of light. One side of the probe emits light of two different wavelengths (one red and one infra-red) that passes through the tissue of the finger and is received by a photodetector on the other side of the probe. A microprocessor analyses the signals received and sends the percentage SaO_2 to the digital display. **Plethysmography** uses light absorption technology to reproduce waveforms produced by the pulsatile flow of blood.

Cardiac cycle

Knowledge of the **cardiac cycle** is essential to understand blood pressure and the electrical activity of the heart. The cardiac cycle, shown in Figure 4.3, lasts approximately 0.8 seconds in a person at rest and represents the contraction and relaxation phases of the heart. The **systolic** (contraction) phase, also referred to as **systole**, commences with the atria contracting, forcing blood from the atria into the ventricles. The ventricles then contract and eject the blood into the aorta and pulmonary arteries. The walls of the aorta expand to take much of the expelled blood and so act as a reservoir. The intra-cardiac pressure falls as the heart enters the relaxation or **diastolic** phase of the cycle. During

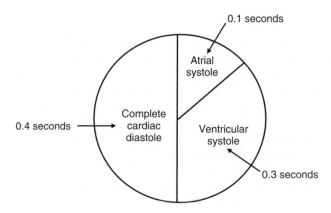

Total period of one cycle = 0.8 seconds

Figure 4.3 The cardiac cycle.

diastole the atrioventricular valves are open and the ventricles fill up with blood from the atria.

Blood pressure

Each heartbeat produces a pressure wave in the arterial circulation. Blood pressure (BP) is the force exerted on the blood vessel wall by the blood as it is pumped around the body by ventricular contractions. In younger people the blood vessels are more elastic so the arteries absorb some pressure. There is a tendency for BP to rise with age because the larger arteries become harder and less elastic. During diastole the ventricular pressure drops to zero but the arterial pressure does not; the closure of the aortic valve and resistance within the arterial system maintains a diastolic pressure.

The BP of an individual can vary dramatically as it is influenced by many factors, such as sounds, talking, recent intake of foods, caffeine, smoking, exertion and arm position. Age, anxiety and fear can all increase the BP, but the diastolic pressure is less likely to be affected by anxiety than the systolic pressure. Measured in the seated, relaxed patient the normal range of arterial pressures may be taken as 100–140 mmHg for the systolic and 60–85 mmHg for the diastolic pressure. Systolic reading is written above the diastolic value, e.g. 120/70 mmHg. Ideally the blood pressure should be less than 120/80; however, the systolic reading does increase with age. A raised BP is called **hypertension**, and patients with a sustained BP of 160/90 mmHg (or greater) should be medically assessed. Patients who may have isolated systolic hypertension (BP >160/<90 mmHg) should also seek medical advice. It should be remembered that dental anxiety can significantly increase BP, so readings should be repeated. Those with repeatedly high readings should be monitored by their doctor. Undiagnosed or poorly controlled hypertension can cause serious health problems such as hardening and narrowing of the arteries (arteriosclerosis), a risk of a cerebrovascular accident (a stroke), myocardial infarction (heart attack) and renal damage. Low BP is called **hypotension** and is usually taken as a systolic BP below 100mmHg; it does not usually cause serious health problems, but patients may be prone to fainting.

Pulse points

A pulse is an impulse transmitted to arteries by the contraction of the left ventricle. The pulse reflects the heart rate. Pulse points can be found in many **peripheral** or **major** arteries; often a pulse can be palpated (felt) when the artery crosses a bony prominence or it can be compressed against firm tissue. The radial and brachial are the commonly used superficial pulses and are detected in arteries that pass close to the surface of the body. The carotid and femoral pulses are major pulses and are used to assess a collapsed patient. In a baby the brachial pulse is used because the neck is poorly developed making the carotid pulse difficult to feel. An average resting pulse rate for an adult is around 80bpm (range 60–100bpm). Children's pulse rates are faster. When the heart rate is slower than 60bpm then the patient has a slow heartbeat – or **bradycardia**. A rapid heart rate of greater than 100bpm is called **tachycardia**. A pulse will increase with exertion, anxiety, fear, fever, acute pain and certain illnesses, and decrease during fainting and in certain heart disorders. Elite athletes may have a normal resting pulse of below 60bpm.

Electrical activity of the heart

The heart is made up of cardiac muscle cells (fibres) which branch and network to form the myocardium. The fibres are arranged to allow a contraction wave to spread quickly across the cardiac muscle; no nerves are involved. The heart contracts regularly because it has areas of specialised tissues that conduct electrical activity in a highly organised manner. The heartbeat originates in the **pacemaker** or **sinoatrial** (**SA**) **node**, situated in the right atrium (Figure 4.4). The SA node sends out electrical signals across both atria, causing them to contract simultaneously and expel blood into the ventricles. The electrical impulses then reach the **atrioventricular node**, situated at the junction of the atria and ventricles. From here the electrical impulses travel down the **bundle of His** (a group of cells that run down the fibrous ventricular septum) towards the apex of the heart. The transfer of electrical activity to the **Purkinje fibres** (which fan outwards and upwards into the ventricles) instigates ventricular contraction, which expels blood into the aorta and pulmonary artery.

Two sets of nerves from the autonomic nervous system can affect the heart rate by influencing the SA node. The sympathetic nerves increase the heart rate, while the parasympathetic system, via the vagus nerve, slows the pacemaker down. A vasovagal attack (faint) is when the heartbeat is too slow and the brain receives too little blood with a resultant loss of consciousness.

The electrical events of the cardiac cycle can be detected by an ECG and displayed as a trace on graph paper or a monitor. An ECG waveform displaying normal heart function in **sinus rhythm**, is shown in Figure 4.5. Various points of the wave are identified by

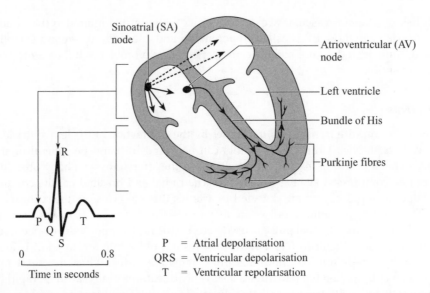

Figure 4.4 The conduction pathway of the heart and a normal ECG trace. (Adapted from Mallett and Dougherty, 2000.)

Figure 4.5 Waveform of sinus rhythm (Mallett and Dougherty, 2000).

letters, starting with the letter P. The whole wave is allocated the letters P, Q, R, S and T (see Figures 4.4 and 4.5). The first wave is called the P wave and represents the electrical activity of the atria during atrial contraction. The time it takes for the electrical impulse to travel down the bundle of His from the atria to the ventricles is represented by the P–Q interval. The QRS complex is the spread of electrical activity through the ventricles. The T wave is the last waveform and represents the preparation (repolarisation) of the ventricles for the next contraction.

Anatomy relevant to venepuncture

When sedative drugs are to be administered intravenously an IV cannula needs to be placed securely into a superficial vein. The nurse needs to be:

- familiar with the relevant anatomy and physiology of the common venepuncture sites
- aware of the criteria used to select a vein and the venepuncture device

- aware of the potential problems that may be encountered (see Table 4.13 in the section on intravenous sedation)
- aware of the importance of cross-infection control, including the safe disposal of sharps. Venepuncture has the potential to introduce micro-organisms into what is normally a closed, sterile circulatory system. Therefore, an aseptic technique must be used to place the IV cannula
- aware of the physical and emotional comfort of the patient
- able to explain the procedure to a patient and answer questions appropriately.

Dentists only use superficial veins of the dorsum (back) of the hand and the forearm for IV access. The main accessible veins are shown in Figures 4.6 and 4.7 and are the metacarpal vein (on the dorsum of the hand) and the median cubital vein (often easier to palpate than to visualise). The cephalic and basilic veins are only occasionally used by dentists for IV access. Venous anatomy is, however, very variable, especially the dorsum of the hands.

The cephalic vein rises from the dorsal vein and runs along the radial border of the forearm until it crosses the antecubital fossa as the median cubital vein. The median cubital vein crosses the brachial artery in the antecubital fossa. As a general rule, arteries tend to be placed more deeply than veins, they have thicker walls, do not tend to collapse and have a pulsatile blood flow. The brachial artery usually lies beneath the median cubital vein deep to the biceps tendon. Aberrant positioning of the brachial artery does occur and can result in a superficial artery. The operator must take care to avoid intra-arterial cannulation.

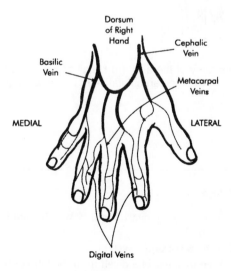

Figure 4.6 Dorsum of the hand (Girdler and Hill, 1998).

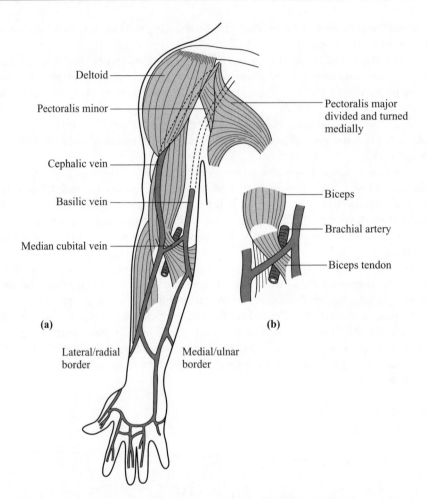

Figure 4.7 (a) Venous anatomy of the arm. (b) Detail of the antecubital fossa showing the biceps tendon lying between the median cubital vein and brachial artery. (Adapted from Ellis, 2002.)

Recommended tasks

(1) Draw a labelled diagram of the heart. Identify which chambers and vessels transport deoxygenated blood.
(2) Draw a diagram of the respiratory system.
(3) Outline the path taken by a red blood cell from the left ventricle to the pulmonary vein. Comment on the variations in oxygen saturation that are likely to occur.

(4) Midazolam is often administered intravenously by injecting a vein on the dorsum of the hand. Describe the main blood vessels that a molecule of midazolam will travel along to reach the brain.
(5) Describe the anatomy of a vein. How do veins differ from arteries and capillaries?

Monitoring

The patient who is to receive sedation must be closely monitored by the dental nurse before, during and after dental treatment. **Monitoring is the continuous observation of data from specific organ systems to evaluate the status of physiological function**. This requires staff to be trained and to have appropriate monitoring facilities. The following variables are important to monitor:

- oxygenation
- breathing
- circulation
- level of consciousness
- level of anxiety.

Temperature has not been included because it is not usually significantly altered by sedation, but it may be taken if a patient is thought to be unwell with an infection (the normal value is 37°C/98.6°F). It is important to remember that a patient may sometimes feel cold during sedation and require a blanket.

Monitoring may be clinical or electromechanical; all patients receiving sedation must be monitored clinically. However, when a patient is receiving IV sedation electromechanical monitoring is also required.

Clinical monitoring

Clinical monitoring is by far the most important method of monitoring the dental patient. There are numerous signs that may be monitored, some are obvious but many are subtle.

- Level of consciousness – response to questions and commands, level of co-operation.
- Respiration – rate and depth (shallow or deep), the amount of effort respiration is taking (the accessory muscles are not required for normal respiration) – any unusual sounds.
- Pulse – rate, regularity and quality.
- Colour of the patient.
- Anxiety – assess the patient's general mood, demeanour, composure and body language to ascertain the extent of relaxation.

At rest, respiration should be regular, effortless and quiet; breath sounds should not be obvious. The number of breaths can be counted over a 30-second period and the respiration rate calculated for one minute. The rate and depth of respiration is often reduced during sedation and should be monitored closely. Respiratory depression is most likely to occur immediately following induction of sedation with IV agents. When there is obstruction on inspiration, increased respiratory signs are seen, such as excessive abdominal movement and noisy breathing. The nurse should immediately inform the dentist to stop treatment if respiratory problems are observed.

Dental nurses learning to assist in the care of the sedated patient should deliberately try to increase their powers of observation. When a patient is receiving dental treatment both the dentist and nurse should be aware of how comfortable or restless the patient is. A restless patient may fidget and appear tense; an anxious patient may have their shoulders hunched and their hands may become clenched or tighten around the armrests (see Table 4.1). It is helpful to monitor the patient prior to sedation and compare the observations with those seen following sedation. Sedated patients should be conscious, co-operative, responsive and relaxed. The nurse should look for signs of under- and over-sedation. Signs of slurred speech, drooping eyelids (**ptosis** or **Verrill's sign**) and impaired psychomotor co-ordination (e.g. **Eve's sign**) are often quoted as being indicative of sedation. These features are not always seen in an adequately sedated patient and can sometimes be signs of over-sedation. Patients respond to sedatives in many different ways, just as patients react in numerous ways to dental treatment without sedation; some patients are very easy to treat while others are extremely difficult. The response of sedated patients to dental treatment is equally variable. The sedated patient is therefore not always as easy to treat as one would like.

Measurement of the radial pulse

- The patient should be comfortable and have rested for five minutes prior to taking the pulse.
- Explain the procedure to the patient.
- Place your second and third fingers in the hollow immediately above the wrist creases at the base of the thumb, and press lightly, do not use your thumb to record a pulse, because it has a pulse.
- Assess the rate (over a minimum period of 30 seconds), calculate the value for one minute. The rhythm and the amplitude may take longer to assess (it is relatively easy to comment on pulse rate and rhythm, and with experience it may become possible to assess the amplitude of a pulse, e.g. weak or strong and bounding).
- Record your findings in the clinical notes.

Electromechanical monitoring

Inhalation sedation with nitrous oxide is usually only accompanied by clinical monitoring. If the patient has cardiovascular or respiratory disease the use of a pulse oximeter can be helpful. When a patient is receiving IV sedation their cardiovascular and respiratory function should also be monitored electromechanically by using a pulse oximeter and a BP device. Pulse oximetry should also be used when undertaking oral and transmucosal sedation. Electromechanical monitoring is essential just prior to treatment and during recovery. Baseline values should have been obtained at the assessment visit. It is not standard practice for fit and well patients undergoing IV sedation solely with midazolam to be monitored with an ECG, but this may be employed in a hospital in patients with cardiac problems who are receiving sedation.

Blood pressure

An average BP in a healthy young adult is around 120/80 mmHg when the patient is relaxed. Anxiety can raise the systolic pressure so it is helpful to take the baseline BP at the assessment visit. This can be taken using a traditional sphygmomanometer or an electronic device.

Sphygmomanometer

A sphygmomanometer consists of an inflatable bladder enclosed in a cuff, an inflating bulb, a control valve and a manometer to read the various pressures applied to the bladder (Figure 4.8). When an artery is subject to varying pressures certain pulsatile sounds can be heard – called **Korotkoff** sounds, after the person who first described them. Taking BP involves locally stopping the arterial blood flow by squeezing the arm with an inflated cuff and then lowering the cuff pressure until the flow of blood can be

Figure 4.8 Using a sphygmomanometer and the appearance and disappearance of Korotkoff's sounds.

felt or heard again. When the pressure in the inflated cuff is being released, the compression on the brachial artery is reduced and blood begins to flow back into the artery, causing turbulence. This turbulence can be heard with a stethoscope, and the detection of this sound represents the systolic pressure. As the pressure is gradually reduced further, a muffled sound is heard and this eventually disappears. The diastolic pressure is recorded at the point when all sound ceases.

A sphygmomanometer has a number of components.

■ **Cuff**: This is an inflatable rubber air bladder inside a cloth cover. The bladder is connected to: (i) an inflation bulb via a control valve; and (ii) tubing that is connected by a metal or plastic connector to the manometer. The cloth cover holds the centre of the bladder in place over the artery. When in place the bladder should nearly or completely circle the arm. A variety of cuff sizes are available for children through to large adults.

■ **Inflation-deflation bulb**: The bulb is used to produce a rapid inflation of the bladder to 20–30 mmHg above the patient's systolic pressure. The control valve allows a controlled deflation of about 2–3 mmHg/second.

■ **Manometers**: There are two types of manometers available.
   □ **Mercurial** – this is the traditional apparatus where pressure forces mercury from a reservoir into a narrow, vertical tube in which the height of the column is measured, hence the BP is recorded in millimetres of mercury (mmHg). The scale is from 0 to 300 mmHg, marked at 2-mm intervals. This method is thought by some to be the most reliable. It is an auscultatory (hearing) method. The sphygmomanometer will need routine maintenance every 6–12 months depending on usage.
   □ **Aneroid** – the pressure is applied to a bellows and spring mechanism that moves a pointer around a dial. This can give accurate measurements, but it needs to be maintained and calibrated more frequently, usually every six months.

■ **Stethoscope**: A stethoscope consists of two earpieces connected by flexible tubing to the chest piece. The earpieces can be rotated to ensure correct positioning in the ear canal and to facilitate sound transmission. Many chest pieces have a flat side (the diaphragm), and a raised side (the bell). The chest piece rotates to activate access to one side only. The diaphragm is most commonly used to detect Korotkoff sounds, but the bell is preferable for faint sounds. It is important to maintain stethoscope hygiene, and the earpieces should be periodically unscrewed and cleaned. The external surfaces of the stethoscope should be routinely cleaned with an alcohol wipe after use.

Suggested procedure for taking a manual BP using an arm cuff, sphygmomanometry and auscultation

(1) **Preparation of equipment**
   Select the correct-sized cuff for the patient and check the equipment. Deflate the cuff by squeezing all the air out of the cuff-bladder. Check the condition of the equipment, e.g. ensure that the rubber tubing has not cracked or perished, stitching on

the cloth cover is still intact and the Velcro fastening is still functional. The valve and connectors should not be leaking air. The mercury column or needle on the aneroid dial should be at zero prior to inflating the cuff. Place the scale of the sphygmomanometer so that it can be read at eye level.

(2) **Preparation of the patient**
Use a quiet room[1] with a comfortable temperature. Ideally the patient should have rested for five minutes and have avoided exertion in the previous 30 minutes. If the patient has not had their BP taken before, explain the procedure and reassure the patient throughout to allay their anxiety. Ensure the patient is sitting in a relaxed upright position, and support the arm at the level of their heart.[2] The palm of the hand should be facing upwards. Locate the brachial artery. Attach the appropriate-sized cuff to the upper arm; there should be a clearance of 2–3 cm between the lower end of the cuff and the antecubital fossa, with the centre of the bladder over the brachial artery. Request the patient not to talk.

(3) **Estimation of the systolic BP**
Palpate the brachial or radial artery (on the thumb side of the wrists) and inflate the cuff until the pulse disappears, deflate the cuff and record this reading – the estimated systolic pressure. Deflate the cuff and wait 30 seconds before re-inflating it.

(4) **Measurement of the systolic and diastolic pressures**
Place the stethoscope, with a light pressure only, over the brachial artery. Locate the brachial pulse by auscultation, rapidly inflate the cuff to about 30 mmHg above the previously estimated systolic BP. With the stethoscope in place, slowly release the cuff pressure (rate 2–3 mmHg/sec), initially no sounds are heard but as the pressure falls a point is reached when repetitive tapping sounds, corresponding to the heart rate, are heard in the stethoscope. When the first audible sharp thud (representing the blood flow) appears, note this reading – the **systolic pressure**. The pressure in the cuff should now be reduced slowly until this repetitive sound becomes muffled and then disappears. The diastolic pressure is measured at the point when sound can no longer be heard. Rapidly deflate the cuff and remove it (unless continuous BP monitoring is required). Thank the patient. This method should usually take around five minutes. If the procedure needs to be repeated, wait one to two minutes to allow for venous emptying.

(5) Record the reading in the patient's notes together with the time when it was taken.

Arterial oxygen saturation

Hypoxaemia can occur before there are detectable changes in vital signs, skin or mucosal colour and symptoms may not become evident until the blood PaO_2 drops considerably.

---

[1] Environmental noise can increase BP and also make it difficult to hear the Korotkoff sounds, also the BP may be increased when a patient is talking or being spoken to.
[2] Support the arm to avoid muscle tension, which can raise diastolic BP.

A **pulse oximeter** will detect impending hypoxia, allowing for early corrective action. Supplemental oxygen should be given if the saturation is below or around 90%.

It must be remembered that pulse oximetry is an aid to patient monitoring and not a substitute. A fall in SaO_2 may be clinically significant but needs to be viewed in conjunction with the patient's general condition. The most common reason for the saturation reading on a pulse oximeter to drop is a poor signal. This may be because the finger probe has become displaced. The probe is also sensitive to patient movement and nail polish. An ill-fitting probe will allow external light to interfere with the reading. A poor blood supply to the fingers can be due to anxiety, low temperatures or systemic disease such as Raynaud's syndrome. Often a fall in oxygen saturation is observed 10 minutes from the start of sedation, when the patient is relaxed and local anaesthesia is being administered. Breath holding is common at this point. Patients should be told by a member of the dental team to take several deep breaths and this usually restores the saturation to baseline values.

Safety checks and preparation of the pulse oximeter

- Ensure that the unit is regularly serviced.
- Clean the probe with a 70% alcohol wipe.
- Check battery.
- Switch on.
- Check the machine by placing the finger probe on yourself.
- Check the alarm limits (pulse rate and oxygen saturation) are appropriately set.[3]
- Check that appropriate probes are available (a toe or ear probe can be helpful for special needs patients who often play with the finger probe).

Use of the pulse oximeter (with a finger probe)

- Remove any nail polish – this can affect light absorption and accuracy.
- Gently place probe on the finger, informing the patient what you are doing.
- Sometimes the probe needs to be secured with tape (if applied too tightly, venous return will be restricted).

If the SaO_2 alarm is triggered

- Stop the clinical procedure.
- Assess the patient clinically to see if there is a problem, if so identify the cause.
- Check if the finger probe is still in place.
- Check that the airway is clear. Any obstruction should be identified, such as poor head position. A foreign body should be removed with suction or forceps.
- Ask the patient to take a few deep breaths.
- Consider if supplemental oxygen is required.
- Consider if reversing benzodiazepine sedation with flumazenil is required.

---

[3]The oxygen saturation alarms on the pulse oximeter should be set at around 92% (but this does vary).

- Choking should be managed according to the guidelines of the Resuscitation Council.
- In the rare event of respiratory arrest, rescue breathing would be required.

Recommended tasks

(1) Observe patients just before they receive sedation and notice how their behaviour, demeanour and pulse rate change after they have been sedated. Make a list of your observations.

(2) Observe the body language of non-sedated patients during treatment. Notice if their legs and feet are still. What are the patient's hands doing? Are their shoulders hunched up? Look for signs of tension and restlessness. Notice the rate of respiration. Extend this to observe a patient's behaviour and demeanour when they present for assessment.

(3) Take the pulse rate and BP of colleagues, friends and family members until you become comfortable and confident with the procedures. Practise explaining to people what you are doing. When measuring BP always enquire if a person has had their BP taken before; if not explain the procedure and what they will experience.

(4) Read the product literature that comes with the monitoring equipment and note how often it should be serviced. If the literature is not available contact the company that made the equipment and ask if they can send you any information.

Pharmacology

Basic knowledge of the principles of applied pharmacology is important in order to understand the sedative and emergency drugs used in dentistry. The term **pharmacokinetics** refers to the effects that the patient has on the drug concentration, while the term **pharmacodynamics** is used to describe the actions the drug has on the body.

Pharmacokinetics

Pharmacokinetics is principally the study of four important processes that influence the concentration of the drug in the body. These are **absorption**, **distribution**, **metabolism** and **excretion** (elimination).

Absorption

There are many different methods of delivering a drug to a patient, but in dentistry only a few are important. The routes of administration for the most frequently used

Table 4.6 Routes of drug administration used in dental sedation and the management of medical emergencies.

Route	Sedative/Hypnotic	Emergency drugs	Onset of action
Oral	Diazepam Temazepam Nitrazepam Midazolam	Aspirin Glucose	30–120 minutes
Sublingual/buccal	Midazolam	GTN# Glucose gel Midazolam	1–2 minutes
Inhalation	Nitrous oxide Oxygen	Oxygen Nitrous oxide & oxygen Salbutamol	1–5 minutes
Intramuscular		Epinephrine* (adrenaline) Glucagon	5–15 minutes
Intravenous	Midazolam Propofol	Flumazenil Midazolam	20–30 seconds
Intranasal	Midazolam	Midazolam**	10–20 minutes
Topical	Dermal anaesthetic creams		30–60 minutes

* IM is the preferred route of administration of epinephrine (1 : 1000) in anaphylaxis.
# GTN, glyceryl trinitrate.
** If a patient has status epilepticus and an IV cannula is in place then the operator may wish to use IV midazolam rather than use buccal or intranasal routes of administration.

sedative and emergency drugs in dental practice are listed in Table 4.6. Two important factors influencing the choice of drug administration are patient acceptability (not all patients will accept an injection or swallow tablets) and the time it takes for a drug to work. The onset of action varies with the different routes of administration (see Table 4.6). In most emergency situations the drug needs to be delivered to the site of action quickly.

The **oral** route is a frequently used method of administration in dentistry, but the onset of action can be slow and unpredictable. The absorption of drugs from the gastrointestinal tract is unpredictable and the formulation of the drug (e.g. liquid preparations have more rapid absorption than most tablet formulations) and the presence of food in the stomach will affect the rate of drug absorption. Circulating drug levels following oral absorption increase more slowly than when a drug is given intravenously. Adverse reactions, including allergic reactions, are thought to be fewer and less severe following oral administration, but a potentially fatal anaphylactic reaction is still possible. Anxiolytics and hypnotics (e.g. diazepam, nitrazepam and temazepam) can be given orally, but fortunately allergic reactions are considered to be exceptionally rare, with only a handful of reported cases. Propofol, however, is more likely to be associated with allergic reactions and this may be due to the drug or the lipid vehicle it is dissolved in. Allergic reactions to propofol are still rare.

Transmucosal absorption is the absorption of a drug across a mucosal surface and this term includes the administration of drugs by the **sublingual**, **buccal**, **intranasal** and **rectal** routes. The rectal administration of sedatives has proved to be a predictable and safe route, especially in children; it is not an accepted route in dental practice in the UK. The absorption of a drug across the mucosal tissues is rapid due to their rich blood supply. The sublingual and buccal routes are used for the administration of glyceryl trinitrate (for angina) and glucose gel (for the conscious hypoglycaemic patient). Midazolam can be administered by the buccal and intranasal routes to achieve sedation, and is especially useful in treating patients with learning disabilities. Buccal or intranasal midazolam may be used as a single sedative agent or in combination with intravenous techniques. Intranasal or more commonly buccal midazolam can be used in the emergency management of status epilepticus. The use of a topical anaesthetic agent, such as benzocaine gel, prior to giving a dental injection is also an example of delivering a drug by the transmucosal route.

Drugs administered by **inhalation** are absorbed across the small bronchioles and the alveolar sacs; the onset of action is rapid. However, the **intravenous** route has the quickest onset of action, taking seconds rather than minutes for the drug to exert an effect. The rate of onset of action following the **intramuscular** (IM) administration of a drug is slower than the IV route. The rate of absorption is dependent on the quality of the blood supply to the injected muscle; the deltoid muscle of the upper arm is a good site because it is easily accessible. The tongue has been suggested as a convenient place for the IM administration of emergency drugs. This route is not advisable because local swelling could increase airway problems. The use of drugs in medical emergencies is discussed more fully later in this chapter.

Topical dermal anaesthetic agents may be used prior to IV access and are discussed later in this section. There are many other methods of administering drugs (e.g. intraosseous, intratracheal and spinal routes) but these are not relevant to dental practice.

Distribution

After a drug has been absorbed into the circulation it is transported around the body, and hopefully delivered to the intended *site of action* – the target tissues. The intended site of action for sedative drugs is the brain. Drugs usually exert their action by binding with a specific **receptor** (molecule) to which that drug has an affinity (attraction).

Metabolism

Metabolism refers to how a drug or chemical is broken down into smaller molecules and made inactive by the body. The majority of drugs are metabolised by enzymes in the liver; however, some drugs such as nitrous oxide are not metabolised and so remain chemically unaltered as they pass through the body Metabolism alters the physical and chemical properties of drugs so that they may be more readily eliminated from the body.

Usually the drug is made water soluble so that it can be eliminated in urine by the kidneys; alternatively, lipid-soluble drugs combine with bile salts and are excreted into the intestine.

The **half-life** of a drug refers to the time it takes to reduce the drug levels to half of its original value, i.e. by 50%. This gives an idea of how long the drug will remain active in the body. The half-life can be represented in various ways, for example the drug levels in serum (blood) or the elimination half-life. In essence, drugs with a short half-life are quickly eliminated from the body so their duration of action is short. In dentistry it is preferable to have a sedative with a short half-life; in this way the pharmacological effects of the drug are short lived. The short half-life of midazolam (around two hours elimination half-life) is a major reason why midazolam replaced diazepam as the IV sedative of choice. Diazepam has an elimination half-life of around 43 hours.

Sometimes the liver converts the drug to another compound that is pharmacologically active – just like the parent molecule. This product is called an **active metabolite**. When a sedative is metabolised to an active metabolite, the period of sedation is prolonged. Diazepam is metabolised to the active metabolite desmethyldiazepam, which has an elimination half-life of around 75–100 hours. Patients with liver disease may have impaired metabolism of drugs; this prolongs a drug's action and the patient is susceptible to prolonged effects of the drug and overdose. The very young and the elderly have reduced liver enzyme function and are therefore not as efficient at metabolising drugs.

Excretion

The excretion (elimination) of drugs occurs mainly in the kidneys, but sometimes drugs or chemicals cannot be made water soluble, so these are excreted into the intestine and eliminated in the faeces. The lungs are also organs of excretion: nitrous oxide, oxygen and carbon dioxide are eliminated by this route. Other minor routes of drug elimination are saliva, sweat and breast milk. It is important to be aware that patients with kidney disease may not excrete drugs efficiently, and that the very young and the elderly have reduced kidney function.

Pharmacodynamics

Pharmacodynamics is the study of how the drug affects the patient; it involves understanding the mechanisms of how drugs act on the body. The body contains many cells that have specialised groups of molecules called **receptors**, and these receptors have the ability to combine with complementary parts of the chemical structure of a drug; in this way a **drug–receptor** complex is formed. When a drug combines with a sufficient number of receptors a change occurs that initiates an activity, and this leads to the pharmacological effect of the drug. To understand the concept of drugs and receptors it is helpful to use the analogy of a *lock and key*, where the drug is the key and the receptor the lock. If a key correctly fits the lock it can enable an action to occur – it can *open the door*. However, if the key fits the keyhole but not the lock, then no action occurs, but the key prevents (or blocks) the activity of other keys/drugs on that lock/receptor. Therefore, some drugs activate receptors (turn the lock) and cause an event (or sequence of actions) to happen; these drugs are called **agonists**. Other drugs merely occupy the receptor and block the site without causing any action (the lock is not opened); these drugs are called **antagonists**.

- An agonist is a drug that combines with a receptor and this causes an effect – the effect may be inhibitory or excitatory. Midazolam is an agonist.
- An antagonist is a drug that interferes with the action of an agonist, and often this drug has no activity of its own. Flumazenil is an antagonist of midazolam.

When considering the pharmacodynamics of sedation agents used in dentistry the reader should appreciate that benzodiazepines (the agonists) combine with benzodiazepine receptors in the body to exert their pharmacological effects. Midazolam therefore activates the benzodiazepine receptors, unlike flumazenil, which merely occupies the receptors.

Pharmacological properties of commonly used sedative agents

In dentistry, the most commonly used sedative drugs are nitrous oxide and midazolam. Nitrous oxide is inhaled, whereas midazolam is most frequently given by the IV route, but can also be administered by the oral, intranasal and buccal routes.

Terminology in sedation can be confusing, as sedative medicines are also used for other pharmacological properties that they possess. When talking about sedation it is the action of reducing anxiety rather than causing drowsiness that is important in the management of the anxious/phobic patient. Achieving anxiolysis is therefore the objective.

- A **sedative** is a drug that is administered to alleviate anxiety. A sedative therefore has a calming effect, relieving anxiety and tension. A better term would be anxiolytic.
- A **hypnotic** is a drug that is administered with the intention of producing sleep or drowsiness. Hypnotics in small doses are often used as sedatives.

Many sedative drugs will achieve anxiolysis at low doses and are more likely to cause drowsiness and even induce sleep at high doses. The reader is to be reminded that the GDC has adopted a strict definition for conscious sedation and when a deeper state of sedation is achieved the GDC will regard this as a state of general anaesthesia.

Nitrous oxide

Nitrous oxide has the following properties and characteristics.

- It is a colourless and virtually odourless, non-irritant gas that is 1.5 times heavier than air.

■ It is compressed to a liquid and supplied in cylinders that are coloured blue. In a full cylinder up to four-fifths of the contents are in the liquid state, the remaining nitrous oxide exists as a gas. The exact amount of nitrous oxide present can only be determined by weighing the cylinder.

■ It is an anxiolytic, analgesic and a weak anaesthetic agent, it produces little if any amnesia.

■ It has a high **minimum alveolar concentration** (MAC) of about 105%. The MAC is the concentration of an inhalation anaesthetic required to abolish the response to a standard surgical stimulus in 50% of the patients; it is a measure of the relative potency of the gas. Nitrous oxide has a relatively high MAC and a low potency; this means that nitrous oxide is potentially safe as a sedative agent. In other words, there is a relatively wide difference between the sedative dose of nitrous oxide and the dose required for GA.

■ It is carried in simple solution in the blood; it does not bind chemically to any components of the blood (unlike oxygen).It places no metabolic demands on the body, it is therefore excreted unchanged by the lungs, with insignificant amounts being excreted via the skin.

■ Nitrous oxide gas has a **blood/gas solubility coefficient** of 0.47 at 37°C – it has poor solubility in blood and tissue fluids and so induction and recovery are rapid. The poor solubility of nitrous oxide means that only small quantities enter the blood and this is rapidly released into the tissues. Therefore:
  □ once the supply of nitrous oxide is stopped it is rapidly released from the tissues into the blood and is quickly excreted by the lungs. The majority of the drug is excreted unchanged via the lungs within minutes after discontinuing nitrous oxide administration. A small and insignificant proportion (around 1%) will be excreted via the lungs and skin over the following 24 hours
  □ the diffusion of nitrous oxide from the blood across the alveolar membrane and back into the lungs is so quick that it has been postulated that this rapid outflow across the alveolar membranes can prevent the normal flow of oxygen from the alveoli into the bloodstream. Thus it is possible that the concentration of oxygen in the alveoli could become dangerously low. This phenomenon is called **diffusion hypoxia** and is prevented by giving 100% oxygen for a minimum of two minutes at the end of nitrous oxide sedation.

■ Long-term (chronic) exposure to nitrous oxide is associated with adverse effects. Prolonged exposure can cause increased incidence of liver, renal and neurological disease, bone marrow toxicity and interference with vitamin B_{12} synthesis. Signs and symptoms similar to those of pernicious anaemia may develop; folic acid supplements can help prevent this. Nitrous oxide can inhibit the reproductive system and an increased number of spontaneous abortions following chronic exposure have been reported. Employing dentists have responsibilities to ensure that staff exposure to any anaesthetic gases should be reduced to the workplace exposure limits (WEL). The

Health and Safety Executive recommends WELs that have been approved by the Health and Safety Commission. The maximum level of exposure to nitrous oxide is 100 ppm (parts per million) over an eight-hour period. Patients and staff need to be protected from environmental pollution with nitrous oxide and scavenging is discussed later in the chapter under Sedation techniques.

■ Nitrous oxide has the potential for abuse and staff should be aware of this risk.

■ Nitrous oxide causes peripheral **vasodilation** (this can be helpful if IV access is required in needle phobic patients).

Nitrous oxide is frequently used in dentistry as a sedative for mild to moderately anxious patients of all ages; but it is particularly useful in paediatric dentistry. Nitrous oxide inhalation sedation (N_2O IS) consists of two components:

■ administration of low-moderate concentrations of nitrous oxide – titrated against patient response from a dedicated relative analgesia (RA) machine
■ verbal reassurance and hypnotic suggestions.

The above elements coupled with the standard safety features of a purpose-built RA machine make N_2O IS a remarkably safe technique. The objective of sedation is to relieve anxiety, and any analgesic effects are a bonus.

RA has been divided into three planes – planes 1 and 2 represent the clinically useful state of sedation called RA, when the patient is relaxed and responsive to commands.

Plane 1, moderate sedation and analgesia: Usually obtained at concentrations between 5 and 25% of nitrous oxide. The patient begins to feel relaxed, fear and anxiety are reduced, and the pain threshold is increased. The patient may experience tingling (paraesthesia), mainly in their fingers and toes, but this can also occur in their cheeks, tongue, head and chest. The skeletal muscles including the facial muscles relax, with a reduction in spontaneous movements.

Plane 2, dissociation sedation and analgesia: Usually seen with concentrations of between 20 and 55% of nitrous oxide. The patient becomes detached from their surroundings, with a sensation of being 'far away', they feel as if they are *floating* or *light headed*. They may laugh or giggle, feel euphoric, warm or drowsy. The senses of hearing, vision and touch are impaired; this can be accompanied by buzzing in their ears and the blink reflex is reduced. Paraesthesia can be profound and may be generalised. There is a reduction in the gag reflex.

Plane 3, total analgesia: Occurs with 50–70% nitrous oxide. Verbal contact may be lost, and the laryngeal reflex impaired, over-excitation and nausea may occur. Plane 3 approaches GA and is therefore unsafe.

The planes of inhalation sedation/RA overlap considerably, and there is a gradual transition from one plane to another; there are no clear boundaries. There is great variation in response to nitrous oxide sedation between patients; some patients may require only 20% nitrous oxide to become adequately sedated, while a few require a concentration of greater than 50%. The operator uses their clinical skills and knowledge to titrate the concentration of nitrous oxide against the patient's response to achieve the appropriate level of sedation. The concurrent use of behavioural management is an integral part of any form of sedation, but especially with N_2O IS.

Entonox

Entonox is a mixture of 50% nitrous oxide and oxygen. It is supplied in blue-coloured cylinders with quartered (chequered) white and blue collars. It is widely used for pain control during labour and is beneficial in terms of analgesia and anxiolysis for patients having a myocardial infarction.

Isoflurane and sevoflurane

Isoflurane and sevoflurane are volatile liquid GA agents. They have been used in subanaesthetic doses alongside oxygen as sedatives but their use is unlicensed. There is currently no commercial device available for the administration of either of these agents with oxygen by a dentist acting as an operator–sedationist. There is also concern over scavenging and there is a lack of safety information available for dental applications.

Benzodiazepines

Benzodiazepines have been used since the 1960s as anxiolytic and sedative drugs. Some are also occasionally used as anticonvulsant agents (clobazam and clonazepam), but their sedative properties are often problematic and they tend to become less effective after weeks and months of continuous use (see Tolerance and dependence below). The benzodiazepines have a wide margin of safety but can cause respiratory depression. The pharmacological properties are as follows.

- **Anxiolytic**: A drug with anxiolytic properties will reduce the distressing feelings of tension, anxiety and panic, so inducing a state of relaxation. Anxiolysis is the most important pharmacological property when considering the management of anxious patients.

- **Sedative/hypnotic**: Benzodiazepines reduce the level of a patient's consciousness, the extent of which is dose dependent; if given in a large dose GA could be induced. Some of the signs of sedation include reduced concentration, a reduction in response time and occasionally slurred speech. Disinhibiting effects can occur and rarely hallucinations of a sexual nature have been reported. This emphasises the need for a chaperone to always be present throughout treatment.

- **Muscle relaxant**: Benzodiazepines relax skeletal muscles (e.g. the relaxation of clenched fists, tensed shoulders and the elimination of anxiety-induced tremors of the limbs). Sedation can therefore be helpful for patients who have conditions that cause tremors, involuntary muscle movements and muscle spasticity (e.g. Parkinson's disease, cerebral palsy). While not all of the tremors may disappear, IV sedation with midazolam can make a significant improvement to safe and effective management.

■ **Anticonvulsant**: Benzodiazepines have anticonvulsant activity. They increase the seizure threshold by preventing the spread of the focus of electrical activity to the surrounding brain tissue. This is useful in patients whose epilepsy is triggered by stress.

■ **Anterograde amnesia**: Benzodiazepines can cause amnesia, preventing recall of events that occurred after the sedation was given but not recall of events that happened before the administration of the drug. Amnesia is more likely to occur following IV administration, it is dose related but is not predictable, therefore the patient should never be promised that they will forget their treatment under sedation. Amnesia is not always considered to be an advantage by the dental team because it would be helpful if patients could remember that their treatment was not painful or distressing. This is an important aspect of behavioural management for the anxious patient.

■ **Respiratory depression**: Benzodiazepines will cause respiratory depression and the effect is more pronounced with high doses. This is why pulse oximetry is mandatory when patients are sedated with benzodiazepines. Respiratory depression is more likely to occur when a sedative cannot be titrated against patient response, so oral and transmucosal benzodiazepines are more likely to depress respiration than an IV drug that has been titrated appropriately. Respiratory depression following benzodiazepine administration can be exacerbated by concurrent use of opioid analgesia, alcohol and other central nervous system (CNS) depressants.

■ **Xerostomia**: A patient often reports a dry mouth (xerostomia) following the administration of a benzodiazepine.

■ **Drug interactions**: Certain medicines that patients may be taking have the potential to interfere with the pharmacokinetics or pharmacodynamics of benzodiazepines. These medicines may be prescribed or bought as over-the-counter preparations. The importance of taking a good medical and drug history cannot be overstated. When patients are taking medicines that are CNS depressants (e.g. tranquillisers, antidepressants, antipsychotic drugs, opioid analgesics, anticonvulsants, alcohol and antihistamines) a lower than expected dose of benzodiazepines could cause profound sedation. In effect, you may see an increase in the sedative actions of benzodiazepines with an associated increased risk of respiratory depression. Over-sedation should be less of a problem with benzodiazepines administered intravenously. This is because, unlike oral or transmucosal routes, the dose of the IV preparation can be titrated, by incremental administration, against patient response. It is possible that some medicines may inhibit liver enzymes and therefore slow down the metabolism of a benzodiazepine (e.g. erythromycin and some antiviral drugs used to treat human immunodeficiency virus). The benzodiazepine antagonist, flumazenil, will inhibit many of the actions of benzodiazepines, by occupying the benzodiazepine receptors and preventing the pharmacological effects of the agonist.

■ **Tolerance and dependence**: Benzodiazepines have the potential to be abused, by both patients and staff. When benzodiazepines are given to a patient regularly for prolonged periods, their pharmacological effectiveness decreases; this phenomenon is called tolerance. This means that dose levels will need to be increased to achieve the same clinical result. Therefore chronic users of oral benzodiazepines may require a larger dose of sedative to provide an acceptable degree of sedation. The long-term use of benzodiazepines can also cause dependence (addiction). Sudden cessation of the medication would therefore lead to profound psychological and physical withdrawal symptoms. It is unlikely that the occasional use of benzodiazepines for dental sedation would reactivate a benzodiazepine addiction.

■ **Metabolism and excretion**: Benzodiazepines are principally metabolised by the liver and excreted by the kidneys. They may pass into breast milk and this has clinical implications when treating a nursing mother. In the elderly and the very young, liver enzyme function may be impaired and there is a risk of prolonged sedation and overdosage.

■ **Paradoxical reactions**: Paradoxical reactions such as an increase in agitation, aggression, restlessness, hyperactivity and disorientation have been reported.

■ **Treatment of overdosage**: The symptoms of overdosage are profound sedation, muscle weakness and rarely paradoxical excitation. Respiratory depression and/or loss of consciousness can occur. Flumazenil is the specific antagonist for use in emergency situations.

■ **Children**: Midazolam is used as a sedative for children in both medical and dental practice. While the evidence base for IV midazolam in paediatric dentistry is growing, it is still poor. Benzodiazepines should be used with caution in children and are not deemed to be the first choice of sedative for dental treatment. The age of the child and the experience of the dental team are important factors when assessing the suitability of a young patient for sedation with benzodiazepines. The physiology and psychology of a 5-year-old will be very different to that of a mature 14-year-old.

Mechanism of action of the benzodiazepines

Benzodiazepines exert their effects by reducing the excitability of certain cells in the CNS which are predominantly situated within the brain. They inhibit (block) some of the incoming (sensory) information that would normally stimulate the brain. This occurs because benzodiazepines enhance the effects of one of the major CNS-inhibitory neurotransmitters called gamma-amino-butyric acid (**GABA**). All benzodiazepines share a common chemical shape or structure that enables the drug molecules to readily bind to and stimulate specific **benzodiazepine receptors**. Benzodiazepine receptors are located on nerve cells in close proximity to GABA receptors, and when benzodiazepines bind to their receptors a **benzodiazepine–GABA–receptor complex** is formed resulting in enhanced GABA activity. As a consequence of this, sensory nerves become less excitable thus reducing the sensory input into the brain. A neurone therefore requires a greater stimulus to trigger a response. The overall effect is inhibition of activity within the brain.

Benzodiazepines enhance or facilitate the action of GABA, which is an inhibitory neurotransmitter of the CNS. This reduces the activity within the brain and makes it less susceptible to excitation.

Diazepam

Diazepam has been used successfully as both a sedative and hypnotic in dentistry since the 1960s, but now its use in dentistry as an IV sedative has been replaced by midazolam. Midazolam has several advantages over diazepam. One major disadvantage is the very long half-life of diazepam. Some practitioners may still prescribe diazepam as a hypnotic to help the patient sleep the night before treatment.

Diazepam preparations are available for use by the oral, IV and rectal route. The latter is often used as a rescue medication for some patients who have poorly controlled epilepsy. Historically, diazepam has been widely known by the former trade name of Valium; however, diazepam has not been marketed in the UK under this brand name for several years.

Presentation

IV use: A glass ampoule containing 10 mg of diazepam in 2 ml. Diazepam is insoluble in water and is available in one of two solvents:

- dissolved in propylene glycol, it forms a clear colourless solution. This is painful on injection and can cause vein damage (**thrombophlebitis**)
- emulsified in soyabean oil, this forms a white emulsion that is non-irritant and unlikely to cause venous problems. It is marketed under the trade name of Diazemuls.

Oral use: Available as 2, 5 and 10 mg tablets and in an oral solution containing 2 mg in 5 ml.

Metabolism

Diazepam is metabolised by the liver and then excreted by the kidneys. Its half-life is approximately 43 hours, but there is great individual variation. In addition, active metabolites are produced and these prolong sedation. One such metabolite is desmethyldiazepam, this has a half-life of up to 100 hours.

Midazolam

Midazolam was initially introduced as an intravenous sedative in the early 1980s and is at least twice as potent as diazepam. It is now the most commonly used IV sedative in dentistry. Midazolam can also be given by oral, buccal and intranasal routes. Midazolam (initially marketed under the brand name of Hypnovel) is currently recognised as the drug of choice for IV sedation in anxious patients. Midazolam is a water-soluble benzodiazepine and should not cause pain on injection. Midazolam is more likely to cause amnesia than diazepam. The duration of action of IV midazolam is up to approximately one hour (but this does vary); the elimination half-life is about two hours and there are no clinically significant active metabolites. Recovery is usually complete within eight hours. The data sheet stipulates that patients should not drive or operate machinery for 12 hours after sedation, but recovery may be longer if patients are taking other CNS depressants or have reduced liver function. In medical practice midazolam is sometimes administered in conjunction with an opioid (narcotic) analgesic such as fentanyl; this is a useful addition if pain relief is required. In dentistry, good anaesthesia can usually be obtained with local anaesthetics and so dentists do not routinely use this combination.

Presentation
IV use: A colourless aqueous solution in a clear glass ampoule. The ampoules come in two sizes:

- 10 mg of midazolam in 2 ml (5 mg/ml). This concentrated solution was initially used for induction of general anaesthesia. This use has been superseded by other drugs such as propofol. This preparation is too concentrated to be used as an IV sedative in dentistry, as it is difficult to give small incremental doses. It is however used in some sedation units and can be administered by the oral, buccal or intranasal route. These methods of administration constitute an *off-licence* use of the product. Intranasal midazolam tends to be used in units of special care dentistry

- 10 mg of midazolam in 5 ml (2 mg/ml). This concentration is favoured for IV sedation as it is easier to titrate small doses of the drug.

Midazolam is preferable to diazepam because:

- it has a faster onset of action
- it does not have clinically significant active metabolites and has a shorter half-life
- the IV preparation is water soluble and does not cause pain on injection – unlike diazepam when it is dissolved in propylene glycol
- it has more consistent and profound anterograde amnesia (but this is not always viewed as an advantage by dentists).

Oral, buccal and intranasal administration of midazolam
In the UK midazolam for injection is licensed for IV use but not for administration by oral, buccal or intranasal routes.

Oral use: The use of midazolam by the oral route in dentistry is well recognised. It is used to treat pre-co-operative children under the care of a specialist paediatric dentist. The dose is calculated according to the weight of the child. Midazolam for injection (10 mg/2 ml or 10 mg/5 ml) is given in blackcurrant or orange juice/cordial to disguise the bitter taste; alternatively, it can be combined with paracetamol elixir. The patient is monitored clinically and with a pulse oximeter. A flavoured preparation of oral midazolam (2.5 mg/14 ml) is available from Special Products.

Adult dental patients are sometimes successfully managed with oral midazolam sedation alone, but others may require further sedation (usually with IV midazolam). Oral midazolam can be useful in patients with special needs who will not allow IV access.

The onset of action of oral midazolam does vary but is around 20–30 minutes.

Buccal use: It has already been mentioned that midazolam for injection can be administered by the buccal route. This preparation tends to be used in status epilepticus; in this emergency situation the taste is not important. Buccal midazolam is also available in a 10 mg/ml preparation (Epistatus), which is a 'special order product'. Epistatus is presented in a bottle that contains 4 ml (40 mg) of midazolam as a clear liquid; four 1 ml syringes are also provided for ease of use. This preparation, as the name suggests, is intended for use in status epilepticus, but it has also been adopted for use as a sedative in many sedation units. The preparation should be placed over the oral tissues and held in the mouth, not swallowed. When used in this way it does tend to increase salivation and sometimes has a tendency to be swallowed. This is certainly the case in patients who are unable to comply with the instructions such as those with learning disabilities. Most patients do not think that this preparation has an acceptable taste.

Intranasal use: In special care dentistry the administration of sedatives by the oral, buccal or IV route is not practical. The intranasal administration of midazolam is often helpful in this situation (Manley *et al*. 2008). The resultant sedation may allow an intra-oral examination to be undertaken or it may allow IV access for further sedation. A mucosal atomisation device is attached to a small syringe and this atomises the solution when it is discharged into a nostril. Patients can find this an unpleasant method of drug administration. Coughing and sneezing can occur and burning of the nasal mucosa has been reported with the 10 mg in 2 ml preparation. It is also a possibility that some of the drug is swallowed or lost into the atmosphere. Some hospital pharmacies may prepare a more concentrated preparation (40 mg/ml) that will allow smaller volumes to be administered intranasally. It is important to remember that respiratory depression remains a risk following the oral or intranasal use of midazolam and monitoring is still required.

Other oral benzodiazepines

Benzodiazepines are available that are licensed for oral use as hypnotics and/or anxiolytics, e.g. temazepam, nitrazepam and diazepam. Temazepam is licensed as a sedative or hypnotic and is available in an oral suspension (10 mg/5 ml) and in 10 mg and 20 mg tablets. Diazepam and temazepam are not now routinely used as oral sedatives for dental treatment; their use has been largely replaced with oral midazolam or titratable sedation techniques (IV sedation or N_2O IS) that are more reliable. These benzodiazepines may occasionally be used as a hypnotic to help anxious patients sleep the night before treatment. Temazepam may be preferable to diazepam as an oral hypnotic because it has a shorter half-life of approximately 13 hours.

Flumazenil

Flumazenil (Anexate) is the benzodiazepine antagonist. Flumazenil is a benzodiazepine but has no significant agonist activity. It is a competitive inhibitor and binds to the benzodiazepine receptors but does not stimulate the benzodiazepine receptor. Flumazenil merely occupies the receptors and prevents other benzodiazepines (agonists) from attaching to the receptors and causing sedation. Flumazenil is effective in reversing anxiolysis, sedation, the respiratory depressant effects and muscle relaxation caused by benzodiazepines, but not the amnesic effects. The pharmacokinetics of benzodiazepines is unaltered in the presence of flumazenil. The plasma half-life of flumazenil is only 50 minutes, significantly less than that of midazolam, therefore patients can theoretically *re-sedate* after the concentration of flumazenil reduces. This is due to the residual sedative effects of any circulating midazolam. However, with the low doses of midazolam used in dentistry this risk is thought to be minimal. Patients who have received flumazenil to reverse the effects of benzodiazepine sedation still require the routine post-operative instructions.

Presentation
Clear glass ampoules containing 500 micrograms flumazenil in 5 ml of an almost colourless solution.

Non-benzodiazepine oral sedatives

Non-benzodiazepine oral sedatives have been used principally in paediatric dentistry. Antihistamines are sometimes used as a hypnotic in small children to help ensure a restful night's sleep.

Propofol
Propofol is a general anaesthetic IV induction agent, but it is also used as an IV sedative agent for adults. It is a phenolic compound that is insoluble in water but highly soluble in lipids and is therefore presented as an emulsion. It is dissolved in a soyabean oil, glycerol and purified egg product; it can sometimes cause pain on initial injection into a vein. As mentioned earlier, propofol can cause allergic reactions. Propofol enhances the effect of GABA in producing CNS depression, but it does not work directly on GABA receptors. Propofol is an anti-emetic (reduces the likelihood of vomiting). It does cause amnesia, although this is less predictable than with IV midazolam. It is rapidly distributed around the body and has to be administered continuously by slow IV infusion during the period of treatment. An automatic electronic pump can be used to control a steady rate of infusion. However, the dose of the drug is still titrated against the patient's response. It can also be administered by patient-controlled (maintained) infusion. This involves the patient administering their own sedation. This is very similar to how morphine and other painkillers are used in patient-controlled analgesia. There is a time-lock mechanism on the device and this reduces the risk of over-sedation. Recovery from

propofol sedation is quite rapid and can be observed shortly after the infusion is stopped. This makes it excellent for short procedures, for example a needle phobic who is only bothered about intra-oral injections. Because it is administered by continuous infusion it is useful in prolonged procedures such as implant placement. There is no reversal agent for propofol; it is metabolised in the liver and excreted by the kidneys. Propofol has a narrower margin of safety than IV midazolam in that there is more of a risk of unintended loss of consciousness and hypoxia. Propofol sedation is not regarded as a standard sedation technique for dentists and should only be undertaken by fully trained and experienced specialist practitioners. Propofol is only licensed for use by anaesthetists.

Propofol is a milky white emulsions and the 1% (10 mg/ml) preparation is used in dental sedation in a clear 20 ml glass ampoule. It is also available in pre-filled syringes.

Miscellaneous drugs

Topical anaesthetic agents

To prevent pain on venepuncture a topical dermal anaesthetic can be applied under an occlusive dressing prior to IV access. Two preparations are frequently used:

■ **Emla** cream is a eutectic mixture of local anaesthetics consisting of lidocaine 2.5% and prilocaine 2.5%). Emla takes at least one hour to work and is not commonly associated with allergic reactions
■ **Ametop** consists of 4% tetracaine (amethocaine) gel and is faster acting than Emla. Tetracaine is an ester local anaesthetic agent and is associated with localised skin reactions such as erythema, oedema and blistering. It should not be left on the skin for more than 30 minutes.

Recommended tasks

(1) Look up the various hypnotic and sedative drugs in the *Dental Practitioners' Formulary* (*DPF*) and identify the drug presentations, indications, cautions and side effects of the different preparations.
(2) Look up the drug information sheets (and patient information leaflets if available) that accompany the sedative drugs that you have in your dental practice.
(3) Ask the relevant drug companies for the data sheets and patient information sheets for those sedative drugs for which you would like to find out more information. The addresses of the drug companies are in the back of the British National Formulary (BNF) (just before the index).
(4) Obtain the regulations and guidelines for the storage of medical gas cylinders. Find out the sizes of cylinders in which N_2O and O_2 are available.

Sedation techniques: practical considerations

Indications and contraindications for sedation

The indications and contraindications for inhalation, IV and oral sedation are outlined in Table 4.7. The contraindications can be absolute or relative. An absolute contraindication means that a procedure definitely should not be carried out under any circumstances (e.g. IV midazolam sedation should not proceed if flumazenil is unavailable, staff are not adequately trained in the sedation technique or equipment required for sedation is faulty). However, in certain circumstances sedation may be undertaken despite there being a relative contraindication; this will depend on the relative risks involved, and such treatment is likely to be carried out in a hospital environment. In this situation the advantages of using sedation will have to outweigh the disadvantages. There are many relative contraindications and most relate to the patient's medical history.

Nitrous oxide inhalation sedation

Inhalation sedation with nitrous oxide is usually called relative analgesia, but this name implies that analgesia is a prominent feature of RA. While nitrous oxide is an analgesic, the pain-relieving properties of this drug are more effective for pain of muscular origin (e.g. pain associated with childbirth or a myocardial infarction) rather than pain caused by dental treatment. The term *nitrous oxide inhalation sedation* is preferred over RA. Members of the sedation team will often abbreviate N_2O IS to inhalation sedation or IS; this is open to criticism because other anaesthetic agents are occasionally used for inhalation sedation. In reality, however, all terminologies are used. For clarity, N_2O IS will be used when referring to this sedation technique; however, when discussing the equipment used for delivering N_2O IS, the term *RA machine* will be used.

The advantages and disadvantages of N_2O IS are given in Table 4.8.

Relative analgesia machine

There are several makes of RA machine dedicated to N_2O IS available on the market, and all machines should conform to British Standards and be maintained according to the manufacturer's recommendations. The service history should be documented. An RA machine has four gas cylinders, two for oxygen (the body of the cylinder is black with a white top) and two blue nitrous oxide cylinders. All cylinders should be appropriately labelled as *in use* or *full/reserve*. A key should be available to switch the cylinders on and off. There are two pressure gauges on the RA machine; the oxygen gauge will give an accurate reading of the oxygen concentration in the cylinder but the nitrous oxide gauge will only measure the partial pressure of nitrous oxide that is in the gaseous phase and is therefore an unreliable measure of how full a cylinder is. This is because nitrous oxide is stored as a liquid under pressure and the liquid present will not be accurately represented by the reading on the pressure gauge. The amount of nitrous oxide present in a cylinder can only be obtained by weighing the cylinder. The weight

Table 4.7 Indications and contraindications of three sedation techniques.

Contraindications	Additional comments relevant to a specific sedation technique		
	Nitrous oxide inhalation sedation	**IV sedation with midazolam**	**Oral and transmucosal sedation with benzodiazepines**
Dental anxiety/phobia	Mild to moderate dental anxiety Patients with needle phobia *Suitable to use in patients who are breast feeding, and those who have liver or kidney disease. A vasodilator so can aid IV access and anxiolysis may help a patient accept IV cannulation*	Moderate to severe anxiety Patients who will not accept a nasal mask	Mild to moderate anxiety An anxiolytic so useful prior to N$_2$O IS or IV sedation
The dental treatment ■ Unpleasant dental procedures ■ Patients with a gag reflex	*Especially useful for simple extractions in children* *Helpful*	*Helpful* Can be helpful in children but for use only by specialists	*Not as reliable and predictable*
Medical conditions ■ Involuntary movement disorders, e.g. cerebral palsy, Parkinson's disease	Not effective	Helpful because of muscle relaxation	Less reliable than IV midazolam
■ Medical conditions that are exacerbated by stress	All techniques may be suitable; the choice will depend on the patient's anxiety, the procedure and the medical condition, e.g. the increased inhaled O$_2$ concentration of N$_2$O IS benefits patients with cardiorespiratory disease; benzodiazepines may help patients with stress-induced epilepsy		
■ Learning disabilities	Any of the techniques may be suitable – it will depend on the extent of the patients' disability and if anxiety is present		

Table 4.7 *Continued*

Contraindications	Additional comments relevant to a specific sedation technique		
	Nitrous oxide inhalation sedation	IV sedation with midazolam	Oral and transmucosal sedation with benzodiazepines
Absolute *Resources*			
■ Poorly maintained or inadequate equipment	e.g. inadequate scavenging systems in place, no O_2 reserve cylinder	No pulse oximeter, BP machine or flumazenil	No pulse oximeter, BP machine or flumazenil. Training in IV sedation is essential for sedation with oral and transmucosal benzodiazepines
■ Untrained staff	This applies to both the dentist and the nursing staff		
■ No responsible escort or carer	Escort/carer is not always required for adults		
Medical conditions			
■ Respiratory problems	Temporary respiratory or nasal obstruction, e.g. common cold Permanent nasal obstruction, e.g. enlarged adenoids		Upper respiratory tract infections
ASA III & IV patients in a primary dental care facility	Patients usually require treatment in a specialist unit		
Allergy		Allergy is extremely rare	
Relative			
Pregnancy	The first trimester (12 weeks)	Throughout pregnancy: benzodiazepines will cross the placenta and are potentially harmful to the unborn baby	
Breast feeding		A small amount of benzodiazepines can pass into breast milk, additional postoperative instructions may be required to minimise risk to the baby	
Phobias	Patients who will not accept a nasal mask	Phobia of needles[1]	

Age	
■ Children	Co-operation is required for successful sedation
■ The pre-co-operative child	Caution; specialist training in managing this group of patients is required, although oral and IV midazolam can be very successful in teenagers when N_2O IS has failed
■ The elderly	Risk of prolonged and over sedation, consider N_2O IS, but titrate doses slowly
Medical conditions	
■ e.g. chronic respiratory disease, multiple sclerosis, severe psychiatric disease	e.g. hepatic or renal impairment Patient response can be unpredictable when alcohol or recreational drugs have been taken, risk of CNS depression Response can be variable and unpredictable in psychiatric patients
Conditions that prevent co-operation or understanding[2]	This technique relies on hypnotic suggestion and patient co-operation May be helpful, caution is required and training in managing this group of patients, who can be unpredictable
Dental procedure	The nasal hood may limit access for surgery to the anterior teeth, and surrounding soft tissues and alveolar bone

[1] Patients might consider accepting IV access if a dermal topical anaesthetic is used pre-operatively, or N_2O IS is given prior to IV access.

[2] In patients with severe behavioural problems, dementia, learning disabilities or certain psychiatric disorders it is often difficult to appreciate the level of co-operation possible until a procedure under sedation is attempted.

Table 4.8 The advantages and disadvantages of nitrous oxide (N_2O) inhalation.

Advantages	Disadvantages
Non-invasive technique	Nasal mask can limit access to anterior maxillary teeth
Rapid onset of sedation, rapid recovery and sedation can be quickly reversed by administering oxygen	Mask may be unacceptable to some patients
Depth of sedation can be easily and quickly altered	Unsuitable for patients unable to co-operate because the technique depends on a high level of psychological reassurance and hypnotic suggestion
Suitable for patients of all ages	Pollution and chronic exposure to N_2O, and the potential for staff to abuse the drug are important health and safety issues
Can use for unescorted adult patients	Equipment is expensive and free- standing machines are bulky
Drug is not metabolised by the liver, excreted by the kidney or into breast milk	
Excellent safety record, RA machine has several safety features	
Some analgesia	

RA, relative analgesia.

of an E-size gas cylinder full of N_2O is 9.07 kg (20 lb) and an empty cylinder weighs 5.44 kg (12 lb).

The yoke or manifold of the RA machine supports the gas cylinders. The gas cylinders fit onto the manifold accurately and in a specific manner because there is a pin index system that ensures that the nitrous oxide and oxygen cylinders are located correctly and cannot be interchanged. Pressure-reducing valves act to reduce the high pressure from each of the gas cylinders as the gases transfer through a series of colour-coded pipelines to the RA machine head. Again these pipes cannot be interchanged between the different gases.

The machine has a flow meter to adjust the rate of flow of gases delivered to the patient and also a dial to alter the percentage of nitrous oxide delivered. The flow rate of each gas can be seen in the two flow meters (calibrated in litres/minute); these indicate the gas flow rate through the delivery tubing to the patient. All machines are fitted with a fail-safe system that will automatically cut off the nitrous oxide supply when the oxygen supply falls to below 30%. Machines in dental practices are usually free-standing but in hospitals and specialist clinics they may be connected to a central supply of gases, which allows for a neater, more compact system. The safety features that are present on RA machines are listed in Table 4.9.

Surgery levels of nitrous oxide should be kept to as low a level as is reasonably achievable, and practical methods are given in Table 4.10. Scavenging of waste gases should

Table 4.9 Safety features built into an RA machine.

Colour coding: N_2O cylinders and pipes that carry N_2O are blue. O_2 cylinders are black with a white top and O_2 carrying pipes are white

Pin index system: prevents the N_2O and O_2 gas cylinder being interchanged (placed onto the wrong yoke)

'O' ring washers (Bodok seal): improves the seal between the cylinder and the yoke

Pressure reducing valves: reduces the pressure of the compressed gases from the cylinder

N_2O and O_2 pressure dials: allows monitoring of cylinder pressures

Minimum flow level: a minimum flow level of 3l/min is set for many machines

Minimum oxygen delivery system: maintains a minimum flow rate of 30% O_2

Oxygen fail-safe: if O_2 flow drops to less than 275.49 kPa (40 psi) the N_2O flow cuts out

Air entrainment valve (automatic air intake valve): this is normally closed but will open to allow room (ambient) air into the breathing circuit when gas flow rates are too low (i.e. when a negative pressure is in the circuit)

Oxygen flush button: when the oxygen button is depressed it can deliver 100% O_2

Reservoir bag: the bag allows the rate and depth of respiration to be monitored and serves as a reservoir of gas for the patient to breathe from

One-way valve to prevent re-breathing of N_2O: RA machines have a non-re-breathing patient circuit; exhaled gases pass into the exit port from the mask and into a scavenging hose. The system has a one-way valve to prevent re-breathing exhaled air and prevent a build up of CO_2 in the breathing circuits. This valve is typically in the scavenging hose but in some systems may be in the nasal hood.

RA, relative analgesia; N_2O, nitrous oxide; O_2, oxygen; CO_2, carbon dioxide.

conform to COSHH (Control of Substances Hazardous to Health) guidelines. Nitrous oxide levels should not exceed the workplace exposure limits of 100 ppm over an eight-hour time-weighted average. The room should always be well ventilated and active scavenging should be employed. The active scavenging equipment should be checked regularly by a member of the dental team (and this should be clearly recorded) and serviced as recommended by the manufacturers. Nitrous oxide pollution occurs mainly from patients' exhaled breath, but can also be due to leaks from the breathing circuits, face mask and connections on the RA machine.

The breathing circuit, reservoir bag and hose can all be obtained in materials that do not contain natural rubber latex. If staff are unsure if products contain latex, accurate information should be obtained from the manufacturer before treating a latex allergic patient.

Sedation with nitrous oxide: role of the dental nurse

When assisting in the care of the sedated patient there are many procedures that are common to all sedation techniques. To avoid repetition, the processes that are shared by the different sedation techniques will only be described once, in the section on N_2O IS.

Table 4.10 Methods to minimise nitrous oxide (N_2O) pollution in the surgery.

Always perform safety checks on a well-maintained and regularly serviced RA machine prior to treatment

Always use the minimum effective dose of N_2O during treatment

Use scavenging:
  Active scavenging involves the removal of waste gas by the application of low-power suction to the expiratory limb of the breathing circuit
  Passive scavenging includes such commonsense methods as opening a window and a door to create a through draft and extending the expiratory limb so that the exhaled gas is voided outside the building or surgery area

Have good room ventilation; an extractor fan placed at ground level is helpful (N_2O is heavier than air)

Use well-fitting nasal masks and ensure the patient is breathing through their nose – the use of rubber dam will also help reduce N_2O pollution and improve sedation by preventing mouth breathing

Discourage the patient from talking

If the patient is persistently crying stop the N_2O flow until the patient is settled

Switch off machine when not in use

Ensure staff are well trained and have defined duties

Monitor the environment for N_2O levels

RA, relative analgesia.

When preparing for the treatment appointment it is helpful to divide the duties of the dental nurse into those associated with the preparation of the surgery, preparation of the patient to receive sedation, administration of sedation and treatment of the patient (this includes monitoring the patient), the recovery and discharge phase, and documentation. Some duties are not unique to treatment under sedation (e.g. no patient should be treated if the emergency drugs are not in date or if emergency oxygen is not available), but have been included for completeness.

Preparation of surgery

(1) Ensure that appropriate emergency drugs and equipment are available.
(2) Check the clinical records for the following:
  (a) a consent form that has been signed appropriately (inform the dentist if one is not available)
  (b) any significant medical history
  (c) what treatment is to be undertaken
  (d) what aspects of dentistry cause anxiety to the patient
  (e) any special considerations (e.g. some patients request that the escort remains in the room, white clinical coats should not be worn for some anxious patients).
(3) Prepare the dental equipment, instruments and materials required for the proposed treatment and place them discreetly in the surgery.

(4) Ensure that there is a suitably trained person available to monitor and assist in the care of the sedated patient. Once the patient is sedated the second appropriate person must stay with the patient and dentist. If radiographs need developing or equipment is required from elsewhere then another staff member (a runner) must be available; this person need not be sedation trained.

(5) Prepare the RA machine. The RA machine must be checked before each session and this is usually carried out by the dental nurse, although it is ultimately the responsibility of the dentist. The nurse should have a set routine for performing the safety checks. Table 4.11 lists all the items that should be inspected. Choose a nasal hood but this will need to be checked on the patient.

Preparation of the patient

■ Have a calm, reassuring and friendly manner throughout.
■ Be aware of the patient's body language and be empathetic.
■ Welcome the patient, check their name and date of birth.
■ Confirm with the patient what dental treatment is planned.

Table 4.11 Pre-procedural safety checks on the inhalation sedation machine.

While checking the machine ensure all connections are secure and tight

Valve block and manifold
pin-index system: check pins for wear periodically and check that Bodok seals are in place

Check oxygen cylinders
check *full* cylinder against pressure gauge – turn off. Flush out O_2 with the O_2 flush button
check *in-use* O_2 cylinder (leave on to check N_2O cylinders)

Check N_2O cylinders
check *full* N_2O cylinder against pressure gauge. Turn off. Clear N_2O out of circuit by having 50% O_2 flow
turn on *in-use* cylinder, read pressure gauge. Leave this cylinder turned on

Check oxygen fail safe
turn off *in-use* O_2 cylinder. Set mixture to 50% O_2 and press oxygen flush to empty O_2 circuit. N_2O
should *cut out* in the absence of O_2

Check machine calibration
turn off 50% O_2 and N_2O and ensure that both flow meters are at the same level

Check reservoir bag and emergency oxygen flush
physically examine it to check for holes, cracks or wear. Inflate reservoir bag with O_2 flush by removing breathing circuit and blocking the gas exit. Check for leaks

Check breathing circuit (including nasal hood)
physically examine circuit. Check the non-return valve (this may be in the expiratory limb or the nasal hood), check that the hoses are intact, not perished or leaking

Scavenging system
check system works

- Check that the pre-operative instructions have been adhered to. Ask the patient when they last had something to eat and drink. There is no need for a patient to starve prior to sedation with the standard techniques. Occasionally, however, patients susceptible to vomiting during N_2O IS may be asked to starve for three hours prior to treatment.
- Ensure that the patient has an escort and confirm their transport arrangements for returning home and that both patient and escort are aware of the postoperative instructions.

Sedation and treatment

(1) Always have a calm and reassuring manner; explain the procedure to the patient (unless otherwise requested by the patient). In any event maintain words of reassurance and encouragement

(2) Remain with the patient and dentist at all times.

(3) Place chair in a supine position, ensuring the patient is comfortable (some patients prefer to sit upright).

(4) Explain to the patient the *stop signal* that is used in your clinic.

(5) Reassure the patient throughout and give positive reinforcement as appropriate.

(6) A well-fitting facemask is connected to a previously checked RA machine and the mixture dial is set to 100% oxygen.

(7) The oxygen flow is turned on to about 5 l/min (approximately the patient's minute volume).

(8) The patient or a member of staff places the nosepiece into position. By monitoring the reservoir bag the oxygen flow rate is adjusted to match the patient's tidal volume. The patient's mouth should be closed throughout. A flow of nitrous oxide (10%) is then introduced; suggest to the patient the sensations they might feel (e.g. light-headedness, tingling of hands and feet, warmth, floating sensation). The concentration is gradually increased by 5 or 10% at one- to two-minute intervals. The concentration that produces adequate sedation is noted. Commonly concentrations of between 20 and 50% are used. During treatment the nitrous oxide can be reduced if this is thought to be appropriate.

(9) Treatment is started. The use of rubber dam for restorations improves the sedation and reduces nitrous oxide pollution. The patient should wear eye protection and the nurse should ensure efficient aspiration when appropriate. A member of the dental team (this may be the nurse) should use hypnotic suggestion to help relax the patient.

(10) While assisting the dentist, the nurse continually monitors:
   (a) **equipment**: gas cylinder gauges, flow meters, movement of reservoir bag, fit and comfort of the nosepiece. The rate and depth of respiration is probably best monitored using the reservoir bag
   (b) **patient**: respiration, skin colour, pulse rate, level of responsiveness/ consciousness and mood. If the patient is becoming increasingly sedated, nauseous, restless, agitated or unresponsive the dentist should immediately

reduce the amount of nitrous oxide. If sedation is inadequate the N_2O flow and the fit of the nosepiece should be checked; ensure the patient is not mouth breathing. Electromechanical monitoring is not normally required as the patient is receiving a constant supply of oxygen during treatment. The development of restlessness and agitation after a period of adequate sedation is usually due to too high a concentration of nitrous oxide.

(11) At the end of sedation, 100% oxygen is delivered for a minimum of two minutes to prevent diffusion hypoxia. Remove the nasal mask (while oxygen is still flowing) and return the chair slowly to an upright position. Within 10 minutes 95% of nitrous oxide will be eliminated following a short sedation session. If the patient is coping well or is only anxious about one item of treatment (e.g. the injections) then the nitrous oxide may be switched off during the treatment phase and the patient remains on oxygen.

Recovery and discharge

- Continue with praise and positive reinforcement. If the treatment went particularly well, inform the patient.
- The patient can remain in the dental chair or be transferred to a recovery area. Patients who have received nitrous oxide sedation recover very quickly, usually around 15 minutes after cessation of sedation. Some dentists ask the unescorted adult patient to remain on the premises for 30 minutes after turning off the nitrous oxide.
- Allow the patient to stand up slowly. Monitor their co-ordination as they stand up and move about. The patient should be able to walk unsupported before discharge. The dentist is ultimately responsible for discharging the patient.
- Give appropriate postoperative instructions verbally and in writing for both the sedation and the treatment undertaken. The escort and patient should be told what treatment was undertaken. A contact telephone number must be given.
- Pain control should be prescribed if appropriate.
- The RA machine should be turned off and any empty cylinders replaced; nasal hoods should be sterilised or discarded as appropriate. Disposable items should be discarded.

Clinical records

When a member of staff reads the patient's notes they should be able to identify what concentrations of sedative were given and the patient's response to the sedation. The following information should be recorded:

- date
- written consent obtained
- escort available
- name of operator, second appropriate person and ideally other personnel present
- any premedication taken by the patient or oral sedation given prior to N_2O IS

- size of mask used, the average flow rate, the maximum concentration of nitrous oxide administered and the minimum if it was reduced at different stages of treatment
- how long oxygen was administered after sedation. Time of administration of nitrous oxide sedation and cessation of sedative
- the quality of sedation achieved and the level of anxiolysis. Any unexpected or adverse reaction to the sedation or any other problems encountered
- details of the dental treatment carried out
- that written and verbal postoperative instructions were given and any special instructions given
- time of discharge.

It is often helpful to have available a proforma with '*tick boxes*' to record details of pre-sedation checks, treatment details and monitoring data.

Intravenous sedation

Midazolam is the drug of choice for IV sedation in dentistry; the advantages and disadvantages are listed in Table 4.12. Propofol is growing in popularity as a sedative agent; however, the administration of this drug necessitates an infusion pump. Propofol is not currently regarded as a standard method of sedation and the methods of administration are outside the remit of this chapter.

The complications associated with IV sedation commonly relate to minor local problems associated with cannulation, and late complications are very rare (see Table 4.13). Failure to cannulate is probably the most significant problem as some patients have few suitable superficial veins. A patient's peripheral circulation reduces when they are anxious and also when they are cold. When a person has had prolonged and extensive therapies involving the administration of IV medicines there may be no suitable veins. Patients who are or have been recreational IV drug users are often unsuitable candidates

Table 4.12 The advantages and disadvantages of sedation with midazolam.

Advantages	Disadvantages
Rapid onset of sedation	Venepuncture is invasive and may be unacceptable to some patients
Surgery pollution is not an issue	Intravenous access may not be easy to achieve in some patients
Midazolam is not administered continuously throughout treatment	Expensive monitoring equipment is required
Mouth breathing does not influence the quality of sedation	An escort and home care are always required
Anxiolytic properties of midazolam make it suitable for patients with severe dental anxiety and phobia	Patient may experience hallucinations and sexual arousal during sedation

Table 4.13 Complications of peripheral venous access.

EARLY COMPLICATIONS	
Failed cannulation	The needle fails to enter the vein lumen, it may be pushed completely through the vein or remain in the wall of the vein
Haematoma	Haematoma can occur because of poor technique, fragile blood vessels (e.g. the elderly or a patient on steroids) or lack of pressure dressing after removal of cannula
Extravasation of drugs	Usually due to a failure to site IV cannula correctly, this results in the painful collection of solution in subcutaneous tissues and a localised swelling
Intra-arterial	The injection of drugs into an artery will cause arteriospasm. This decreases the blood supply to the limb distal to the injection site. Cannulation is painful and there is a problematic leaking of blood during cannulation. The blood flow is pulsatile and the colour is bright cherry red as opposed to the darker venous blood. Pain occurs during injection (typically radiates distally – down the limb – away from the site of the injection). An intra-arterial injection is more likely in the antecubital fossa than the back of the hand
Damage to local structures	Often due to poor technique. The risk of damage to adjacent vital structures is increased in the antecubital fossa because of the local variation in anatomy
LATE COMPLICATIONS (exceptionally rare)	
Thrombophlebitis	This is inflammation of the vein – larger veins are less susceptible
Cellulitis	Usually associated with poor aseptic technique

for IV sedation due to the lack of adequate veins for cannulation. The patient will let you know the best available vein and may actually site their own cannula. Interestingly, a significant number of ex-IV drug users are needle phobic. General complications include:

■ **over-sedation** – this is discussed later
■ **paradoxical reactions** – a small number of patients appear to sedate normally with standard doses of sedative but appear to become extremely distressed when treatment is started. Treatment is usually abandoned in such circumstances.

Considerations for IV sedation at the treatment visit

■ When preparing the surgery for IV sedation, it can be helpful to place the equipment in two trays, one tray containing the items required for administering midazolam and the other for emergency use only (Table 4.14). Check that the packaging around sterile equipment (e.g. syringes, cannula) is intact. The dental nurse can draw up the drugs under supervision from the dentist. Drugs for injection should be drawn up in a clean and designated area using an aseptic technique and the syringe should be labelled **immediately**. Hands should be washed prior to drawing up drugs.

Table 4.14 Preparation of equipment for the administration of intravenous midazolam.

Tray 1	Tray 2
Tourniquet	*Contents to be used only if reversal of sedation is required*
Ampoule of midazolam (10 mg/5 ml)*	5 ml syringe
5 ml syringe† (eccentric nozzle)	Drawing up needle
Drawing up needle (blunt, long, wide bore)	Napkin/ampoule breaker
23/25 g cannula‡	25 g cannula
Napkin/ampoule breaker	Non-allergenic sticky tape
Alcohol skin wipe or suitable skin disinfectant	Ampoule of flumazenil*
Non-allergenic sticky tape	
Cotton wool roll/swab for a pressure dressing to venepuncture wound	
Saline/water for injection	
Stopwatch to time the increments	

* All drugs should be checked (e.g. label, expiry date). The glass ampoule should be seen to be intact and the drug solution should be clear.
† Some clinicians dilute the midazolam (usually with 5 ml water for injection to achieve a concentration of 1 mg/ ml), in which case a 10 ml syringe is required. This allows smaller increments of midazolam to be used for titration.
‡ Butterfly needles are not recommended because they do not give secure venous access (they can cut-out of the vein) and they require regular flushing with saline to prevent coagulation).

■ Ensure that monitoring equipment (pulse oximeter and BP device) are fully operational.

■ Patients having IV sedation should have their BP, pulse and SaO_2 measured pre-operatively. Patients wearing nail polish should remove it prior to treatment.

■ The technique used for the administration of IV midazolam sedation is given in Table 4.15.

■ The patient should be allowed to recover from sedation until they can stand and walk unaided; they should not feel or appear to be unstable whilst walking. The **Romberg test** can be used to determine recovery after sedation. The patient is asked to stand up, place their feet together, close their eyes and then touch their nose with an index finger. If the patient sways or has difficulty maintaining this position they are not fit for discharge. Alternatively, the patient may be asked to stand up and walk unaided. Asking a patient to put their coat on also demands quite a high degree of co-ordination. The escort and patient should both feel confident about being ready to go home.

■ The patient can remain in the dental chair or be transferred to a recovery area.

Table 4.15 The administration of intravenous midazolam sedation.

(1) Explain to the patient when you are about to attach the finger probe of the pulse oximeter and place it gently on to a finger

(2) The dental nurse occludes venous return from the hand or arm by using their hands or a tourniquet, while the dentist selects a suitable vein for cannulation, usually on the dorsum of the hand or the antecubital fossa

(3) The cannulation site is swabbed with a suitable antiseptic (e.g. isopropyl alcohol wipe) and allowed to dry. A cannula is inserted into the vein and the nurse secures the cannula to the skin with a dedicated sterile dressing or hypoallergenic tape. If the cannulation has been unsuccessful at that site, the nurse will apply pressure with a swab at the injection site, this prevents bleeding after removal of the cannula. The swab is then taped securely to the skin

(4) The midazolam is injected into the vein in increments – titrated against patient response. The patient is told that this might feel cold. If the patient experiences pain at the cannulation site then the drug is probably escaping into the tissues, and administration of midazolam should cease until a new cannula is inserted. Pain radiating down the arm or hand is indicative of an arterial injection and another cannula should be inserted. It is common practice for 2 mg to be administered over a 30-second period. Ask the patient if the limb is comfortable during the initial administration of midazolam – there should not be any pain. The effect on the patient is observed over a two-minute period.* If further sedation is required incremental doses of 0.5 mg to 1 mg are given, with 30 seconds* between each increment, until the desired sedation is achieved. The nurse or dentist should maintain verbal contact with the patient during this time

(5) Commence treatment but monitor the patient. The duration of sedation will vary between individuals but usually there will be a window of approximately 30–60 minutes treatment time

(6) Supplemental oxygen is not used routinely but it should always be readily available

*This time may be increased for the elderly or medically compromised patient.

- When a patient has received IV sedation it is often stated that a period of one hour should elapse between the last increment of sedative and the discharge of the sedated patient. While this is a reasonable guide, there is great variation in recovery from midazolam sedation. Discharge instructions remain the same irrespective of whether or not flumazenil has been given to reverse the sedative; except that when flumazenil has been administered, the possibility of residual sedation should be mentioned.

- The cannula is left *in situ* until the patient is ready to be discharged. When the cannula is removed, a dry sterile cotton gauze, cotton roll or plaster is placed over the cannulation site. The cannula is removed swiftly and firm pressure applied to the site for two to three minutes ensuring that there is no subcutaneous leakage of blood, then a pressure dressing is secured with tape. The cannula should be checked to ensure that it is intact and then disposed of in the clinical waste.

- Prior to discharge the patient's escort should be told what treatment was undertaken and it should be made clear that the patient did not have a general anaesthetic. The escort should be warned that patients may not remember what happened during treatment and this might lead them to think that they had had a general anaesthetic.

■ Following IV sedation the tray containing the used ampoule, syringe and needles is retained until the patient has been discharged and the patient's notes written up as soon as possible after the treatment. The needles, syringes and glass ampoules should be safely disposed of into suitable receptacles. In addition to the treatment undertaken and the quality of sedation and anxiolysis obtained, the following information should be documented in the notes:

□ expiry date
□ pre-operative BP
□ batch numbers of the drugs used, some clinicians also record expiry dates
□ site of cannulation (number of attempts at IV access)
□ the amount of drug used
□ monitoring details
□ time of administration of midazolam and time of discharge.

Reversal of benzodiazepine sedation with flumazenil

Should reversal with flumazenil be required an initial dose of 200 micrograms (2 ml) is given over 15 seconds. If the desired level of reversal is not achieved within 60 seconds, further increments of 100 micrograms may be injected every minute to a maximum total dose of 1 mg (two ampoules).

Over-sedation

Over-sedation is a risk with any sedation procedure. Over-sedation with midazolam may occur when the drug has been given too quickly or too much midazolam has been administered. Titrating the drug incrementally against the patient's response usually prevents this. Over-sedation can result in reduced co-operation from the patient, loss of consciousness, hypoxia, respiratory depression and ultimately respiratory arrest. It is important to realise the difference between sedation and anxiolysis. Sometimes it is possible to have a patient who is well sedated but still anxious and perhaps not as co-operative as one would like. Further sedation could cause over-sedation in this situation.

When over-sedation occurs with N_2O IS the concentration of N_2O can be reduced and the over-sedation is quickly reversed. With benzodiazepines, no matter what the route of administration, over-sedation is prolonged and if left untreated will only resolve when the drug levels in the blood reduce. This will depend on the rate of metabolism and excretion of the drug. The dental team should therefore be prepared to manage the over-sedated patient. Respiratory depression and loss of consciousness can occur with over-sedation; however, a patient who is only mildly over-sedated needs only to be stimulated while treatment is being undertaken. This can be done by talking to the patient and asking them to breathe more deeply. Patients may not want to keep their mouth open so a mouth prop may also be necessary, but monitoring needs to continue to ensure the patient is still conscious. The use of a mouth prop should never be routine practice in managing the sedated patient. Always ensure that the pulse oximeter is accurately recording the oxygen saturation – it could have been displaced or even fallen off the finger. Some patients play with the pulse oximeter. It is important to monitor the patient and not solely rely on electromechanical monitoring. Sometimes the over-sedated patient will drop their chin or move their head forward and cause airway obstruction. In this situation the airway can be improved with a head tilt or chin lift. Alternatively, a jaw thrust can be used.

Monitoring is important and if there is any significant steady fall in oxygen saturation by 5% that does not respond to the above methods then supplementary oxygen is indicated. If supplementary oxygen is given, when it is turned off, the oxygen saturation levels should be closely monitored to ensure that they are stable before the patient is discharged. Flumazenil may be used in the over-sedated patient, but prolonged monitoring is required as re-sedation is a possibility. The likelihood of re-sedation will depend on the dose of midazolam used, the depth of sedation achieved and the time the last increment of midazolam was given.

A severely over-sedated patient (with a reduced respiration rate) may require assisted ventilations, with a bag-valve-mask-reservoir attached to an oxygen supply, to restore an effective respiration rate. Respiratory arrest remains a possible outcome in a grossly over-sedated patient and this is managed by following the Basic Life Support (BLS) algorithm. Therefore there is a graded response to managing over-sedation that depends on the severity of the problem. Always ensure that the finger probe of the pulse oximeter is fitted correctly, observe the patient's colour, breathing pattern and their level of consciousness. Ask the dentist to stop treatment. Then consider the following, depending on the extent of the problem, while remembering to monitor the patient:

- ask the patient to take a few deep breaths
- open the airway
- supplementary oxygen
- administration of flumazenil[4]
- assisted ventilations
- call emergency services
- start cardiopulmonary resuscitation (CPR) algorithm if the patient is in respiratory arrest.

The technique of IV cannulation
IV cannulation should achieve a **secure** venous access, the cannula should not allow clotting and a needle should not be left in the vein. IV access is necessary for the administration of drugs and emergency drugs. The most popular method of achieving venous access is with a plastic cannula mounted over a needle, the bevel of the needle extends beyond the cannula. Cannulae come in different sizes. A 16-gauge cannula is used by paramedics in an emergency situation. In dental sedation a 21- to 23-gauge cannula is commonly used. The sterile tubing of the cannula should not be touched.

---

[4]Administer flumazenil by IV injection – initial dose 200 micrograms IV over 15 seconds with a further dosage of 100 micrograms at one-minute intervals until consciousness returns, up to a maximum total dose of 1 mg (the usual dose required is 300–600 micrograms).

■ Universal cross-infection precautions apply. Wash hands first and wear gloves because:
  □ the cannula will breach the body's natural barrier (the skin) and provide an entry site for bacteria
  □ there is a risk of contact with body fluids.
■ Select the venepuncture site (superficial veins in the upper limb are most commonly used) and apply tourniquet pressure (proximal to the site) to obstruct venous return but not arterial flow (approximately 20 mm/Hg below systolic pressure).
■ A vein is chosen by visual inspection but principally by palpation. Time is required to select a suitable site and both arms may need to be inspected prior to choosing a vein. The selected vein should be straight, feel bouncy and spring back when depressed.
■ Venous filling can be improved by:
  □ asking the patient to alternatively open and close their hand into a fist
  □ lightly tapping the vein
  □ lowering the arm to below heart level
  □ ensuring the hand is warm.

■ Ensure that the skin is cleaned at the site of cannulation. Alcohol wipes (70% isopropyl alcohol) or chlorhexidine wipes are commonly used. Many trusts will have a cannulation policy with clearly defined protocols on skin preparation and how to secure a cannula with sterile dressings.
■ The tourniquet should be released once the cannula has been successfully inserted into the vein.
■ The cannula should be secured firmly with a dedicated sterile dressing or low-allergenic adhesive tape.
■ It can be confirmed that the cannula is correctly positioned by injecting 0.9% sodium chloride through the cannula. The cannulation site should be inspected for signs of leakage or swelling. The dentist may feel confident that the cannula is in the vein and administer the sedative straight away. Nevertheless, the site of cannulation should be observed during the initial drug administration.

Oral and transmucosal sedation with benzodiazepines

Oral and transmucosal sedation in dentistry is a simple and non-invasive method of achieving anxiety control. Oral sedatives are used in dentistry either as **hypnotic** or **anxiolytic agents**. Both methods may be employed for the anxious patient.

Oral and transmucosal sedation is given to a patient under direct clinical supervision with the intention of reducing their anxiety such that they will accept dental treatment. Oral or transmucosal midazolam is the oral sedative of choice, but historically oral benzodiazepines such as temazepam and diazepam have been used. These drugs have a much longer half-life than midazolam and so have prolonged sedative effects. Some patients will still need further sedation (IV or N_2O IS) to enable them to accept dentistry. The dose used for midazolam sedation will vary according to the patient's previous

Table 4.16 Advantages and disadvantages of premedication and oral sedation.

Advantages	Disadvantages
Orally administered drugs are usually well accepted and tolerated by patients	Onset of action is unpredictable
A quick, convenient and cost- effective method of drug administration	The desired anxiolytic or sedative effect may not be achieved
	Patients may become restless and agitated in the clinic while waiting for the sedation to work
	The clinician should only prescribe the required amount of pre-medication to safeguard against the potential for drug misuse
	Monitoring is still required

sedation experiences, medical history and age. A frequently prescribed dose is 10 mg in a healthy adult patient of normal stature. Care should be taken if patients are very small or have a complex drug or medical history; in this case the dose should be reduced. The time taken for the drug to act will also vary and depend on the methods of administration. The advantages and disadvantages of pre-medication and oral sedation are given in Table 4.16.

Oral, buccal and transmucosal midazolam do not have a UK product licence to use as sedatives and so is given *off-licence*; patients should be told about this during the process of obtaining consent. Details of the presentations of these preparations are given in the section on pharmacology. Buccal midazolam may be used to produce sedation in the same way as oral midazolam; the onset of action should be quicker – around 10 minutes; sometimes, however, the preparation is swallowed and then in effect becomes an orally administered drug. A frequently used dose is 10 mg.

Intranasal midazolam can be of value in special care dentistry (Manley *et al.* 2008) and the onset of action can be very quick, taking just a few minutes to notice an effect. A mucosal atomisation device is required to produce an aerosol to aid administration and absorption. A patent nostril is required for application. When the 10 mg/2 ml concentration is used the dose can be divided between two nostrils, but this is not required if a more concentrated preparation (40 mg/ml) is used. It is advisable to obtain IV access as soon as is practicable following administration of oral and transmucosal midazolam. Over-sedation is a recognised risk with these techniques as the dose is not being titrated against patient response. While dosage varies considerably in all of these techniques, 10 mg is a frequently used dose in an adult.

Considerations for oral and transmucosal sedation at the treatment visit

- Consent must be obtained prior to administration of the oral sedative. Once the patient has received oral/transmucosal sedation informed consent cannot be obtained because judgement is likely to be impaired and the patient cannot therefore be considered to be competent to give consent.

■ The sedative should be administered while the patient is under the direct supervision of a member of the dental team in an environment where the patient can be adequately monitored. A patient who has been given oral/transmucosal sedation should be monitored as for IV sedation as they may become heavily sedated. An IV cannula and flumazenil need to be readily available. Many dental clinicians will want to place an IV cannula when the patient is sufficiently sedated. If oral sedation is used then the patient may be asked to wait in a separate area to the dental surgery; this is often preferable for anxious patients who dislike the surgery environment. The room should be quiet, the patient should be monitored and pulse oximetry should be used. A wheelchair may be necessary to transfer the patient to the dental surgery.

■ Dental treatment is undertaken in much the same way as for the other methods of sedation. Comprehensive monitoring is always required. It is, however, possible for a patient to become more deeply sedated after the treatment has been completed because peak blood levels of the sedative agent may not be achieved until one or two hours after administration. The patient should be constantly monitored clinically throughout the visit. At all times the patient should be able to respond to verbal commands. It is also important to appreciate this when discharging the patient.

■ The postoperative instructions for oral/transmucosal sedation are the same as for IV sedation.

■ Details of the sedative drug, method of administration, the time interval between drug administration and the start of treatment should be noted.

Premedication with benzodiazepines

Premedication is the use of a small dose of a sedative drug that is taken by the patient *outside* the surgery environment. Sometimes a patient presents for treatment having already self-medicated with benzodiazepines. The drug is prescribed to achieve the following objectives.

■ Anxiolysis – reducing the patient's anxiety concerning their appointment.
■ Hypnotic – to assist sleep on the night prior to the appointment; dental anxiety can cause insomnia.

Essentially, premedication is given to make it easier for the patient to attend for treatment. Premedication may be beneficial in a number of situations.

■ A hypnotic would be useful for patients who require sedation for dental treatment but who have disturbed sleep the night before treatment. Sleep deprivation can reduce a patient's co-operation.

■ An anxiolytic would be helpful for patients who find the process of travelling to the dental surgery exceptionally traumatic.

■ Patients with learning difficulties who become anxious in clinical or unfamiliar environments may also benefit from premedication.

Diazepam has been a commonly used for premedication. The usual dose is in the range of 5–10 mg, taken prior to going to bed on the evening before the appointment and on waking on the morning of the dental appointment. When the appointment is in the afternoon a further dose may be taken one to two hours before treatment. The use of a shorter-acting sedative such as temazepam may prevent the patient from experiencing the prolonged sedative effects of diazepam. An alternative regime is 10–20 mg of temazepam at bedtime followed by 10–20 mg one hour prior to treatment. It can be difficult to keep rigidly to recommended drug regimes with oral benzodiazepines because of the variation in patient response. When a patient has experienced successful treatment using one drug regime it may be prudent to keep to it, unless of course there are good reasons for changing it. Some dentists prefer the general medical practitioner to prescribe hypnotics prior to treatment; this is a prudent approach in patients who are taking numerous medications already, especially if several are CNS depressants.

Titration end point

The clinician has to decide when the patient is sufficiently sedated such that they can start treatment. This point is called the titration end point. It is difficult to define this point concisely because there is a great variation in patient response to sedative agents; this decision is based on experience. The patient should have a relaxed demeanour, be able to maintain verbal contact, respond to commands and maintain mouth opening on request. During N_2O IS the eyes usually have a glazed appearance. The patient may have poor neuromuscular co-ordination (e.g. failure to accurately place their finger on the tip of their nose), delayed eye movement and blinking, and delayed response to commands. However, these signs cannot be relied on, and some patients appear and respond no differently to when they are not sedated. Signs such as slurred speech and Verril's sign (ptosis – when the upper eyelids drop down to bisect the pupils) may be indicative of over-sedation in some patients. One important point is never to ask the patient if they would like more sedation, as invariably the answer will be yes!

Recommended tasks

(1) Compare and contrast the advantages and disadvantages of N_2O IS, IV sedation and oral sedation with GA. Try to use a table to summarise the key points. Remember to consider age, medical, drug and social history.

(2) Obtain technical information on an RA machine from the manufacturer and study the information sheets.

(3) Inspect the pin index system on an RA machine and identify why the oxygen and nitrous oxide cylinders cannot be interchanged, and identify the Bodok seals.

(4) Approximately how long will it take for a patient to become sedated with oral, intranasal, buccal and IV sedation with midazolam? Compare this with the time it would take to sedate a patient under N_2O IS.

Medical emergencies

It is essential that the dental team is trained in the management of medical emergencies, irrespective of whether or not sedation is carried out. Regular checks should be undertaken on all emergency equipment and emergency drugs to ensure that each is fit for purpose and complies with contemporaneous guidance. These checks should be recorded. While sedation courses have historically included the management of medical emergencies, it should be appreciated that conscious sedation techniques, when used appropriately by a trained dental team, are not associated with an increase in medical crises. This section is included as it forms part of the NEBDN examination in sedation.

Life-threatening emergencies are rare in dental practice and may occur anywhere on the premises. The casualty may be a patient, staff member or visitor. The dental team in any dental practice must be able to recognise an unwell patient and be prepared to provide acutely ill patients with potentially life-saving measures prior to the arrival of specialist help. The GDC recommend that continuing professional development (CPD) in medical emergencies is undertaken on a yearly basis. It is therefore essential that all staff regularly update their knowledge and skills in this mandatory core topic. This has traditionally involved rehearsal of CPR for respiratory and cardiac arrest using manikins. While this is valuable it does not equip the clinical staff to manage an unwell patient. The team should develop and practise scenarios for other conditions that may be encountered in dental practice (Table 4.17). An immediate life support course, tailored for the dental team covering the scenarios listed in Table 4.17, gives valuable training for the assessment and systematic management of the sick patient.

Table 4.17 Medical emergencies that may be encountered in dental practice.

■ Vasovagal attack (faint/syncope)	■ Chest pain (angina, myocardial infarction)
■ Panic attack (hyperventilation)	■ Anaphylaxis
■ Seizures	■ Respiratory arrest
■ Hypoglycaemia	■ Cardiac arrest
■ Asthma attack	■ Unwell deteriorating patient with no diagnosis
■ Cerebrovascular accident (stroke)	

It is not unusual for a patient with dental phobia or anxiety to have a vasovagal (fainting) or panic attack at the assessment or treatment visit. In addition, some anxious/ phobic patients are medically compromised. Illnesses such as hypertension, angina, asthma and epilepsy may be triggered or exacerbated by stress and sedation is often beneficial for these patients.

Fainting (vasovagal attack/syncope) is the most frequently encountered cause of collapse in dental practice. The brief loss of consciousness that occurs is due to an abrupt fall in cardiac output that leads to a reduction in cerebral blood flow. The dental team should recognise the characteristic signs that precede syncope and take appropriate action; this may prevent loss of consciousness. Very occasionally syncope may not have a benign cause and can be associated with serious cardiac arrhythmias (irregular heartbeat) or a transient ischaemic attack (TIA or mini-stroke).

When a patient is feeling unwell or has lost consciousness the team needs to constantly assess and monitor the patient's **airway**, **breathing** and **circulation**; this sequence of actions has traditionally been abbreviated to '*ABC*'. This enables the rescuer to quickly ascertain if the patient is breathing and if they still have a cardiac output (a pulse). A respiratory arrest occurs when there is no spontaneous breathing but there is a pulse. A cardiac arrest occurs when cardiac function comes to an abrupt halt: there is no arterial pulse present. This condition may be reversed in some instances with appropriate prompt treatment. If either of these conditions is diagnosed then the algorithm for CPR should be followed.

A patient may remain conscious and feel unwell and it is not always possible for the dental team to diagnose the cause of the problem. In this situation it is equally important that the team recognises an unwell or deteriorating patient and seeks emergency assistance. In this way hopefully a cardiorespiratory arrest can be avoided. The Resuscitation Council advises a systematic approach which is an extension of the *ABC* algorithm to assess the sick patient, irrespective of loss of consciousness. They advocate an *ABCDE* approach. A course on *immediate life support* explains this approach and an explanation can be found in the Resuscitation Council's guidance on medical emergencies and resuscitation (2006) and Balmer and Longman (2008). The following section is a brief overview of the management of acute medical problems in dental practice, it is not a comprehensive guide; this is covered extensively in the references just given. Table 4.18 lists some principles that can be used in the management of the medical emergencies.

Basic life support

The objective of basic life support (BLS) is to maintain adequate ventilation and circulation until a specialist team arrives to undertake post-resuscitation care. BLS comprises patient assessment, airway maintenance, expired air ventilation and, if required, chest compressions. The dental team should supplement BLS with simple airway adjuncts (an adjunct is something used to help you with the task in hand) such as an oropharyngeal airway, which would facilitate airway management in BLS. BLS is a holding operation – it buys time. Failure of the brain to receive oxygen for longer than three minutes will result in irreversible brain damage. The purpose of chest compressions is to circulate the

Table 4.18 Common principles to follow in the management of medical emergencies.

Use the following information to assess the severity of the patient's condition and to decide if expert assistance is required.

Assessment	Actions	Comments
	Stay calm Assess the level of consciousness – *Is the patient confused or alert? If unconscious try and rouse the patient* Reassure the conscious patient and assess their level of consciousness, ask them how they feel	*Shout for a colleague to help if you are alone with the patient** *Ensure a safe approach if you have just come across a collapsed patient* *If conscious make them comfortable, always consider the chair position, in an unconscious patient lie them flat*
Airway	Look for signs of airway obstruction Open the airway (head tilt, chin lift or jaw thrust, airway adjuncts if patient is unconscious) Suction Oxygen	*If the patient is talking to you normally their airway is OK* *A patent airway must be maintained,* *Use mask with oxygen reservoir – 10 l/min*
Breathing	Look, listen and feel Any signs of respiratory distress (noises, accessory muscles of respiration, cyanosis)? What is the respiration rate: No breathing: then give rescue breaths following algorithm for respiratory arrest Use a pulse oximeter	*Normal rate of respiration in an adult = 12–20 bpm* *If a respiratory wheeze consider giving salbutamol* *If the respiration rate is very high or low call an ambulance, unless you think it is a panic attack. Assisted ventilation may be required for respiration rates of around 5 bpm*
Circulation	Assess quality of peripheral and central pulses (rate, rhythm, regularity) Is the patient appearing cyanosed? What is the capillary refill time? What is the blood pressure? Chest pain? Any signs of bleeding	*A patient in shock will have peripheral shut down, limbs will feel cold. Cover the patient with a blanket* *If low BP and circulatory collapse put patient flat* *GTN? Aspirin? Place the patient in a comfortable position.*
Disability	Level of consciousness Blood glucose levels Response of pupils to light	*If unconscious lie the patient flat* *Hypoglycaemia? Give glucose or glucagon?* *Patient may have taken a drug overdose?*
Exposure	Rashes Ankle oedema Shivering, tremors	*Anaphylaxis? Give adrenaline?* *Cover the patient with a blanket if they are cold*

*If you are on your own you must leave the patient to ring for specialist help. If you have help, send a person to call the emergency services and ask them to clearly state the problem (e.g. the casualty has had a cardiac arrest) and give clear instructions as to your location. The person who alerts the emergency services should report back to you to confirm that this has been done. If a person is available send them to meet the emergency team at the entrance to the building or clinic you are in.

Figure 4.9 The chain of survival.

oxygenated blood around the body. Even when this is performed under optimal conditions, it is not possible to achieve more than 30% of normal cerebral perfusion. The best method of treating cardiac arrest is to follow the chain of survival as shown in Figure 4.9. The chain of survival describes the ideal sequence of interventions that contribute to survival after a cardiac arrest. The survival prospects following cardiac arrest decrease every minute even when BLS is being performed. Defibrillation is the most important determinant of success or failure. It delivers a massive electrical shock to the heart in an attempt to synchronise or '*kick start*' the heart into its normal (sinus) rhythm. In the UK, the majority of adult cardiac arrests are associated with ventricular fibrillation, a rhythm that is amenable to defibrillation.

Algorithms for CPR are constantly being revised and the dental team needs to be aware of current protocols. An algorithm is a term used to describe a pathway, a recommended sequence of events or a set of rules. The reader requires an in-depth knowledge of BLS and they should also understand the different algorithms for children. You are therefore advised to obtain the current BLS algorithms, with supporting information, including the recovery position, from the Resuscitation Council (UK) website (www.resus.org.uk). Table 4.19 lists the minimum requirements for emergency equipment in dental surgeries.

When a patient is being artificially ventilated the oxygen should be delivered at the maximum flow rate (10–15 l/min). The amount of oxygen actually delivered to the patient will vary, depending on the type of mask used. Expired air ventilations from the rescuer, with or without a pocket mask, delivers only 16% oxygen. If a pocket mask is connected to high-flow oxygen then approximately 40% oxygen can be delivered to the patient; this figure rises to 80–90% when a self-inflating bag, valve and mask with reservoir is used with oxygen. If a self-inflating bag, valve and mask are used without the reservoir bag attached then only around 40% oxygen will be delivered.

Signs of airway obstruction

The dental team should be able to recognise airway obstruction, which can be partial or complete and can occur at any level in the respiratory tract. In the unconscious patient

Table 4.19 Emergency equipment required in the dental surgery.

Pocket mask with one-way valve and oxygen inlet (e.g. Laerdal mask)
Self-inflating bag, valve and mask with reservoir (e.g. Ambu bag) in various sizes
Oropharyngeal airways (sizes 1, 2, 3 and 4)
Nasopharyngeal airways (various sizes)
Oxygen therapy masks with tubing and appropriate connectors to attach to oxygen cylinder
Syringes and needles to deliver emergency drugs by a parenteral route
IV cannulae and adhesive tape*
Independently powered portable suction apparatus with wide bore aspiration tips
Blood pressure monitor*
Blood glucose monitor#
Pulse oximeter*
Automated external defibrillator#

Ideally equipment should be free from natural rubber latex. Appropriate equipment must also be available in children's sizes.
* Essential in a practice that carries out intravenous (IV) sedation.
# **These items of equipment have been recommended by the Resuscitation Council UK (2006)**.

the most common cause of pharyngeal obstruction is the tongue, but blood, vomit or foreign objects may be responsible. Airway obstruction can be recognised by adopting a look, listen and feel approach. The use of the accessory muscles of respiration, causing a '*seesaw*' movement of the rib cage and abdominal movements, is a sign of airway obstruction. Partial airway obstruction is usually noisy due to reduced airflow. Sounds that can be heard are wheezing, gurgling, snoring and crowing. A gurgling sound suggests the presence of liquids or semi-solid material. Snoring is common when the tongue partially occludes the pharynx. Crowing is a sign of laryngeal spasm (**laryngospasm**), which is often as a result of irritation by foreign bodies or secretions. **Bronchospasm** is a contraction of the smooth muscle of the bronchial airways; it can occur in asthma and in allergic reactions.

Once airway obstruction is suspected, immediate action should be taken to maximise the airway and identify the cause of the problem. All treatment should be stopped; the mouth should be examined for debris and suction used if necessary. The airway should be improved by a chin lift or jaw thrust. This will displace the tongue anteriorly, away from the posterior pharyngeal wall.

All members of the dental team should be able to recognise choking and manage the condition according to the protocol detailed on the Resuscitation Council (UK) website. In the rare event of complete airway obstruction above the level of the larynx, a surgical airway will need to be created below the obstruction. In an emergency situation this entails performing a needle cricothyroidotomy as a temporary measure.

Administration of drugs

The administration of emergency drugs has been discussed previously in the section on Pharmacology and the reader is advised to review Table 4.6. In general dental practice, the oral, inhalation, intramuscular and transmucosal (buccal, sublingual and possibly intranasal) routes are the most important for the administration of emergency drugs. Table 4.20 lists the drugs that are commonly recommended for use in medical emergencies that may occur in the dental surgery together with their indications and

Table 4.20 Emergency drugs: indications and mechanisms of action.*

Drug (route)	Indications (dose)	Mechanism of action
Oxygen (Inhalation)	Oxygen can be used for most emergencies	To prevent cerebral hypoxia
Epinephrine† (IM)	Anaphylactic shock (0.5 mg of 1:1000 (1 mg/ml), repeat at 5-minute intervals if required)	This sympathomimetic agonist: – reverses peripheral vasodilation and preserves blood flow to essential organs – relaxes bronchial smooth muscle (dilates the airways) – increases coronary blood flow and the force of myocardial contraction – suppresses histamine release
Glucagon (IM; can also use IV or SC routes)	Unconscious hypoglycaemia (1 mg)	This hormone increases serum glucose by converting glycogen stores into glucose
Salbutamol (inhalation)	Asthma (100 micrograms)	Relaxes bronchial smooth muscle
Glyceryl trinitrate (sublingual spray)	Cardiac/chest pain (400 micrograms metered dose)	Vasodilation of the coronary arteries
Glucose (oral)	The conscious hypoglycaemic (10–20 g)	Rapid absorption – elevates serum glucose levels
Midazolam (oral, buccal or intranasal)	Status epilepticus (10 mg)	Anticonvulsant action. They are CNS inhibitors by virtue of their action on GABA receptors
Aspirin (oral)	Myocardial infarction (300 mg)	The anti-thrombotic effect of aspirin reduces mortality after infarction
Flumazenil (IV)	Over-sedation with a benzodiazepine	The antagonist of benzodiazepines, the antagonism is reversible and competitive

*Drug protocols are constantly being updated and modified as new scientific information becomes available; it is the duty of the clinician to keep up to date with current guidance. Please note that only adult doses are given in this table.

†Epinephrine is also known as adrenaline, it is available in 1 ml glass ampoules containing 1:1000 epinephrine, but pre-loaded 1 ml syringes are preferred by most dentists. Please note that an Epipen contains only 300 micrograms.

IM, intramuscular; IV, intravenous; SC, subcutaneous; CNS, central nervous system; GABA, gamma-amino-butyric acid.

mode of action. The signs and symptoms and management of collapse are outlined in Table 4.21.

Paramedic transfer

When a patient is transferred to the paramedics a summary of events leading up to the medical emergency is required. The acronym **MAPLES** (or SAMPLES) can be helpful in remembering what information is required.

Medicines
Allergies
Past medical history (including allergies and drug history)
Last oral intake (if known)
Events leading up to the incident
Symptoms and signs.

Duties of a dental nurse in an emergency

The dental nurse is a valuable member of the dental team and should have a well-defined role in an emergency. The nurse would be expected to undertake the following tasks providing that appropriate training has been received.

- Know and be familiar with all the emergency equipment and drugs and be able to access them quickly.
- Notice if a patient is unwell or deteriorating and inform the dentist.
- Administer oxygen to an unwell patient.
- Monitor the unwell or collapsed patient.
- Manage a faint, administer glucose if appropriate.
- Help an unwell patient to administer their prescribed drugs, such as bronchodilators and preparations for the relief of angina.
- Prepare emergency drugs for use if requested to do so by the dentist. This may include drawing up drugs for injection.
- Initiate and perform BLS (with airway adjuncts) and administer oxygen under intermittent positive pressure, irrespective of whether a dentist is present or not.
- Manage a choking patient.
- Call the emergency services when a patient is in need of urgent specialist medical treatment if the dentist is not available.
- Liaise with the paramedic team when transferring the patient to their care.

Dental nurses are not usually expected to administer emergency drugs by injection; however, if the nurse is the only member of the team around and there is an emergency situation the nurse may decide to utilise their training and administer appropriate drugs.

Table 4.21 The management of medical emergencies.

Emergency Predisposing factors	Signs and symptoms	Management*
Faint/syncope/vasovagal attack Predisposing factors include hypoglycaemia, anxiety, fear, pain, hunger, stress and fatigue	Patient may feel unwell, light-headed, weak, confused, dizzy, nauseous Skin pallor, sweating, tachycardia followed by a bradycardia, loss of consciousness. Minor convulsions or incontinence can occur	Lay patient flat with legs elevated. Alternatively a sitting patient may lower their head by placing it between their knees, this is not as effective as lying a patient down. Lay a pregnant patient on her side Administer oxygen Reassure the recovering patient, a glucose rich drink may be helpful When a member of the dental team recognises that a patient is likely to faint the patient should be placed in a supine position – this may prevent loss of consciousness *If the patient fails to regain consciousness promptly then other causes of loss of consciousness must be considered*
Hypoglycaemia Precipitating factors may be known diabetic, anxiety, infection and fasting	Cold and clammy skin, trembling Irritability, confused, double vision, slurring of speech, behaviour changes (e.g. aggression and unco-operative behaviour) Drowsiness and disorientation	*Conscious*: 10–20 g of glucose as a drink, tablets, sugar cubes or gel *Unconscious*: 1 mg of IM glucagon Administer oxygen, monitor patient and maintain airway Call emergency services if patient does not recover or they are newly diagnosed or their diabetes is poorly controlled
Epileptic seizure Predisposing factors include known epileptic who is poorly controlled or not-compliant with drug regime, stress	Patients may have an aura (e.g. altered sensations, mood change) and realise that they are about to have a seizure. Loss of consciousness. Muscle rigidity followed by jerking movements, tongue may be bitten, incontinence may occur. Confusion may be present during recovery. The clonic phase consists of jerking movements of the limbs and body, it is during this phase that the patient may bite their tongue and injure themselves	Note the time. Protect patient from injury (remove potentially harmful objects, place pillows around patient if these aid their protection). Maintain airway and administer oxygen if possible. If the patient can be discharged home ensure that they are accompanied home – they might have post-ictal confusion. If they sustained injuries during the attack or had an atypical attack the patient may need to go to hospital Status epilepticus is likely if a seizure continues in excess of 5 minutes, therefore call the emergency services. If status epilepticus is diagnosed midazolam (10 mg) by the buccal or intranasal routes may be given. If the patient is already cannulated then IV midazolam may be considered.# Benzodiazepines are not always effective and other anti-epileptic drugs may be required

Table 4.21 *Continued*

Emergency Predisposing factors	Signs and symptoms	Management*
Asthma Pre-existing disease that is poorly controlled, anxiety, infection, exercise, exposure to an antigen	Breathlessness with wheezing on expiration. Restlessness, difficulty in talking, tachycardia, low peak respiratory flow, using accessory muscles of respiration, cyanosis. If untreated breathing may become increasingly difficult and respiratory arrest is possible	Administer a bronchodilator (e.g. salbutamol) as an inhaler and give oxygen Place the patient in a comfortable position; if there is no improvement summon emergency services If a nebuliser is available then use this to administer a bronchodilator combined with oxygen Status asthmaticus is a life-threatening condition
Angina Occurs because a coronary artery is blocked and the heart is deprived of oxygen (ischaemia)	Usually a crushing chest pain, may travel down left arm or into neck and jaw, irregular pulse, patient may experience breathlessness, nausea or vomiting. Breathing shallow. Can lead to a myocardial infarction	Administer patient's usual medication; if this is not available offer sublingual GTN spray, administer oxygen. Place patient in a comfortable position – consult with the patient; if they have a known history of angina ask if the symptoms are typical. Call emergency services if pain does not subside in 3 minutes (possibility of a myocardial infarction – MI) Consider administration of oral aspirin (300 mg) if an MI is suspected
Myocardial infarction(MI) Pre-existing cardiac disease, non-compliance with drug therapy, stress	Usually a crushing chest pain not relieved by GTN	Call emergency services, place patient in a comfortable position, administer oral aspirin (300 mg) and oxygen. Nitrous oxide and oxygen sedation, if available, can be helpful to reduce pain and anxiety. Monitor; if loss of consciousness follow the protocol for cardiopulmonary resuscitation
Hyperventilation Stress, pain or expectation of pain. This is often a response to unfocused fears. Can be associated with chronic generalised anxiety disorder	Rapid breathing, tachycardia, trembling, dizziness, faint, sweating Paraesthesia, muscle pain/stiffness Can lead to tetany. Patients can complain of chest pain	Reassure Ensure comfortable position Stop treatment Rebreathe expired air

Anaphylaxis
Exposure to an antigen to which the patient has been sensitised, commonly drugs (most notably penicillins), insect bites/stings or natural rubber latex. Hypersensitivity to local anaesthetic is exceptionally rare

Initial flushing of the skin may occur followed by oedema of the head and neck. Altered sensations such as paraesthesia around the mouth and fingers. Pallor, cyanosis will accompany acute breathing difficulties with bronchospasm and possible laryngeal oedema, severe hypotension
Loss of consciousness and cardiac arrest can occur if untreated. Hypotension and/or bronchospasm must be present for a diagnosis of anaphylaxis

Lay flat, elevate legs, maintain airway and administer oxygen via a facemask
Call for expert assistance
Immediate epinephrine (0.5 ml of 1:1 000) IM, repeat if necessary
Intravascular fluid replacement will be required and the paramedics will normally do this

Cerebrovascular accident
(stroke)

Partial or total weakness on one side of the body and possible loss of consciousness

Administer oxygen, maintain airway, place patient in a comfortable position
Call emergency services, monitor patient

Local anaesthetic toxicity
Maximum safe drug values may be considerably reduced in patients with liver or kidney disease, and in extremes of age

Light-headedness, visual or hearing disturbances. Agitation, confusion, seizures, respiratory distress. Loss of consciousness, respiratory and cardiac arrest can occur (this is **not** anaphylaxis)

Lay flat and administer oxygen, maintain airway, monitor
Summon expert help. Some authorities suggest that an IV benzodiazepine should be given to the patient who has seizures following overdose of local anaesthetic. This is not advised because it carries the risk of respiratory depression

Respiratory arrest
Status asthmaticus, airway obstruction

No breathing, central pulse present initially – if untreated it will proceed to a cardiac arrest

Follow BLS algorithm (this includes summoning expert help)

Cardiac arrest
Myocardial infarction
Circulatory collapse
Anaphylaxis
Hypoxia
Respiratory arrest

Unconscious
No central pulse

Follow BLS algorithm (this includes summoning expert help)

* It is assumed that if the nurse is alone with a patient at the time of the emergency then other members of the dental team are called immediately to assist.
# If midazolam is administered for status epilepticus that occurs in a patient who has just received IV sedation then the clinician should be aware of the potential risk of inducing respiratory depression.

Recommended tasks

(1) Identify the expert committees/organisations that issue advice on the emergency drugs and equipment that should be held in dental practice and study their recommendations. Ascertain how frequently the drugs and equipment are checked in the clinical environment in which you work.

(2) Download (i) the Resuscitation Council's guidance on medical emergencies and resuscitation from www.resus.org.uk/pages/MEdental.pdf; (ii) the Scottish Dental Clinical Effectiveness Programme (section 2 on medical emergencies) and compare the guidance offered in these two documents with that summarised in the British National Formulary

(3) Describe the methods you would use to manage choking; check your answer with the algorithm described by the Resuscitation Council (UK) (www.resus.org.uk).

(4) How are the emergency drugs presented in your dental practice and what different presentations are available for these drugs?

Medico-legal issues

This section highlights some of the clinical governance and medico-legal considerations that are important in the practice of sedation in dentistry

Standards of practice and regulatory bodies

The dental team must follow current established standards of care issued by respected bodies; failure to do so means the team may deliver poor-quality patient care and will be vulnerable to adverse outcomes and litigation. Standards of dental care are influenced by expert reports, guidance and recommendations issued by authoritative bodies. Such bodies include the GDC, specialist societies, surgical colleges, the Department of Health and other interested parties such as the British Dental Association and defence societies. Employing trusts may also have local policies on sedation and governance issues. This information is constantly being updated.

The GDC is the regulatory body of the dental profession in the UK; its role is to protect patients and to maintain standards within the dental profession. The GDC gives ethical guidance, monitors and upholds clinical standards of practice for dentists, dental nurses and dental undergraduates. The GDC has stated in its guidance document *Standards for Dental Professionals* (GDC, 2009) that it supports and expects dentists to follow the guidance set out in *Conscious Sedation in the Provision of Dental Care*, a Standing Dental Advisory Committee report of an expert group on sedation for dentistry (Standing Dental Advisory Committee, 2003). Those who fall short of the standards expected could be found guilty of serious professional misconduct. The GDC has the authority to prevent a registered member of the dental team from practising within the UK by having their name removed from the Dental Register.

Over the past two decades there have been many national reports that have advised on the provision of sedation in dental practice; some have been more successful than others in instigating change in clinical practice. The *Poswillo Report* (1990) and *A Conscious Decision* (Department of Health, 2000) are two widely quoted documents that have promoted sedation within the dental profession.

Negligence

Patients have a right to expect a high standard of advice and care from dental professionals. They must be given relevant and accurate information regarding any condition they have and the treatment they require. Patients therefore expect quality care. Errors of judgement and accidents do happen in dentistry, this is acknowledged legally, but the clinician needs to take appropriate action to remedy the error. The majority of medico-legal problems are associated with issues relating to consent and negligence. Accurate and up-to-date dental records are essential, as these will be used to help clarify events.

To prove negligence the patient (called the claimant) must show that:

- a duty of care was owed
- the duty of care was breached (broken)
- harm resulted to the patient as a result of this breach in care.

An example of negligent treatment would be when a dentist treats a patient under IV sedation, discharges the patient without an escort and the patient falls over and sustains injuries on their journey home.

When a clinician provides sedation there must be an indication for sedation; this should be noted in the patient's records and the patient should have been fully assessed (as described earlier). While a patient's preference for sedation is important it must not be the over-riding consideration. The dentist should prescribe a treatment in consultation with a patient but should not allow the patient to insist on a technique about which the dentist has reservations. Advice should be given to the patient concerning the sedation technique, both verbally and in writing. The benefit of any dental intervention should substantially outweigh any risks associated with the procedure. When procedures carry risks the patient should be informed about those risks prior to giving their consent. It is the dentist's responsibility to ensure that the patient understands the instructions and is able to follow them. Lack of communication is probably the most common cause of medico-legal problems in dentistry. The sedation technique used must be appropriate and dental treatment delivered under sedation must be of a satisfactory standard. Adequate clinical records should be maintained and these should include any particular risks that have been discussed with the patient. Standards of clinical practice change with the availability of new research and technology. All members of the dental team must therefore keep themselves up to date with current standards of care.

Dentists are accountable to their patients. A dentist may be found guilty of negligence when they have failed in their duty of care to the patient and this resulted in harm to the patient. It is necessary to show that the standard of care fell below what would be reasonable and acceptable. What is reasonable and acceptable is usually judged in comparison to normal practice by a recognised body of practitioners.

The **Bolam** principle recognises the fact that many professionals may disagree in their opinions. For example two different clinicians may come up with differing management strategies for the same patient. The dentist can be defended against inappropriate care providing that they are supported by 'a responsible body of dental opinion'; this allows for alternative and contrary views.

The dentist also has a responsibility towards their staff and any visitors to their premises. The control of hazards to the staff, patients and the public is the professional and legal duty of the practitioner. The Health and Safety Executive is an important regulating body and employers must comply with the Health and Safety at Work Act 1974.

Confidentiality

Information gained by the dental team in the course of a professional relationship with a patient is confidential. It should not be conveyed to a third party as a breach of confidentiality may lead to a charge of professional misconduct.

Consent

Consent is a complicated area and can be confusing because of the terminology used. In legal terms, every adult of sound mind has the right to decide and to consent to what is being done to their own body. The dental team, therefore, can do nothing to a patient without their consent. Case law has established that touching a patient without their consent may constitute a civil or criminal offence of battery. Consent can be implied or expressed, oral or written. In the case of an adult, for consent to be valid it must be given voluntarily. The patient must, however, be informed and have the capacity to consent. It should be remembered that consent is a process, not a one-off event. Obtaining consent can be described as a three-stage process involving the exchange of information, an opportunity for the patient to seek clarification and then a confirmation of consent. The consent process should therefore be started at the assessment appointment when the patient is often less anxious. All questions should be answered truthfully. The relationship between the patient and the dental team must be both open and honest.

For the patient to give consent they should be able to understand and retain the information given with regard to the reasons for, the nature, benefits, risks and discomfort of the proposed treatment, the alternatives to and the consequences of not accepting the proposed treatment. Any associated risks of the procedure should be explained if the incidence is 0.5% or greater (e.g. the risk of nerve damage is discussed prior to removal of mandibular third molars). The severity of the risk is also important. The patient should therefore be informed about any possible serious risks, even though they may only occur rarely.

The dental team should always seek consent for any treatment that is to be carried out under sedation. All the relevant treatment options should be discussed with the patient, including alternative methods of pain and anxiety control. When sedation is recommended to adult patients, they should be told that sedation can be provided in a number of ways, usually by administering a drug orally, intravenously or by inhalation. Endeavours should be made to differentiate sedation from GA.

A patient[5] has a basic right to either grant or withhold consent prior to treatment or even an examination. For consent to be valid the patient should be capable of making an informed choice regarding their treatment. This implies that the following has been discussed with the patient and in terms that the patient understands:

- the reasons for the procedure recommended (what is wrong with the patient)
- the nature of the procedure
- the benefits of the procedure
- the risks of the procedure
- the discomforts of the procedure
- the alternatives to the procedure
- the consequences of the patient not having the procedure.

The extent of information given to the patient is often difficult to assess. In the UK, the Bolam test can be applied to the amount of information given to a patient prior to a procedure, i.e. the information that would be given by a 'responsible body of professional opinion'. However, the law appears to be shifting to take into account the 'prudent patient'. Here the emphasis is on what a reasonable patient would want to know rather than what the clinician should disclose. Patient information leaflets can be helpful in obtaining informed consent.

If a specific piece of information has the potential to influence a patient's decision then withholding such information is likely to invalidate the consent. Dentists do not obtain written consent for many procedures. The fact that a patient sits in the dental chair and, for example, opens their mouth to receive an injection and remains in the chair to receive a filling is evidence that this patient has **implied** their consent to have treatment. When a patient is having treatment under sedation, consent should **always be obtained in writing** and a copy kept with the patient's record card. Obtaining the patient's signature on a consent form is not proof that consent is informed, it merely provides some evidence to the effect that the patient has agreed to the proposed treatment. Written consent is unacceptable if the form is filled in inappropriately or the written contents are illegible. It should also be remembered that consent is a process, not a momentary event, and patients have the right to withdraw their consent at any stage.

The age of the patient is also important in consent. The law defines an adult from the date of a person's eighteenth birthday; minors are under 18 years of age. However,

---

[5]The patient should have the ability to believe, weigh up and decide upon the information received. Where you believe the patient lacks intellectual capacity to give informed consent then treatment may be performed in the best interest for that patient.

children aged 16 or 17 years are entitled to give consent for surgical or medical procedures providing they have the capacity to make decisions. Children under the age of 16 years may be capable of giving informed consent in which case their wishes must be respected above those of their parents (**Gillick competence**). Nevertheless, it is good practice to obtain consent from both the child and the parents whenever possible. A parent cannot over-ride a child's consent but a court of law can.

When adult patients do not have the intellectual capacity to *understand, use and retain* the information you are giving them to help them make a decision they are unable to give consent. It is not possible for another adult to give consent on their behalf, unless another adult has been legally given that authority. It is, however, always good practice to involve the relatives and carers in the decision-making process in order that they can understand and therefore see the need for any necessary treatment. Treatment should then be carried out in the **best interests** of the patient and should fall within what would be reasonably expected by a responsible body of the profession. It is prudent in such cases to obtain a second dental opinion.

It is also important to remember that patients suffering from mental illness (e.g. schizophrenia) do not necessarily lack the capacity to consent. When undertaking treatment under best interests the clinician should comply with the 2005 Mental Capacity Act (MCA). The MCA provides a statutory framework for decision making in people (over 16 years) who lack capacity. One significant change is the introduction of the Independent Mental Capacity Advocate (IMCA) whose role is to support and represent the person without capacity. When a patient without capacity does not have a relative or an unpaid friend or carer who is able to be consulted about the treatment, then an IMCA will need to be involved in serious medical treatment decisions. The administration of a GA would be categorised as a serious medical intervention. The use of standard sedation techniques would not always be regarded as a serious procedure, but the risks would need to be assessed in individual cases; for example, sedation in a patient who is ASA group IV may be considered as a serious intervention.

It is inappropriate to ask patients who are sedated for consent, as their competence to do so would be questionable. When treatment options are unpredictable (e.g. restoration of a tooth may not be possible and an extraction might be required) patients should be warned of this pre-operatively and consent obtained for the possible and appropriate treatment plans.

Record keeping

Records must be kept of all dental procedures that are undertaken, irrespective of the use of sedation. Record keeping is important not only for delivering quality care to the patient but also for audit and medico-legal reasons. Poor record keeping prevents the successful defence of allegations of clinical negligence and professional misconduct. All entries in a patient's clinical notes should be written in ink and should be current, accurate, complete, clear and legible.

Documentation on the assessment visit should include what is normally required during a consultation appointment but should also identify why sedation is indicated, and that the proposed treatment plan and options were discussed with the patient as were any warnings about the risks of treatment. The pre- and postoperative instructions given and whether any patient information leaflets were used should also be noted. The details of what information should be recorded at the treatment visit are discussed in the section on Sedation techniques. It is helpful to have a separate sedation assessment and treatment proforma as this can be used to prompt the dental team to capture all the relevant information on: ASA status, monitoring, types of sedatives used (including dose, administration route, the quality of sedation achieved) and it can also include a checklist to ensure that all the relevant equipment is available and that it has undergone appropriate safety checks, that written consent has been obtained and that appropriate postoperative instructions have been given.

Staff resources and training

All members of the dental team using sedation must ensure that they are suitably trained and experienced. This requires theoretical, practical and supervised clinical training in each conscious sedation technique that is used. These should be regularly updated.

The dental nurse is always an important member of the dental team, but the nurse has extra responsibilities when assisting in the care of the sedated patient. A dentist who is acting as both the operator and sedationist must be assisted by a second **appropriately trained** person. A trained dental nurse can act as a second appropriate person and their role is to:

- be present throughout the treatment, thus acting as a chaperone to both dentist and patient
- assist the dentist during dental treatment
- monitor the sedated patient (this has been discussed in depth earlier)
- assist the dentist in any complication or emergency
- give appropriate postoperative instructions to the escort.

It is always best practice for a dentist to be accompanied by a member of staff whenever they are treating a patient, but it is *essential* when a patient is receiving treatment under sedation. While all sedative agents have side effects, some are known to induce fantasies, sometimes of a sexual nature, and it is possible that a patient could make accusations of assault.

Dental nurses, like dentists, should receive both theoretical and supervised hands-on clinical training. Nurse training should follow the syllabus and recommendations for entry to the NEBDN Certificate in Dental Sedation Nursing. This will involve keeping a logbook of clinical activity. It is also advisable for the trainee to keep a portfolio of lectures/tutorials/courses attended during training. Ideally all sedation-trained nurses should be encouraged to obtain the national post-certificate qualification in Dental Sedation Nursing. This examination is organised by the NEBDN and is open to registered dental nurses.

When sedation is undertaken by a second dental or medical practitioner, the operating dentist must be satisfied that the sedationist has undergone appropriate relevant post-graduate education, training, experience of conscious sedation in dentistry and adheres to the GDC's definition of sedation.

It is a requirement for all dental teams, irrespective of the use of sedation, to practise their emergency resuscitation skills on a regular basis. Traditionally, this has meant practising CPR. However, it would be prudent for the dental team to use scenario training for the management of sedation-related complications such as the over-sedated patient.

A special mention of sedation in children is warranted because there has been much debate over the use of various sedation techniques in children. Nitrous oxide inhalation sedation is the method of choice for most children. However, this may be unsuitable for very young children who have limited understanding and co-operation. In these patients a general anaesthetic may be the safest method of achieving adequate pain and anxiety control. In the older child or teenager, IV, oral or transmucosal methods of sedation may be appropriate if nitrous oxide inhalation sedation has not been effective. These alternative methods should only be used in children if the dental team has appropriate training and levels of expertise.

This chapter has discussed some of the medico-legal implications and governance issues around the practice of sedation; many of these considerations are summarised in Table 4.22. The regulation of conscious sedation techniques is subject to change with the introduction of new knowledge and techniques. The dental team should have a commitment to undertake relevant continuing education and training to ensure that the team keeps up to date with new developments and adheres to current regional and national standards.

Risk assessment

It is prudent for clinicians to minimise the incidents of untoward events that can occur in clinical situations. The identification and management of such issues is called risk assessment and it should be undertaken to prevent mistakes from happening. It is a pro-active rather than a re-active process. However, if untoward events do occur the dental team should review their procedures and put safeguards in place to prevent, whenever possible, reoccurrence of the problem. This often involves the formulation of protocols and standardised procedures. Risk management can be divided into risk awareness, risk control, risk containment and risk transfer. Other issues that fall under the heading of risk assessment are patient information leaflets, consent, staff skill levels, complaints and satisfaction policy, referral mechanisms, standard of facilities, rehearsal of medical emergencies and training updates.

In December 2008 a rapid response report was issued from the National Patient Safety Agency (NPSA) entitled *Reducing the Risk of Overdose with Midazolam Injection in Adults* (NPSA/2008/RRR011). This was in response to 498 midazolam patient safety incidents between November 2004 and November 2008 where the dose prescribed to the patient was inappropriate. The report has five points for implementation from June 2009 and

Table 4.22 Clinical governance: considerations for the practice of conscious sedation in dentistry

All sedation techniques	■ Patients should have adequate pre-operative assessment and be given written and verbal pre and postoperative instructions ■ All staff should be appropriately trained in the theory and practice of the sedation techniques they use and in the management of the possible complications of these techniques ■ Patients should only be given sedation when there is a positive indication to do so ■ The drugs and techniques that are chosen for conscious sedation must be appropriate for that patient, taking into account the patient's age, lifestyle, medical and drug history ■ Written consent must be obtained for sedation and the procedures carried out under sedation ■ Patients who are having sedation should be escorted by a responsible adult and should have arranged appropriate postoperative care (however, this may not be necessary for adults who have received inhalation sedation) ■ Prior to administering sedation the medical history should be checked to see if it has changed ■ While a patient is having sedation the dentist must be chaperoned at all times ■ All procedures and techniques should be recorded accurately in the patient records ■ All drugs must be stored in appropriate conditions and safely but emergency drugs should be readily available. Accurate stock control records must be kept for all medicines
■ Monitoring	■ Clinical monitoring is required for all sedation techniques and pulse oximetry is essential for IV sedation and oral and transmucosal sedation. It is not mandatory whilst administering inhalation sedation
■ Maintenance of equipment	■ All equipment should be well maintained, checked and serviced regularly
IV midazolam sedation	■ Invoices for midazolam must be kept for 2 years ■ The midazolam must be titrated against patient response ■ When preparing drugs the contents and expiry dates should be checked with another person and all syringes must be clearly labelled ■ IV sedation is thought to be unpredictable in children. The GDC and expert bodies have been concerned about governance issues around the use of IV sedation in children
Inhalation sedation	■ Scavenging of waste gases must conform to COSSH standards ■ Relative analgesia machines should undergo safety checks prior to use
Discharge	■ The patient must be assessed fit for discharge (e.g. be able to walk unaided) when they are transferred to the care of the escort

this guidance remains best practice. It has advised a risk assessment in areas that use 10 mg/2 ml and 10 mg/5 ml ampoules of midazolam (referred to as high strength midazolam in the report). It is possible that 1 mg/ml preparations will be used instead of the 2 mg/ml; 1 mg/ml preparations are available for import from Europe.

Storage of drugs

It is a good idea to store all medicines in a locked cupboard that is not subject to direct sunlight, extremes of temperature or damp, because medicines can be subject to physical or chemical deterioration when stored in poor conditions. Certain medicines will have specific storage requirements and the manufacturer's instructions should be followed. Emergency drugs should not be locked away as they need to be readily available for use. The storage of medical gas cylinders is controlled by legislation and stocks of gas cylinders should be kept as low as possible; flammable gases should be kept away from sources of ignition. Stock control should be stringent and records should be accurate. Out-of-date drugs should be disposed of safely. Medical oxygen has a shelf-life of three years and the cylinder should be replaced or refilled during this time period.

The legal status of midazolam changed on 1 January 2008 changing midazolam to a Schedule 3 controlled drug from a Schedule 4 controlled drug. The change in regulations mean that:

- requisitions for midazolam must comply with the full Controlled Drugs Regulations
- invoices for midazolam need to be kept for two years.

Midazolam is exempt from the safe custody requirements and so does not legally have to be stored in a controlled drugs cabinet, nor will records of midazolam usage need to be kept in a controlled drugs register. However, for the dental teams who work in a trust, especially those on hospital premises, directors of pharmacies may require that sedation departments treat midazolam as a Schedule 2 drug (e.g. diamorphine, morphine and pethidine), and therefore subject to full controlled drug regulations. This is not because of legal constraints but because it makes the overall management of such drugs easier within a large trust from operational and clinical governance standpoints.

Recommended tasks

(1) Access the GDC website (www.gdc-uk.org) and read the following guidance documents:
- □ *Patient Consent* (2006) www.gdc-uk.org/News+publications+and+events/Publications/Guidance+documents/Patient+consent.htm
- □ *Standards for Dental Professionals* (2005) www.gdc-uk.org/News+publications+and+events/Publications/Guidance+documents/Standards+for+dental+professionals.htm

(2) Read the executive summary of *A Conscious Decision*. This is a report of an expert group produced by the Department of Health 2000 and is available from the Department of Health website: www.dh.gov.uk/en/Publicationsandstatistics/ Publications/PublicationsPolicyAndGuidance/DH_4074702

(3) Access the internet and download a copy of *Implementing and Ensuring Safe Sedation Practice for Healthcare Procedures in Adults* (2001) by the Academy of Medical Royal Colleges. It can be obtained from: www.rcoa.ac.uk/index.asp?PageID=119. This gives a good overview of training and governance issues around sedation in the medical specialties.

(4) Access the internet and read the rapid response report issued by the National Patient Safety Agency (NPSA) entitled *Reducing the Risk of Overdose with Midazolam Injection in Adults* (NPSA/2008/RRR011) plus the supporting information paper: www.npsa.nhs.uk

References and further reading

Balmer C and Longman L (2008) *The Management of Medical Emergencies*. London: Quay Books.

Cohen SM, Fiske J and Newton JT (2000) Dental phobics – how does dental treatment affect their lives. *British Dental Journal* **189**: 385–390.

Department of Health (2000) *A Conscious Decision: a review of the use of general anaesthesia and conscious sedation in primary dental care*. London: Department of Health.

Ellis H (2002) *Clinical Anatomy (12e)*. Oxford: Blackwell Publishing.

Faculty of Dental Surgery (2002) *Non-pharmacological Behaviour Management*. Available at www.rcseng.ac.uk/fds/clinical_guidelines

General Dental Council (2009) *Standards for Dental Professionals*. London: General Dental Council.

General Dental Council (2008) *Continuing Professional Development for Dental Care Professionals*. Available at www.gdc_uk.org

General Dental Council (2006) *Patient Consent*. Available at www.gdc-uk.org/News+publications+ and+events/Publications/Guidance+documents/Patient+consent.htm

General Dental Council (2001) *Maintaining Standards*. London: General Dental Council.

Girdler NM and Hill CM (1998) *Sedation in Dentistry*. Oxford: Elsevier Science & Technology Books.

Hollins C (2008) *Levison's Textbook for Dental Nurses* (10e). Oxford: Wiley-Blackwell.

Hosey MT (2002) UK National Clinical Guidelines in Paediatric Dentistry. Managing anxious children: the use of conscious sedation in paediatric dentistry. *International Journal of Paediatric Dentistry* **12**: 359–372. (These can be downloaded from the UK national clinical guidelines on the use of conscious sedation in paediatric dentistry (2002) www.rcseng.ac.uk/fds/clinical_guidelines).

Humphris GM, Freeman RE, Tutti H and De Souza V (2000) Further evidence for the reliability and validity of the Modified Dental Anxiety Scale. *International Dental Journal* **50**: 367–370.

Humphris GM, Morrison T and Lindsay SJE (1995) The Modified Dental Anxiety Scale: validation and United Kingdom norms. *Community Dental Health* **12**: 143–150.

Mallett J and Dougherty L (2000) *The Royal Marsden Hospital Manual of Clinical Nursing Procedures (5e)*. Oxford: Blackwell Science.

Manley MCG, Ransford NJ, Lewis DA, Thompson SA and Forbes M (2008) Retrospective audit of the efficacy and safety of the combined intranasal/intravenous midazolam sedation technique for the dental treatment of adults with learning disability. *British Dental Journal* **205**, E3–E3 (doi: 10.1038/sj.bdj.2008.521).

Naini FB, Mellor AC and Getz T (1999) Treatment of dental fears: pharmacology or psychology? *Dental Update* **26**: 270–276.

National Patient Safety Agency (2008) *Reducing the Risk of Overdose with Midazolam Injection in Adults*. Available at: www.npsa.nhs.uk

Poswillo Report (1990) General Anaesthesia, Sedation and. Resuscitation in Dentistry. Report of an expert working party prepared for the Standing Dental Advisory Committee. London: Department of Health.

Poswillo DE (1991) Principal recommendations of the Poswillo Report. *British Dental Journal* **170**: 46–47.

Resuscitation Council (2006, revised 2008) Medical Emergencies and Resuscitation – standards for clinical practice and training for dental practitioners and dental care professionals in general dental practice. Available at: www.resus.org.uk/pages/MEdental.pdf

Report of an Intercollegiate Working Party chaired by the Royal College of Anaesthetists. (2001) *Implementing and Ensuring Safe Sedation Practice for Healthcare Procedures in Adults*. London: Royal College of Anaesthetists.

Scottish Dental Clinical Effectiveness Programme (2006) *Conscious Sedation in Dentistry*. Available at: www.sdcep.org.uk/index.aspx?o=2331

Scottish Dental Clinical Effectiveness Programme (2008) *Prescribing for Dentistry*. Available at: www.sdcep.org.uk/index.aspx?o=2334

Standing Dental Advisory Committee (2003) *Conscious Sedation in the Provision of Dental Care*. Available at: www.dh.gov.uk/en/AdvanceSearchResult/index.htm?searchTerms=Concious+sedation+in+the+provision+of+dental+

Useful websites

Dental Sedation Teachers Group: www.dstg.co.uk
Society for the Advancement of Anaesthesia in Dentistry: www.saad.org.uk

5 Orthodontic Dental Nursing

Jayne Harrison and Kathleen O'Donovan

Orthodontics is the branch of dentistry concerned with facial growth, development of the dentition and occlusion and the prevention and correction of occlusal anomalies.

Anatomical structures relevant to orthodontics

Muscles of mastication

There are four muscles of mastication which are all supplied by the mandibular division of the trigeminal nerve (Figure 5.1).

Masseter

The masseter muscle elevates the mandible to close the jaws. It originates from the lower border of the zygomatic arch. It inserts on the outer surface of the ramus and angle of the mandible.

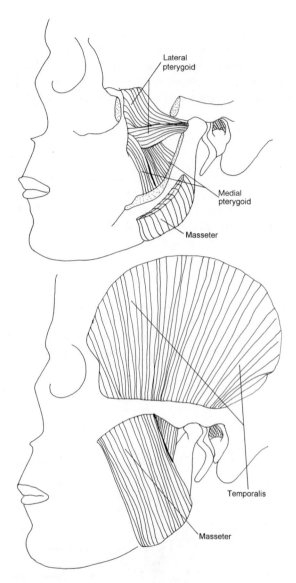

Figure 5.1 The muscles of mastication.

Temporalis

The anterior fibres of the temporalis elevate the mandible and the posterior fibres retract it. This muscle therefore closes and pulls back the mandible. It originates from the temporal fossa on the lateral surface of the temporal bone. Its insertion is via a narrow tendon that is attached to the coronoid process and the anterior border of the ramus of the mandible.

Lateral pterygoid

The lateral pterygoid pulls the mandible forward and downwards and thus initiates opening of the jaws. It originates by two heads from the infra-temporal surface of the greater wing of the sphenoid and lateral surface of the lateral pterygoid plate. Its insertion is into the neck of the mandible and the intra-articular disc of the temporomandibular joint.

Medial pterygoid

The medial pterygoid elevates the mandible and pulls it forward, thus assisting in closing the jaw. It originates by two heads that wrap around the lateral pterygoid muscle attaching from the medial surface of the lateral pterygoid plate, the palatine bone and tuberosity of the maxilla. It is inserted into the medial surface of the ramus and angle of the mandible.

Facial muscles

The orifices of the face, which are the orbits, nose and mouth, are protected by the eyelids, nostrils and lips. The facial muscles serve as sphincters and dilators of these openings (Figure 5.2). The muscles also modify the expression of the face. They are derived from the second pharyngeal arch and are supplied by the facial nerve.

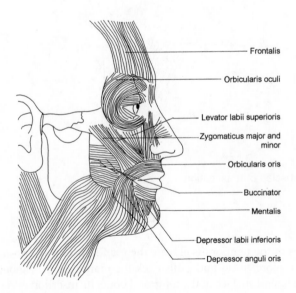

Figure 5.2 The facial muscles.

Forehead

The frontalis muscle does not have a bony attachment but blends with the orbicularis oculi anteriorly and occipitalis posteriorly. It lifts the forehead and raises the eyebrows.

Eyelids

The sphincter muscle, orbicularis oculi, surrounds the opening of the orbit and has two parts. The central palpebral fibres lie within the eyelids and are attached, via the medial palpebral ligament, to the frontal process of the maxilla. The peripheral orbital fibres surround the orbital margin and are attached medially to the medial palpebral ligament and directly to the frontal process of the maxilla. The palpebral part closes the eyelids when sleeping, winking or blinking and the orbital part produces a more forceful closure of the eyelids thus screwing the eyelids together. They are also used in frowning. The dilator muscles, levator palpebrae superioris and the occipitofrontalis raise the upper eyelid and thus open up the eye.

Cheeks

The buccinator muscle forms the greater part of the cheek. Its lateral attachment is into the pterygomandibular raphe and the outer surfaces of the maxilla and mandible next to the third molar teeth. Its fibres then pass forward and medially and span out at the angle of the mouth to blend with the obicularis oris. The buccinator exerts lateral pressure to keep the food between the teeth while chewing.

Nostrils

The compressor and dilator nares muscles pass from the maxilla to the nasal cartilages. They are vestigial in humans.

Lips

The sphincter muscle, orbicularis oris, and the dilator muscles (of which there are many – mentalis, depressor and levator anguli oris, zygomaticus major and minor to name just a few) form the greater part of the lips. When they contract they produce a small orifice, as in whistling, and are responsible for movement of the lips.

Tongue

The tongue is a mass of striated muscle, covered with mucous membrane. The anterior two-thirds lie in the mouth and the posterior third in the pharynx. The muscles of the tongue are divided into two groups – the **intrinsic** (contained within the tongue) and the **extrinsic** (which originate outside the tongue and are inserted into it). A median fibrous septum divides the tongue into left and right. The tongue can also be divided into front and back portions by the V-shaped **sulcus terminalis**. The main function of the tongue is to assist swallowing by directing food into the pharynx. It also assists with speech. The position of the teeth is influenced by the pressure of the tongue versus the pressure of the cheeks.

Intrinsic muscles

The intrinsic muscles of the tongue are arranged in vertical, horizontal and transverse bundles. The intrinsic muscles alter the shape of the tongue.

Extrinsic muscles

The extrinsic tongue muscles attach the tongue to the styloid process and the soft palate above and below to the mandible and the hyoid bone. They are responsible for altering the position of the tongue, that is they move the bulk of the tongue around the oral cavity (Figure 5.3).

Genioglossus

This muscle is attached to the mental spine on the lingual surface of the mandible from which it passes backwards and spans out through the whole length of the tongue.

(a)

(b)

Figure 5.3 (a) The extrinsic muscles and (b) dorsal view of the tongue.

Hyoglossus

This is a thin muscle that passes from the body and greater horns of the hyoid bone upwards and forwards into the dorsum of the tongue.

Styloglossus

This muscle passes anteriorly from near the tip of the styloid process into the side of the tongue.

Palatoglossus

This muscle passes from the soft palate into the side of the tongue.

Blood and nerve supply

The tongue receives blood from the lingual artery, which is a branch of the external carotid artery. It is drained by the lingual vein which drains into the internal jugular vein.

The mucous membrane of the anterior two-thirds of the tongue is supplied by the lingual nerve. Taste fibres to the anterior two-thirds are from the chorda tympani and travel with the fibres of the facial nerve. Taste and sensation to the posterior third of the tongue are supplied by the glossopharyngeal nerve. All the intrinsic and extrinsic muscles of the tongue are supplied by the hypoglossal nerve, except the palatoglossus, which is supplied by the vagus nerve.

Maxilla

Each maxilla consists of a body and four processes (Figure 5.4).

Body

This contains the maxillary air sinuses and has four surfaces. Medially it forms part of the lateral aspect of the nose. The anterior surface contains the infra-orbital foramen and forms part of the facial skeleton. The posterior surface is separated from the pterygoid process of the sphenoid bone by the pterygomaxillary fissure. The superior surface forms the majority of the floor of the orbit.

Processes

- The zygomatic process extends laterally to join the zygomatic bone and form the cheek bone.
- The alveolar process projects downwards and develops in response to the presence of maxillary teeth. The rounded posterior border that extends behind the terminal molars forms the maxillary tuberosity.
- The horizontal (palatine) process extends medially and forms part of the hard palate.
- The frontal process extends superiorly to articulate with the frontal bone and form part of the medial wall of the orbit.

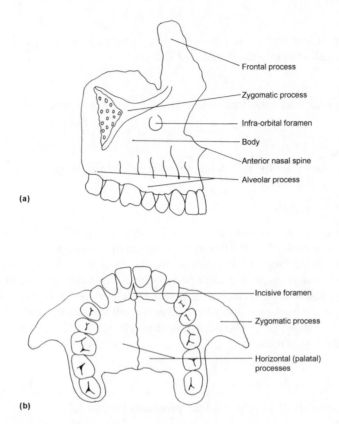

Figure 5.4 (a) The lateral view of the right maxilla and (b) palatal view of right and left maxillae.

Basal bone and alveolar bone

Basal bone is stable and undergoes little remodelling during orthodontic treatment. It determines the skeletal pattern of the individual.

Alveolar bone is dependent on the existence of teeth and is readily remodelled during tooth movement. Extracting teeth causes loss of the alveolar bone. Teeth are attached to the alveolar bone at the periodontal ligament. The parts of this ligament that attach into the bone and cementum are known as **Sharpey's fibres**.

Embryology

The maxilla derives from the maxillary process of the first pharyngeal arch and from the frontal process. During foetal development ossification is intramembranous and starts lateral to the nasal cartilages. Initially there are left and right maxillae which later (at puberty) fuse in the midline at the palatal suture.

Growth

Growth of the maxilla occurs by three methods:

- fill-in growth at the sutures
- drift
- periosteal remodelling.

The deposition of bone at the tuberosities allows the maxilla to enlarge in the antero-posterior direction. This lengthens the dental arch and allows for the eruption of the teeth.

Downward growth is by development of the alveolar process and eruption of the teeth. Bone is deposited on the inferior of the hard palate and removed by resorption from the superior surface. The whole palate moves downwards and forwards by a process of remodelling.

Maxillary growth ceases at approximately 15 years of age in girls and 17 years of age in boys.

Mandible

The mandible consists of two halves that join in the midline. Each half has a body and a ramus that form the angle where they meet (Figure 5.5).

Body

The body has a smooth lower border. The upper margin is irregular and formed from alveolar bone in response to the development of teeth. The mental foramen opens on the lateral surface between the roots of the premolar teeth. From it emerge the mental nerve and mental vessels. The mental nerve is a branch of the inferior dental (alveolar) nerve that supplies sensation to the chin and lower lip.

The lingual surface provides attachment for several muscles, including the mylohyoid, anterior belly of the diagastric and genioglossus muscles.

Ramus

The ramus is flat and rectangular in shape and has two processes (coronoid and condylar) that extend superiorly and are separated by the mandibular notch. The coronoid process extends anteriorly and gives attachment to the temporalis muscle. The condylar process extends superiorly to the articular head that is supported by a narrower neck. The head articulates with the base of the skull at the temporal fossa to form the temporomandibular joint. The lateral surface of the ramus provides attachment for the masseter muscle. The medial surface provides attachment for the sphenomandibular ligament and the medial pterygoid muscle.

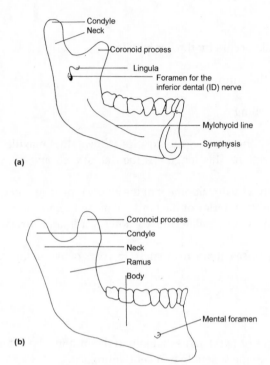

Figure 5.5 (a) The medial surface of the left side of the mandible and (b) the lateral surface of the right side of the mandible.

The inferior dental (alveolar) nerve enters the mandible via the mandibular foramen, which lies in the middle of the lingual surface of the ramus.

Basal bone and alveolar bone

As in the maxilla, the basal bone is stable and undergoes little remodelling during orthodontic treatment and determines the skeletal pattern of the individual. However, alveolar bone is dependent on the existence of teeth and is readily remodelled during tooth movement.

Embryology

Each half of the mandible ossifies in mesenchyme from a centre that appears in the sixth week of intrauterine life and lies lateral to **Meckel's cartilage** (the cartilage of the first pharyngeal arch). Secondary cartilages develop later for the condyle, coronoid process and the midline area, and ossify from the adjacent mesenchyme bone. The mandible is therefore a membranous bone with secondary growth centres in the cartilages. Bony union of the two halves in the midline occurs at about the age of two years.

Growth

The length of the body is increased by apposition of the bone from the anterior border of the ramus and deposition along the posterior border. Vertical growth of the body occurs with deposition of bone along the alveolar process. This is largely determined by the development and eruption of the mandibular teeth.

Growth at the condylar cartilage elongates the mandible causing anterior displacement, while the shape is maintained by remodelling of the anterior and posterior borders of the ramus. Most mandibular growth occurs by periosteal activity with development at the angle and coronoid process in response to muscular attachments, while the alveolar process grows in response to the development of the teeth.

The increase in width of the mandible is brought about by remodelling. Lengthening of the mandible and anterior remodelling are responsible for the increase in prominence of the chin. This feature of maturation is more apparent in males.

Mandibular growth ceases later than maxillary growth at about 17 years of age in girls and 19 years in boys.

Growth rotations

It was originally thought that growth of the jaws was linear in a downward and forward direction. However, studies where implants were placed in the surface of the facial bones demonstrated rotation as well. The effect of these rotations is most obvious in the mandible. The rotations are the result of different amounts of growth of the posterior and anterior face heights. Forward growth rotations, where growth of the posterior face height is greater than the anterior face height, are more common than backward growth rotations. Forward growth rotations tend to result in reduced anterior vertical proportions and an increased overbite (see Incisor relationship later), whereas posterior growth rotations tend to result in increased anterior vertical proportions and a reduced overbite or anterior open bite.

Growth rotations are important in the diagnosis and outcome of treatment of some malocclusions. Unfavourable growth (backward rotation) can prejudice the outcome of treatment resulting in loss of anterior contact and the development of an anterior open bite. This is compounded by the extrusive effect of most orthodontic treatment, which tends to increase the anterior face height.

Development of the dentition

Knowledge of the sequence of eruption, calcification times and root development, together with the ability to identify discrepancies in the eruption time of teeth in contralateral sides, are important when assessing whether development is progressing normally or not.

Table 5.1 Development of the deciduous dentition.

Tooth	A	B	C	D	E
Calcification of crown starts (months in utero)	3–4	3–4	4–5	4	5–6
Average age of eruption (months of age)	6–7	7–8	18–20	12–15	24–36
Root development complete 12–18 months after eruption					

Deciduous dentition

The first teeth to erupt into a baby's mouth are usually the lower central incisors (see Table 5.1). This occurs at approximately six months of age, but there is considerable variation in this as they may put in an appearance any time in the first year. The deciduous dentition is usually complete by the age of three years, with the incisors upright and spaced. There are also usually spaces mesial to the upper deciduous canines and distal to the lower ones that are known as **primate spacing**. If the primary dentition is not spaced by the time it is complete, then it is very likely that a significant amount of crowding will exist in the permanent dentition when it erupts. The overbite gradually reduces as the child grows so that by the time the deciduous incisors are lost they are usually in an edge-to edge relationship, which can lead to a considerable amount of tooth wear.

Mixed dentition

The first permanent teeth to erupt are usually the first permanent molars at about the age of six, although as with the eruption of the deciduous dentition, there is considerable variation in this. The next teeth to erupt are the incisors, with the lowers usually coming first. The permanent incisors develop lingually to their deciduous counterparts and the lower permanent incisors, in particular, often erupt in a lingual position, but this usually corrects spontaneously as space becomes available and the forces from the tongue move them labially. The upper incisors erupt on to a larger arch of the circle to gain some space, which allows the larger permanent teeth to be accommodated. The upper incisors tend to be tipped distally and spaced due to pressure on the lateral incisor roots from the developing canine. This is a normal developmental phase commonly known as the **ugly duckling** phase and does not need any active intervention as it will correct itself when the permanent canines start to erupt. The upper permanent canines also start their development palatal to the deciduous dentition but then move buccally so that they can be felt in the buccal sulcus by the age of 10. If the upper permanent canines can't be palpated or the deciduous canines are not mobile by the age of 10, then suspicions should be raised and radiographs taken to locate the permanent canine. If the permanent canine is found to be lying palatally at this stage, then evidence suggests that if the deciduous canine is extracted, the permanent canine is likely to improve its position sufficiently to allow normal eruption to occur. The amount of improvement seen will depend on how displaced the permanent canine is and the amount of crowding in the rest of the arch. If the

Table 5.2 Development of the permanent dentition.

Maxillary	Average age of eruption (years)	7	8	10	11	12	6	12	18–24
	Calcification of crown starts (months)	3–4	10–12	4–5	18–21	24–27	Birth	30–36	7–9 years
Tooth		**1**	**2**	**3**	**4**	**5**	**6**	**7**	**8**
Mandibular	Calcification of crown starts (months)	3–4	3–4	4–5	21–24	27–30	Birth	30–36	8–10 years
	Average age of eruption (years)	8	9	12	11	12	6	12	18–24

Root development complete 2–3 years after eruption

deciduous canines and molars remain intact until their successors erupt then there should be a small amount of excess space as the combined mesiodistal width of the deciduous canines and molars is greater than the combined widths of the permanent canines and premolars. This space is called the **leeway space** and amounts to 1.5 mm in the maxillary arch and 2.5 mm in the mandibular arch.

Permanent dentition

The first permanent teeth to erupt are the first molars, at about six years of age, and the last the third molars. There is a slight variation in the order of eruption between the arches, with the mandibular first premolar erupting before the mandibular canine and vice versa in the maxillary arch. In general, the mandibular teeth erupt slightly in advance of the maxillary teeth (Table 5.2).

Arch dimensions

The **arch width** (measured between the lingual cups of the second deciduous molars or second premolars) increases gradually until the primary dentition is established (age three years) but then only increases another 2–3 mm by the age of 18 years. The **arch circumference** (between the distal surface of the second deciduous molars or second premolars through the buccal cusps and then incisal tips/edges of the canines and incisors) changes very little in the maxilla once the deciduous dentition is established and reduces in the mandible as the permanent dentition erupts due to the leeway space. The **intercanine width** (between the cusp tips of the canines) increases by 1–2 mm during the deciduous dentition and another 2–3 mm during the mixed dentition but is essentially established by the age of nine years. Growth continues **posteriorly** until the terminal molar has erupted, but there is very little change in the dimensions of the anterior segments once the deciduous dentition has become established.

Biology of tooth movement

Teeth are suspended in their sockets by the **periodontal ligament**, which connects the cementum to the alveolar bone. The periodontal ligament consists of collagenous connective tissue, blood vessels and tissue fluid. It therefore:

- acts as a cushion to sudden forces
- has proprioceptive properties
- plays an important role in tooth eruption and orthodontic tooth movement.

Types of tooth movement

Tipping

Tipping movement occurs when a point force is applied to the tooth. This is the only type of tooth movement that removable appliances can bring about. Teeth tip at a point near the junction of the middle and apical thirds of their root. Tipping can be brought about by a light force (30–60 g) depending on the root surface area (RSA) of the tooth (Figure 5.6a).

Bodily movement

Bodily movement occurs when there is an equal amount of root and crown movement in the same direction. Ideally, a force needs to be applied through the centre of resistance of a tooth to bring about true bodily movement (Figure 5.6b). However, in orthodontic treatment this is not possible as the centre of resistance of most teeth lies two-thirds of the way down the root. Bodily movement therefore needs a couple to resist the rotational effects of the force applied via the crown. This can only be brought about by fixed appliances. A **couple** is two equal forces acting in opposite directions that limit rotation and

xxx	Areas of compression and bone resorption
- - -	Areas of tension and bone deposition
⟶	Force
●	Fulcrum

Figure 5.6 Tooth movement: (a) tipping and (b) bodily movement.

result in bodily movement. The applied force is spread over the whole root surface and therefore requires greater amounts of force to bring about tooth movement than tipping. Typically 70–120 g is required, but again this is dependent on the RSA of the tooth.

Torquing

Torquing (root uprighting) is the movement of the root in a buccolingual direction with either minimal or no movement of the crown in the opposite direction. It requires a couple and a force to be applied to the tooth, and can only be brought about by rectangular wires via a fixed appliance. Consequently, it is usually applied towards the end of active orthodontic treatment.

Rotation

Rotation can only be brought about by fixed appliances. Although rotation of teeth occurs relatively easily and requires low forces (35–60 g) it is not a very stable movement due to the recoil of the periodontal fibres that tend to return the tooth to its original position once the appliance is removed.

Extrusion

Extrusion of teeth can only be brought about by fixed appliances. It is relatively easy to extrude teeth, requiring a force of 35–60 g. However, it is not a very stable movement as the stretched periodontal fibres tend to recoil once the appliance is removed thus taking the tooth back towards its original position.

Intrusion

True intrusion of a tooth is difficult to bring about and requires a great deal of care. When an intrusive force is applied to a tooth it is concentrated at the apex of the tooth. If the force is excessive it can occlude the apical vessels, thus leading to pulpal damage, root resorption or pulpal death. It is therefore important to keep forces low at about 10–20 g per tooth, depending on the RSA of the tooth.

Histological changes during tooth movement

Ideal force

When an ideal force ($20–25 \, g/cm^2$) is applied to a tooth, areas of pressure (compression) and tension develop in the periodontal ligament (Figure 5.6). In the areas of pressure, alterations in the blood flow to the periodontal ligament and adjacent alveolar bone cause conditions within the cells to change and hormones (prostaglandins) to be released. This results in cell proliferation and movement of **osteoclasts** (bone-resorbing cells) into the area from surrounding blood vessels. The osteoclasts line the socket wall and initiate bone resorption. Initially this is seen as shallow depressions in the bone known as **Howship's lacunae** which then join to produce a larger area of resorption. The periodontal fibres become re-attached once the resorption has stopped so that the periodontal ligament remains intact.

In the areas of tension, the periodontal fibres become stretched and within a few days cell proliferation occurs. **Osteoblasts** (bone-forming cells) are then stimulated to move into the area and lay down **osteoid** (young, immature bone) on the socket wall in the areas of tension. The osteoid is then calcified and remodelled into mature bone to support the tooth in its new position.

Excessive force

If an excessive force is applied to a tooth continuously, areas of pressure and tension will build up. However, in this situation the blood vessels within the periodontal ligament become compressed and crushed in the areas of pressure. This results in death of the cells in the periodontal ligament and necrosis of the adjacent bone (hyalinisation). Initially tooth movement is inhibited, but after two to three weeks indirect (or undermining) resorption starts in the alveolar bone adjacent to the hyalinised areas. Once this has occurred the tooth moves rapidly into the resorbed areas.

In areas of tension the periodontal fibres may become so stretched that they may be torn and the blood vessels may rupture. Although traumatic, this does not inhibit the deposition of new bone which occurs in the same way as under optimal forces.

It is not advisable to use excessive forces to bring about tooth movement during orthodontic treatment because it is potentially damaging. Application of excessive force:

- slows down tooth movement (rather than speeds it up)
- is more painful for patients
- may damage the dental pulp
- increases the chance of root resorption
- increases tooth mobility during treatment.

Optimal tooth movement

Optimal tooth movement during orthodontic treatment depends on the level and duration of the force applied. The ideal force to bring about orthodontic tooth movement is about 20–25 g/cm² of the tooth's RSA but depends on the type of movement being carried out (Table 5.3).

The chemical changes that initiate tooth movement appear in the areas of pressure and tension within a few hours, and tooth movement will occur if a force is applied for as little as six hours per day. However, for optimal tooth movement to occur the force needs to be applied continuously.

Table 5.3 Suggested ideal forces for orthodontic tooth movement.

Type of movement	Force
Tipping movement	30–60 g
Bodily movement	70–120 g
Torquing	50–100 g
Rotation	30–60 g
Extrusion	35–60 g
Intrusion	10–20 g

Classification of occlusion and malocclusion

Few people have an *ideal* occlusion and for the majority of people with a *normal* occlusion this usually means that they have a variation from the *ideal* occlusion that is acceptable in terms of its impact on dental health and aesthetics.

A malocclusion is therefore defined as a deviation of the teeth or malrelationship of the dental arches beyond the accepted range of normal. It can be attributed to one or more of the following:

- abnormal jaw size or shape
- congenitally missing teeth
- malformed teeth
- supernumerary teeth
- retained, unerupted or impacted teeth
- abnormalities in embryonic development, e.g. cleft lip and/or palate
- environmental factors, e.g. digit sucking, premature loss of teeth, trauma.

Skeletal classification

The skeletal pattern can be assessed in three planes of space and classified as follows (Figure 5.7).

Antero-posterior

Class 1 – a normal, balanced profile with the mandible 2–3 mm posterior to the maxilla (Figure 5.7a).
Class 2 – the mandible is retruded relative to the maxilla (Figure 5.7b).
Class 3 – the mandible is protruded relative to the maxilla (Figure 5.7c).

Vertical

Two vertical relations can be assessed and classified (Figure 5.8).

Lower face height (LFH) – in the normally proportioned face the lower anterior face height (base of chin to base of nose) equals the upper anterior face height (base of nose

Figure 5.7 Assessment of the antero-posterior relationship: (a) Class 1; (b) Class 2; and (c) Class 3.

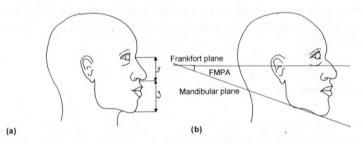

Figure 5.8 Assessment of the vertical relationship. (a) Vertical proportions of the upper and lower face height and (b) the Frankfort mandibular plane angle (FMPA). y, upper face height; z, lower face height, y + z, total face height.

to mid-point between the eyebrows). If it is less or more than that, the LFH is classified as being reduced or increased, i.e. the LFH is approximately 50% of the total face height (Figure 5.8a).

Frankfort mandibular plane angle (FMPA) – this is the angle between the **Frankfort plane** (lower border of the orbital margin to the external auditory meatus) and the lower border of the mandible. This is normally 27° ± 5° and is classified as increased or decreased when outside the normal range (Figure 5.8b).

Transverse

Transverse discrepancies may be **unilateral** or **bilateral**, depending on whether one or both sides of the face are affected.

A **true** transverse discrepancy exists when it is present when the patient is in retruded contact position (RCP) and intercuspal position (ICP). A **pseudo** (false) transverse discrepancy exists when it is present when the patient is in ICP but absent in RCP.

Occlusal classification

Incisor relationship

The British Standards Institute classification is widely used to refer to the relation of upper and lower incisors in occlusion.

Class I
The lower incisor edges occlude with, or lie immediately below the cingulum plateau of the upper incisors (Figure 5.9a).

Class II
Class II incisor relationship has two official subdivisions.

Division 1 – the lower incisal edge bites behind the cingulum plateau of the upper central incisors and the upper incisors are proclined (Figure 5.9b).

Division 2 – the lower incisal edge bites behind the cingulum plateau of the upper central incisors and the upper incisors are retroclined (the lateral incisors may be proclined) (Figure 5.9c).

A third subdivision has also been suggested to aid the classification of borderline cases. This is called the Class II intermediate subcategory and exists in cases where the upper incisors are upright and the overjet is increased to 4–6 mm.

Class III
The lower incisal edge bites in front of the cingulum plateau of the upper incisors (Figure 5.9d).

Molar relationship

Angle's classification is commonly used to describe the relationship of the molars in occlusion (Figure 5.10). This is as follows.

(a) (b) (c) (d)

Figure 5.9 Incisor classification: (a) Class I; (b) Class II division 1; (c) Class II division 2; and (d) Class III.

Figure 5.10 Buccal segment relationship: (a) Class I; (b) Class II; and (c) Class III.

Class I
The mesiobuccal cusp of the upper first molar lies in the buccal groove of the lower first molar (Figure 5.10a).

Class II
The mesiobuccal cusp of the upper first molar lies anterior to the buccal groove of the lower first molar (Figure 5.10b).

Class III
The mesiobuccal cusp of the upper first molar lies posterior to the buccal groove of the lower first molar (Figure 5.10c).

Canine relationship

The relationship of the canines is important when assessing a malocclusion and determining the space requirements to correct it (see Figure 5.10). The relationship is classified in a similar way to the relationship of the incisors and molars.

Class I
The tip of the upper canine occludes between the lower canine and first premolar (see Figure 5.10a).

Class II
The tip of the upper canine occludes between the lower lateral incisor and canine (see Figure 5.10b).

Class III
The tip of the upper canine occludes between the lower first and second premolars (see Figure 5.10c).

Diagnostic terms

Overjet – the overjet is defined as the horizontal distance between the labial surface of the tips of the upper incisors and the surface of the lower incisors.

Overbite – the overbite is the vertical overlap of the incisor teeth.

Anterior open bite – an anterior open bite (AOB) exists when there is no vertical overlap of the lower incisors by the upper incisors.

Crossbite – in the normal relationship the upper teeth occlude labially/buccally to the lower teeth. A crossbite exists if any upper tooth is positioned so that it occludes palatal to a lower tooth. An anterior crossbite involves the upper incisors and a buccal crossbite involves the teeth in the buccal segment.

Scissors bite – a scissors bite exists if any tooth in the upper buccal segment is positioned so that its palatal cusp occludes buccal to the buccal cusp of a lower tooth.

Indications for orthodontic treatment

The main indications for orthodontic treatment are to improve oral function, aesthetics and general dental health. However, treatment should not be started unless there is a reasonable chance that the patient will benefit from it.

Function

Temporomandibular joint disorders

There are only a few specific malocclusions where orthodontic treatment may help treat or reduce the risk of temporomandibular joint disorder (TMD). There is some evidence that these malocclusions cause or predispose the patient to TMD in later life. However, TMD has many causes and it should not be attributed directly to a malocclusion. Orthodontic treatment should therefore not be started for the sole reason of treating TMD. These specific malocclusions include crossbites, either anterior or posterior, that cause a significant displacement on closing, anterior open bites and Class III malocclusions.

Trauma

Orthodontic treatment is indicated in cases where there is an increased overjet because there is a direct relationship between the size of an overjet and the risk of trauma to the upper incisors. Evidence suggests that children with an overjet of more than 3 mm are at about twice as much risk of injury to their anterior teeth and that the risk of injury increases with increasing overjet. Surprisingly, the risk of injury for boys was found to be less than for girls with the same overjet.

Pathology

There is a strong indication for orthodontic and/or surgical intervention for unerupted impacted teeth, e.g. upper canines, because they may predispose the patient to pathology.

Such teeth can cause resorption of the roots of adjacent teeth. This usually stops once the canine has been moved away from the affected tooth or teeth but may prejudice their life expectancy. In these situations, it may be preferable to remove the affected tooth and allow the unerupted canine to erupt into its position. The follicle surrounding an unerupted, impacted tooth can undergo cystic change and then enlarge. The cyst may damage adjacent teeth or cause the unerupted tooth to become severely displaced as it expands.

Aesthetics

The aesthetic impact of a malocclusion is not usually the primary indication for orthodontic treatment from the clinician's point of view. However, it is one of the key motivating factors for patients to seek orthodontic treatment. There is evidence that severe malocclusions and dentofacial abnormalities do have a negative effect on a patient's psychosocial well-being. However, there is little evidence to suggest that minor irregularities of the teeth have a negative effect. Rather, it is the patient's overall attractiveness that is more important when it comes to social interactions and their psychosocial well-being.

Dental health

Dental caries

No association of malocclusion with caries has been found so there are no indications for orthodontic treatment to help prevent or treat dental caries. This is because the primary cause of dental caries is the patient's diet combined with plaque accumulation and exposure to fluoride. Unlike modifications in diet and the use of fluoride toothpaste, orthodontic treatment has not been shown to be associated with a reduced level of caries. However, if dietary control and oral hygiene are poor, orthodontic treatment can increase the level of decalcification and/or caries so should not be started in patients whose general mouth care is poor.

Periodontal disease

Again, there is little evidence to suggest that malocclusion is associated with periodontal disease in all but a few specific situations. This is because the primary cause of periodontal disease is plaque accumulation, which is related to oral hygiene rather than tooth position alone. However, there are a few situations where the occlusion can have a traumatic effect on the gingivae. They include the following.

■ Increased overbites where either the lower incisors are biting into the palate or junction between the teeth and gingivae or the upper incisors are biting on to the labial mucosa. Both these situations are traumatic and can lead to gingival stripping, which may cause the patient discomfort

■ Anterior crossbites, which can displace one or more of the lower incisors labially causing dehiscence of the labial alveolar bone and associated gingivae.

Orthodontic treatment

Aims of orthodontic treatment

■ Improve facial and dental aesthetics.
■ Align the teeth and eliminate stagnation areas.
■ Eliminate premature contacts which can give rise to mandibular displacement and may predispose a patient to TMD.
■ Eliminate traumatic irregularities of the teeth.
■ Align tipped or tilted teeth prior to bridgework or crowns.
■ Align, level, or decompensate teeth and co-ordinate the dental arches prior to orthognathic surgery.
■ Assist the eruption and alignment of displaced or impacted teeth.

Benefits of orthodontic treatment

If orthodontic treatment is to be of benefit to a patient then the advantages that it can offer must outweigh the potential for any damage it might cause. The benefits of orthodontic treatment can be assessed by considering the impact that malocclusion has on the dental health and psycho-social well-being of an individual.

Dental health

The relationship between malocclusion, orthodontic treatment and general dental health is controversial and can be considered in terms of general dentofacial conditions, dental caries and periodontal disease. It would not be unreasonable to think that straighter teeth would be easier to clean than crowded teeth and that in turn this would lead to less plaque retention and therefore less caries and periodontal disease. However, there is only weak evidence that orthodontic treatment produces a measured benefit to patients' oral health.

General dentofacial conditions

The evidence suggests that, with the exception of some extreme malocclusions, the disadvantages of many malocclusions in terms of general dentofacial health, are modest. Orthodontic treatment can be beneficial for patients with excessively prominent incisors. Early reduction of an overjet can reduce the risk of trauma in childhood and the potential for prominent incisors to procline and space in adulthood. Early orthodontic intervention also has the potential to reduce the likelihood of pathology associated with unerupted, impacted teeth.

The benefit of orthodontic treatment in terms of reducing the risk of developing TMD or treating TMD are limited as there is only a very weak association between most malocclusions, TMD and orthodontic treatment.

Correction of very deep overbites can be beneficial by reducing the effects of trauma to the palatal mucosa or gingivae and/or labial mucosa of the lower incisors.

Dental caries

The benefits of orthodontic treatment in terms of reducing or preventing dental caries are limited and most studies that have investigated the link between malocclusion and caries have failed to show any association. This is probably because caries has a multi-factorial aetiology and malocclusion has only a minor part to play when compared with diet and exposure to fluoride.

Periodontal disease

The benefits of orthodontic treatment in terms of reducing or preventing periodontal disease are debatable. It has been shown that some malocclusions make it difficult to clean the teeth, but studies looking at the association between malocclusions and periodontal disease have come up with conflicting results. Again this may be because periodontal disease, like caries, has a multifactorial aetiology and malocclusion has only a minor part to play when compared with oral hygiene, social class and gender.

Psychosocial well-being

Psychosocial research suggests that people with an unattractive physical appearance fare poorly in many areas of social interaction. There is evidence that unattractive children are more likely to be bullied and their teachers have lower academic expectations of them. However, the significance of malocclusion in the overall attractiveness of an individual and the impact on their social interactions is less clear.

Several studies have investigated the impact of malocclusion on nicknames and teasing, self-esteem and social attractiveness. Although other physical attributes, e.g. weight and height, were more commonly the subject of teasing, children who were teased about their teeth found these comments more distressing and hurtful than comments made about other features. Investigation into the effect of dentofacial appearance on social attractiveness suggests that the background facial attractiveness of an individual is more important than the dental appearance in determining first impressions, an individual's popularity and ability to form friendships. Although children rated as more attractive do not appear to have greater self-esteem, evidence suggests that teachers rate attractive children more favourably in many respects.

The potential benefits of orthodontic correction of malocclusions on an individual's psychosocial well-being ought not be underestimated and need to be considered carefully. The negative effects of teasing and bullying may persist into adulthood so the potential benefits that orthodontic treatment in childhood/adolescence can offer may have a far-reaching impact on an individual's quality of life.

Risks of orthodontic treatment

As with most medical and dental interventions, orthodontic treatment does carry risks. These include tissue damage, increased susceptibility to disease or dysfunction following treatment and the failure to achieve the aims of treatment.

Tissue damage

Decalcification and dental caries
When patients are wearing an orthodontic appliance there is an increased tendency for plaque to accumulate. This is especially so when wearing a fixed appliance that cannot be removed to clean. If plaque accumulates, the acid produced from it can cause decalcification of the enamel surface.

Decalcification appears as a chalky, white spot and is most common in the gingival third of teeth especially on the upper lateral incisors and all premolars. If this progresses then cavitation can result. Evidence suggests that about half of all patients who have fixed orthodontic treatment have some degree of decalcification. However, less than 10% will have cavitation. This is disappointing because decalcification and caries are preventable.

If patients practise good oral hygiene and control their diet by limiting the frequency of sugar intake and the consumption of carbonated drinks, the risks of decalcification or cavitation can be limited. Other preventive measures can supplement this, for example daily fluoride mouthwashes. However, compliance with mouthwashes is likely to be poor in the patients who will benefit most from the exposure to additional topical fluoride, i.e. the patients with poor oral hygiene.

Clinicians can minimise the risk of decalcification/cavitation by ensuring that patients do not start orthodontic treatment until their oral hygiene is adequate. They can also ensure that the potential for plaque accumulation is minimised by removing excess composite from around the brackets, advising patients on how to clean around their fixed appliances, e.g. with bottle brushes, and using **glass ionomer cement** (GIC) to cement molar bands. GIC has the advantage that it will release fluoride during treatment which will reduce the risk of decalcification. In addition, if the band becomes loose, failure usually occurs at the band/cement interface. This leaves the enamel surface protected by a coating of GIC rather than being exposed to acid produced by plaque that accumulates very quickly under a loose band.

Gingival and periodontal problems
Most gingival and periodontal problems that can arise during or after orthodontic treatment are related to plaque control. The most common gingival problem occurring during orthodontic treatment is gingivitis. The gingivae become inflamed and swell, which makes oral hygiene even more difficult, leading to more plaque accumulation, etc. Again, good oral hygiene is the key to minimising the risk of gingivitis.

Mouthwashes that inhibit plaque accumulation, e.g. chlorhexidine, attention by the orthodontist to the removal of excess composite from around brackets and minimising the use of auxiliaries that may increase plaque accumulation can also help to reduce the potential for gingivitis to develop. Once orthodontic appliances are removed and normal oral hygiene procedures are re-established any gingival inflammation or swelling resolves. There may be 1–2 mm loss of attachment following orthodontic treatment but this is not usually of any clinical significance.

Gingival recession can occur before orthodontic treatment, for example as the result of a traumatic occlusion (deep overbite), or during treatment if a tooth is moved out of the labial cortex of the alveolar bone, for example following decompensation of the lower incisors prior to orthognathic surgery (see p. 312) or expansion to correct a crossbite. In both situations good oral hygiene can prevent further loss of attachment.

If a patient's oral hygiene is particularly poor and they smoke, there is a risk that acute ulcerative, necrotising gingivitis may develop. Improving the oral hygiene can usually control this but a course of metronidazole (200 mg three times a day for three to five days) may be required.

Root resorption

Some root resorption is inevitable during orthodontic treatment. It is usually in the order of 1–2 mm and is not of any clinical significance. However, a small proportion of patients will experience excessive root resorption that may prejudice the life expectancy of a tooth. Factors associated with root resorption include the amount of root movement that takes place, long or narrow roots, atypically shaped roots and the use of elastics. If root resorption does occur during treatment, patients can be assured that it will stop and not progress once the appliances have been removed.

Allergies and trauma

Many of the metals used to make orthodontic appliances, such as wires and auxiliaries, contain nickel. It is a common metal allergen and although many patients are sensitive to nickel in jewellery or zips and other fastenings, it is very unlikely that they will react to nickel-containing components within their mouth. However, headgear can initiate an allergic reaction on the skin that it comes in contact with.

The most common cause of trauma during orthodontic treatment is ends of wires or ligatures that catch the lips, cheeks or tongue causing ulceration. Such trauma is easily prevented by the orthodontist ensuring that the ends of the archwires are turned under or cut short and that ligature ends are tucked under the archwire.

There have been isolated case reports of trauma to the face or eyes resulting from headgear that has become displaced while the patient has been asleep or during play. The most serious of these injuries has resulted in the loss of an eye that had been injured by the end of a facebow. For this reason it is now recommended that two safety mechanisms be used when headgear is used during orthodontic treatment. Safety features include snap-away headgear straps, safety neck straps, locking facebows and round-ended facebows. Patients need to be warned not to play in their headgear, report any instances when the headgear becomes dislodged at night and seek immediate medical attention if any facial or eye injury results from the headgear.

Pulpal damage may occur during orthodontic treatment. This can be caused if the forces applied to a tooth are too heavy. However, even with normal force levels, teeth that have suffered trauma in the past have an increased chance of this happening. One of the first signs of pulpal damage having occurred is that the tooth appears grey. At this stage the tooth is usually vital and if forces are removed from the tooth for three months the pulp often recovers and remains vital. If vitality is lost then the pulp needs to be extirpated and the root canal dressed with calcium hydroxide until orthodontic treatment is complete after which a permanent root filling can be placed.

Increased susceptibility to disease or dysfunction

Periodontal disease

There is little evidence to suggest that orthodontic treatment predisposes patients to periodontal disease later in life. There is some evidence to suggest that patients who have had orthodontic treatment as adolescents have better oral hygiene than those who have not.

Temporomandibular joint disorders (TMD)

As described previously, there is some weak evidence to suggest that some occlusal traits predispose patients to TMD. Although orthodontic treatment aims to correct such pre-existing occlusal anomalies, it is also possible for orthodontic treatment to create such occlusal interferences. However, the risks appear to be minimal. Long-term studies in Europe and the USA have demonstrated that patients who had received orthodontic treatment suffer from TMD to the same degree as a matched group of patients who had not previously had orthodontic treatment.

Failure to achieve the aims of treatment

One of the greatest risks when starting orthodontic treatment is that the aims of treatment are not met and that a worthwhile improvement is not achieved for the patient. In some cases the patient may end up worse off after orthodontic treatment than before.

Failure to achieve the aims of treatment can be due to inappropriate treatment planning or poor patient compliance. It is therefore very important for the orthodontist to consider all aspects of the patient's history and presenting malocclusion when planning treatment, and to select carefully the patients for whom treatment should be provided. As stated previously, patients need to be willing and able to wear the appliances for the prescribed time, maintain good oral hygiene, take care of the appliances and attend regularly for adjustments of the appliances. Failure of any of these requirements can lead to treatment having to be terminated prematurely and before all aims have been achieved.

There is some evidence that milder malocclusions are more at risk from being no better or worse off after treatment. For this reason patients with relatively mild malocclusions require careful counselling before they start treatment to ensure that they are aware of the risks if they are not compliant.

Phases of orthodontic treatment

The progress of most orthodontic treatment falls into quite well-defined phases. There are subtle variations on this basic format and patients may be treated with other types of appliances before or as part of their fixed appliance therapy.

Two-phase treatment

When correcting some malocclusions, e.g. Class II division 1 in a pre-pubertal child, there is often a preliminary phase with a functional appliance to correct the overjet. This is then followed by re-assessment to determine the need for extractions and/or further treatment to detail the occlusion with a fixed appliance.

Bonding and banding

This is normally completed over two or three visits. A typical pattern is to place the brackets on the anterior teeth and separators between the molars at the first visit. At the second visit the bands can then be selected and fitted and the archwires placed.

Levelling and aligning

Levelling and aligning involves levelling the **curve of Spee** (the curve in the occlusal plane in the antero-posterior plane) and aligning the teeth. Alignment is usually carried out over several visits using flexible nickel titanium (e.g. 0.014″ and then 0.018″ × 0.025″) or stainless steel (e.g. 0.017″ Twistflex) archwires to align the teeth. Initially it is usually not possible to ligate fully all the brackets to the archwires because some of the teeth are very displaced or rotated. At the start of treatment some brackets may, therefore, only be partially ligated and as the teeth gradually align they are tied in more tightly to the archwire with wire ligatures or elastic modules. Progression to a stiffer archwire does not take place until the present archwire is fully tied into all the brackets and is level.

Levelling starts at the beginning of treatment when the bracket slots start to level. However, complete levelling of the curve of Spee requires the use of stiffer archwires (e.g. 0.019″ × 0.025″ stainless steel) and does not occur until the later stages of treatment.

Lacebacks are often used at this stage of treatment. They are metal ligatures (0.010″ soft stainless steel) that are tied from the molars to the canines under the main archwire. They help to maintain the arch length and prevent the lower incisors from proclining as the canines upright. Lacebacks are usually kept in place until the labial segments are aligned. They can be used unilaterally to help centreline correction.

Overbite reduction

Overbite reduction is a key stage in most courses of orthodontic treatment because it is impossible to obtain a Class I incisor relationship unless the overbite is fully reduced.

Overbite reduction can be initiated by an **upper removable appliance** (URA) used in conjunction with a lower fixed appliance at the start of treatment. In this situation the patient continues wearing the URA until a stiff archwire (e.g. 0.019″ × 0.025″ stainless steel) is in place to maintain the overbite reduction that has been obtained. Once this has been achieved the upper fixed appliance can be placed so that levelling and aligning of the upper arch can take place.

If upper and lower fixed appliances are used from the outset there is a tendency for the overbite to increase in the early stages of treatment as the canines upright. This often results in some extrusion of the incisors and so the overbite deepens. Effective overbite reduction needs stiff archwires and only starts to occur when in stainless steel archwires of at least 0.016″ diameter. However, 0.019″ × 0.025″ stainless steel archwires are most effective and bring about most of the overbite reduction.

Overbite reduction can be aided by placing curves in the wire to level the curve of Spee. In the upper arch an increased (or an upward) curve of Spee is placed and in the lower a reverse (or a downward) curve is placed. These curves do have a tendency to procline the incisors so the wires are often tied back (e.g. a wire ligature tied from the molar to a ball hook on the archwire between the lateral incisor and canine) to maintain the arch length and minimise incisor proclination. Alternatively, torque can be placed in the archwire to retrocline the incisors.

Overjet reduction

Overjet reduction is usually achieved by retracting the upper labial segment. This can be assisted by forward mandibular growth, maxillary restraint, distalisation of maxillary molars and/or advancement of the lower labial segment. Overjet reduction can be brought about using a combination of space-closing mechanics and is usually carried out on a 0.019″ × 0.025″ stainless steel archwire – the working archwire. A variety of auxiliaries can be used alone or in combination to reduce the overjet. These include active tie-backs or springs between the maxillary molars and canine hooks, Class II elastics and/or headgear. Correcting the molar relationship is closely related to overjet reduction, with the molar relationship at the start of overjet reduction influencing the type or combination of mechanics that can be used. For example, if the molars are already Class I at the start of overjet reduction the case cannot withstand further mesial movement of the maxillary molars relative to the mandibular molars. This means that mechanics have to be used to either restrict the mesial movement of the maxillary molars, e.g. by using headgear, or encourage mesial movement of the mandibular molars, e.g. with Class II elastics.

Space closure

Once the overjet has been reduced any residual space needs to be closed. Several auxiliary attachments may be used to bring this about, e.g. active tie-backs, nickel titanium closed coil springs, elastomeric chain and Class II or III elastics. They all have their advantages and disadvantages, but from the evidence of clinical trials that have been undertaken to assess the effectiveness of each method, it would appear that the nickel titanium closed coil springs are the most efficient. They are more expensive than other methods, but this may be offset by a shorter treatment time.

Again consideration has to be given to the molar and canine relationships at the start of space closure so that the correct mechanics can be used. For example, if the overjet is not fully reduced and there is space remaining in the upper and lower arches at the start of space closure, it is useful to be able to use space closing auxiliaries in conjunction with Class II elastics that will close the space in the upper arch by retracting the upper labial segment and the space in the lower by mesial movement of the mandibular molar.

Finishing and detailing

Once the desired incisor, canine and molar relationships have been achieved it is usually necessary to finish and detail the occlusion to achieve the best possible occlusion with all the teeth at their correct inclination and angulation and well interdigitated. At this stage careful attention is paid to the position of the brackets and bands, because if the brackets or bands are incorrectly positioned the teeth will not be in their ideal position. It is therefore quite common for brackets or bands to be repositioned at this stage. If this is undertaken then it usually means that a more flexible archwire, e.g. 0.018″ × 0.025″ braided stainless steel or nickel titanium, has to be placed to regain alignment of the brackets.

Intermaxillary elastics can be used to achieve a well-interdigitated occlusion at the end of treatment. The elastics can be placed in a variety of patterns depending on the requirements of the individual case. It is quite common to run a triangular or rhomboid arrangement of elastics to seat the premolars and molars. The elastics can be run from attachments placed directly onto the bracket, e.g. Kobayashi hooks or power pins, or from ball hooks placed on the archwires. Again more flexible archwires are required to allow the desired tooth movements to take place.

Debond

Once the best possible occlusion has been achieved, arrangements are made to remove the fixed appliance and provide the patient with retaining braces. The debond can be undertaken on a single day (if there is a laboratory on site or nearby) or over two appointments.

When same-day retainers are provided, the fixed appliances are usually removed and impressions taken at the start of the day or session and the retainers are fitted later that day. This means that there is minimal time during which any relapse can occur before the retainers are fitted. If local laboratory facilities are not available it is common for the debond to be carried out over two appointments. At the first appointment, the molar bands are removed and impressions taken to make study models on which the retainers are made. Then, at the second appointment, the brackets are removed, teeth cleaned and retainers fitted.

When removing a fixed appliance the archwires are left *in situ* with the modules/ligatures still in place. This acts as a safety precaution so that all the brackets are held onto the archwire and the risk of a bracket being swallowed or inhaled is minimised. The brackets and bands are removed with specifically designed debonding pliers or a lift-off debonding instrument (LODI). When the brackets and bands have been removed there is usually some residual adhesive left on the tooth. This can then be removed by the orthodontist using either instruments, e.g. a Mitchell's trimmer, or a slow-speed handpiece with a tungsten carbide bur. Any remaining plaque or debris can then be removed by undertaking a full mouth polish with prophylactic paste or pumice.

Retention

Following active orthodontic treatment it is important that the teeth are held in their new position so that relapse does not occur. This stage of treatment is called retention. Retainers maintain the teeth in the position achieved by active orthodontic treatment while the gingival tissues and bone around the teeth heal. Retainers can be removable or fixed to the teeth.

Removable retainers come in a variety of designs. The most commonly used retainer is the **Hawley retainer**, which consists of Adam's cribs on the molars, a labial bow around the canines and incisors, and an acrylic baseplate. Initially retainers are worn full time. This is then reduced, after a period of about six months, to night-time-only wear. After about a year the gingival tissues and supporting bone have healed and the retainer wear can be reduced to two to three nights a week if the patient wishes to maintain the alignment achieved by active orthodontic treatment. Alternatively, the retainers may be discarded but the patient must be made aware that minor tooth movements, especially in the lower labial segment, occur throughout life so there may be some relapse of the alignment if retention is abandoned.

In some cases, e.g. where teeth were rotated or very displaced at the start of treatment, it may be preferable to use a fixed retainer to maintain alignment. Fixed retainers can be made from a stainless steel wire, e.g. 0.017" Twistflex, or as joined prefabricated pads that are then bonded to the lingual surface of the teeth with composite. Bonded retainers provide excellent retention, but occasionally debond. If this occurs the teeth are then free to move (relapse) and become susceptible to caries if the debond is not detected and repaired. It is therefore important that patients report any debond of a fixed retainer immediately so that arrangements for a repair can be made.

Orthodontic assessment

Before any treatment plan is drawn up it is very important to reach a diagnosis. In order to do this the orthodontist must take a history from the patient and parent (if appropriate) and undertake a thorough examination of the hard and soft tissues of the face and mouth. Special investigations such as radiographs, study models and photographs are also required before arriving at the final treatment plan.

History

The history from the patient and parent (if appropriate) is important in establishing the motivating factors and attitude towards treatment. It is also a time when other factors that may have an influence on the proposed treatment may come to light, e.g. difficulty in attending. The history will probably need to be taken from both the patient and parent but it is important that most of the questions are addressed directly to the child rather than via the parent. The history will typically include the following.

■ Patient's presenting complaint – what the patient thinks is wrong with their teeth and/or face and why they think they have come to see the orthodontist. This is the time for the patient to voice their opinion about what they think is wrong. It is important to encourage children to be active at this stage rather than rely on the parent to express their opinion.

■ Patient's past medical history – for children this is best taken from the parent. It needs to include details of:
   □ heart or chest problems
   □ history of congenital heart defect or rheumatic fever
   □ jaundice, diabetes, fits or blackouts
   □ any allergies
   and whether they:
   □ are on any regular drugs or medicines;
   □ are under the care of a hospital consultant;
   □ have been into hospital for any reason.

■ Past dental history – again for children this is best taken from the parent. It needs to include details of:
   □ how often the patient attends their general dental practitioner
   □ previous dental treatment, including restorations or extractions
   □ whether any of their teeth have been subjected to trauma
   □ the patient's ability to cope with treatment.

■ Patient's willingness to wear different types of appliance.

Extra-oral examination

The position of the teeth is largely determined by the lips, tongue and cheeks. To aid the diagnosis and treatment planning for the orthodontic patient, it is important to examine outside as well as inside the mouth. The extra-oral examination of a patient needs to include assessment of the:

■ skeletal pattern (in all three planes of space)
■ the soft tissues (including the lips and tongue)
■ temporomandibular joints.

Skeletal pattern

The skeletal pattern is assessed by examining the patient sitting in an upright, unsupported position, looking straight ahead in all three planes of space. The patient's head is positioned so that the Frankfort plane (see Figure 5.8) is parallel to the floor and the teeth are in occlusion.

Antero-posterior

The skeletal pattern is assessed from the side of the patient using the index and middle fingers. The tips of the fingers are placed in the concavities between the base of the nose and the upper lip and between the lower lip and chin. The skeletal pattern (see Figure 5.7) can be classified as *Class 1* when the index finger is horizontal during the examination (a normal, balanced profile with the mandible 2–3 mm posterior to the maxilla); *Class 2* when the index finger slopes down during the examination (the mandible is retruded relative to the maxilla); or *Class 3* when the index finger slopes upwards during the examination (the mandible is protruded relative to the maxilla).

Vertical

The vertical proportions of the face are again best assessed from the side of the patient. Two relationships can be assessed.

FMPA (Frankfort mandibular plane angle) – by positioning the index finger along the lower border of the mandible, the angle that it makes with the Frankfort plane can be assessed. In a patient with an average FMPA, the two lines will join at the back of the head (occiput). In a patient with an increased FMPA, the lines will cross in front of the back of the head and when the FMPA is reduced they will cross behind the head (see Figure 5.8).

LFH (lower facial height proportion) – again this can be assessed using the index and middle fingers. Their tips can be placed on a point midway between the eyebrows (**glabella**) and where the nose meets the upper lip in the midline (**columella**) and then moved and placed on the columella and the lower border of the chin. The distance from glabella to columella and from columella to the lower border of the chin are about equal when the LFH is of normal proportion. However, if the distance from columella to the lower border of the chin is more than from glabella to columella the LFH is increased, and decreased if glabella to columella is longer than columella to the lower border of the chin (see Figure 5.8).

A lateral cephalometric radiograph can also be used to aid the assessment and diagnosis of the antero-posterior and vertical skeletal pattern.

Transverse

The transverse relationships of the face are best examined from directly in front of the patient or from above and behind the patient. Examination of the transverse relationships identifies any asymmetry in the face. The glabella, columella and the midpoint of the

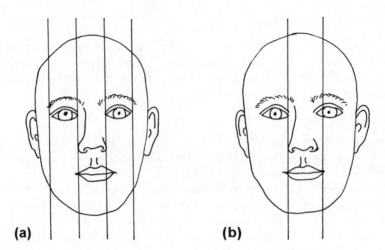

Figure 5.11 Assessment of the transverse relationship: (a) fifths of the face and (b) right line indicates width of the base of the nose (= inter-inner canthal width); left line the width of the mouth (= width between the medial edge of the irises).

chin normally lie in the midline of the face and are in line with each other. The face can also be divided into fifths that are all equal in a symmetrical face. These fifths are from the edge of the face to the outer canthus of the eye; the outer to the inner canthus of the eye; the inter-inner canthal distance; the inner to outer canthus of the eye and the outer canthus to the edge of the face (Figure 5.11a).

In a normally proportioned face, the width of the base of the nose is the same as the inter-inner canthal width, and the width of the mouth is the same as the distance between the medial side of the irises (Figure 5.11b).

Soft tissues

Lips
Several features of the lips need to be assessed. These include the following.

Lip competency – competent lips meet together at rest without there being any undue strain of the lip or chin muscles. If a patient's lips are apart at rest they are said to be **incompetent**. This may be related to the length of the lips, especially the upper or to an increased LFH proportion.

Lower lip position – the relationship of the lower lip to the upper incisors is important in determining their position. Normally the lower lip covers the incisal third of the upper incisors at rest. If the lower lip covers more than this the upper incisors may become retroclined, e.g. Class II division 2 malocclusion. In patients with a severe Class II division 1 incisor relationship the lower lip may lie behind the upper incisors, which leaves the incisors more vulnerable to trauma.

Length of the upper lip – normally the upper lip reveals 2–3 mm of the incisal tip at rest and the entire upper incisor when smiling in girls and a little less in boys. Excessive show of the gingivae or teeth may be due to a short upper lip or vertical maxillary excess (VME). The lips lengthen as patients get older so that the lip competency and length increase with age.

Intra-oral examination

The intra-oral examination of a patient for orthodontic reasons is similar to that performed for routine dental patients but puts more emphasis on the inter- and intra-arch relationships.

Teeth present

This includes recording all teeth that are erupted, partially erupted or palpable, whether they are deciduous or permanent teeth. A note also needs to be made of any teeth that may have compromised prognosis, e.g. due to trauma or caries.

Inter-arch relationships

The following inter-arch relationships are of interest to the orthodontist.

Molar relationship
This usually is taken from the first permanent molars and includes an assessment of whether the teeth occlude in a Class I, II or III relationship (see Figure 5.10) and to what extent. It is possible to have a(¼, ½ or ¾ unit Class II or III relationship depending how far mesial or distal the inter-arch relationship is. For example:

- ½ unit Class II – the buccal cusps of the molars meet tip to tip
- ½ unit Class III – the mesiobuccal cusp of the upper first molar occludes against the distobuccal cusp of the lower first molar.

Canine relationship
This assessment is similar to that of the first permanent molars in that it includes an assessment of whether the teeth occlude in a Class I, II or III relationship and to what extent. For example:

- ½ unit Class II – the upper and lower canine tips meet tip to tip
- ½ unit Class III – the tip of the upper canine occludes against the cusp of the lower first premolar.

Overjet
An overjet (see Diagnostic terms, p. 264) is usually positive but may be negative, i.e. in a Class III incisor relationship where the lower incisors occlude labially to the upper

incisors. The overjet is measured using a metal ruler held parallel to the occlusal plane. It is usual to measure the most prominent part of the central incisors, but in some situations where the incisors are not well aligned, the overjet on other incisors can be measured. For example, in a Class II division 2 incisor relationship it is common for the overjet on the central incisors to be minimal (2 mm) but that on the lateral incisors to be increased.

Overbite

The overbite can be described as:

■ average – the upper incisors overlap the lower incisors by a third of their height
■ reduced – the upper incisors overlap the lower incisors by less than a third of their height
■ increased – the upper incisors overlap the lower incisors by more than a third of their height.

An overbite is also described as:

■ complete – there is contact between the lower incisors and either the upper incisors, dentogingival junction or the palate
■ incomplete – the lower incisors do not contact any hard or soft tissue.

An anterior open bite (AOB) exists when the upper incisors do not overlap the lower incisors.

Centre-line relationship

The upper and lower centre-lines are assessed in relation to each other and the midline of the face. Any discrepancy between the upper and lower centre-lines is measured in millimetres or expressed as a proportion of the lower incisor width (e.g. ¼, ½ or ¾ or full tooth). The relationship of the centre-lines to the midline of the face can be viewed from above and behind the patient. It can be described as:

■ co-incident – dental centre-lines line up with the midline of the face
■ deviated – dental centre-lines are displaced to the right or left of the midline of the face.

Crossbite and scissors bite

In the normal relationship, the upper teeth occlude labially/buccally to the lower teeth. A crossbite exists if any upper tooth is positioned so that it occludes palatal to a lower tooth (Figure 5.12) and can involve one or more teeth, a whole segment or whole arch. A crossbite can involve anterior or posterior teeth. It can involve a single tooth, a segment or the whole arch and can be unilateral or bilateral.

When a crossbite is found, the occlusion needs to be checked for premature contacts and displacements on closing from the RCP to the ICP. Patients with a unilateral crossbite often have a premature contact and displacement on closing, which may predispose them

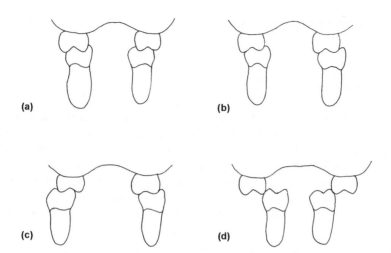

Figure 5.12 Buccal crossbite: (a) normal relationship; (b) unilateral buccal crossbite; (c) bilateral buccal crossbite; and (d) bilateral scissors bite.

to TMD (see Risks of orthodontic treatment, p. 269). A scissors bite exists if any tooth in the upper buccal segment is positioned so that its palatal cusp occludes buccal to the buccal cusp of a lower tooth and can involve a single tooth or a whole segment and can be unilateral or bilateral.

Although typically crossbites and scissors bites are due to a discrepancy in the transverse width of the dental arches, they may also be related to the antero-posterior relationship of the dental bases. In a Class III case, crossbites are more common because the mandible is relatively more anterior than normal so that, at any point, a wider part of the mandibular dental arch occludes with the maxillary dental arch than in a Class I situation. Similarly, in a Class II case, scissors bites are more common because the mandible is relatively more posterior than normal so that, at any point, a narrower part of the mandibular dental arch occludes with the maxillary dental arch than in a Class I situation.

Intra-arch relationships

When assessing the intra-arch relationships, the contact displacement, both mesiodistally and vertically, between adjacent teeth needs to be measured as this gives an indication of the degree of crowding/spacing. The inclination (buccolingual tip), angulation (mesiodistal tip) and any rotations of the teeth also need to be assessed. For this purpose each dental arch is usually divided into three segments. This allows the assessment to give an indication of whether there is a general problem or if it is localised to a particular segment. The segments are the:

- labial segment – canine to canine
- buccal segments (right and left) – first premolar to the last molar.

The degree of crowding/spacing can be described as:

- mild – 1–2 mm
- moderate – 2–4 mm
- severe – more than 4 mm.

Assessment of the inclination and angulation of the teeth is important to determine the most appropriate extraction to provide adequate space to relieve any crowding, and also what type of appliances might be required to bring about the desired tooth movements. When simple tipping movements are required, e.g. if the upper incisors are very proclined or the canines mesially tipped, it may be possible to bring these about using removable appliances. However, if the teeth are upright or distally inclined, bodily movement will be required which can only be brought about by fixed appliances.

Soft tissues

Gingival condition
The gingival condition is closely related to the level of oral hygiene and may be a better reflection of it than the amount of plaque on the teeth at the time of the assessment. This is because it is quite common for patients to make a special effort with their oral hygiene on the day of the visit so that the teeth appear clean. However, this may not be their usual practice and if there is a difference, the effects of poor oral hygiene will be reflected in the gingival condition, e.g. there will be gingivitis in areas that are not normally cleaned or abrasions where the toothbrushing has been particularly vigorous. A patient's level of oral hygiene is important because poor plaque control is the main contributing factor to the most common side effect of orthodontic treatment, namely decalcification.

It is rare for children to have more advanced periodontal problems but all adults need to be assessed for their periodontal state prior to orthodontic treatment because it can accelerate the progression of periodontitis leading to bone loss around the affected teeth.

Tongue
The tongue normally lies behind the lower incisors at rest. However, in some malocclusions its position is different. It is debatable whether an abnormal tongue position has caused the malocclusion or whether the tongue position is an adaptation to the malocclusion. This is best illustrated in patients with an AOB where the tongue often protrudes to fill the gap. Has the anteriorly positioned tongue caused the AOB or has the tongue had to protrude to form an anterior seal?

Fraenal attachments
Occasionally fraenal attachments can contribute to a malocclusion. The most common situation is a median diastema associated with a low or fleshy upper midline fraenum. There is debate about whether a **fraenectomy** (surgical removal of the fraenum) is required and if so when it is carried out. The advantage of carrying out surgery before

orthodontic treatment is that the surgical access is easier, but some argue that if the surgery is carried out once the diastema is closed, the resulting scar tissue may help to prevent relapse. However, others suggest that the use of a bonded retainer to prevent relapse is necessary even following a fraenectomy and so surgery is unnecessary if the patient is to be provided with one.

Occasionally a fraenum may be in a position that prevents adequate oral hygiene, pulls on the gingival margin or is so large that it is unsightly. In these situations there may be another justification for performing a fraenectomy rather than solely to prevent orthodontic relapse.

Oral hygiene

As stressed in other sections of this chapter, good oral hygiene is a prerequisite to orthodontic treatment so as to minimise damage to the gingivae and enamel surface. The most common side effects of orthodontic treatment are gingivitis and decalcification of the enamel. Gingivitis usually reduces once the appliances have been removed, but areas of decalcified enamel remain. For these reasons every effort needs to be made to minimise these risks if orthodontic treatment is going to be of net benefit to patients. Advice and instruction on oral hygiene needs to start before any appliances are placed, and reinforced throughout treatment. This advice may be given by the orthodontist but may be more effective if given by a specialist dental nurse or hygienist who may have more time available and be able to convey the necessary message in a less intimidating environment, e.g. in a specially designated dental health education area away from the chairside (see Chapter 2).

Special investigations

Study models

Study models are used to record the treatment from start to finish and are used to observe the changes that take place throughout the orthodontic procedure.

Impressions of the upper and lower jaws are taken and reproduced as study models. Each impression needs to include all teeth in the jaw and have full extension of the sulcus. The impression ought to be cast as soon as possible, and a model made and the impressions removed from the models as soon as the stone has fully set. The models are trimmed so that they can be articulated in any position that may be required for observation purposes (Figure 5.13).

Radiographs

Radiographs are a valuable addition to the information gathered during the examination of a patient. They are used to assess facial and dentoskeletal relationships and to identify any missing, unerupted or impacted teeth. Radiographs require the use of ionising radiation and for this reason they must be used sparingly. The British Orthodontic Society has

Figure 5.13 Orthodontic study models: (a) in occlusion; and (b) occlusal view.

produced *Guidelines for the use of Radiographs in Clinical Orthodontics* (Isaacson *et al.*, 2008) that are designed to help the clinician choose and take the most appropriate radiographs at the most appropriate time. The guidelines strongly advise against the routine use of radiographs for screening purposes and stress the need for radiographs to provide information that will benefit the patient and that the management of the patient's condition depends on information contained in the radiograph. The most commonly used radiographs in orthodontics are the orthopantomograph (OPG/OPT; panoramic radiograph), lateral cephalogram and intra-oral views of the teeth in the upper labial segment, e.g. periapical radiographs of *3–/–3* or a standard midline occlusal (SMO).

Orthopantomograph
This radiograph is very useful for screening. It is a rotational view and uses the technique of tomography whereby a *slice* view is taken through the mandible and maxilla. The OPG can be used to identify the presence and position of unerupted teeth, root development

and pathology associated with the teeth, mandible or maxilla. It is possible to detect large carious lesions but intra-oral radiographs, e.g. bitewings or periapicals, are more appropriate to detect caries.

Lateral cephalogram

The cephalometric radiograph (ceph) is a widely used diagnostic tool in orthodontics. It was developed by Broadbent in the 1930s and provides a two-dimensional, standardised, lateral (side on) image of a patient's facial bones and the base of the skull.

A lateral ceph is taken with a specially adapted x-ray machine called a **cephalostat**. The machine has the x-ray camera positioned at a certain distance away from the patient, and the patient is placed at a set distance from the x-ray film. The patient's head is held in a fixed position by two ear rods that fit into the patient's external acoustic meati (earholes). As the camera and patient are always in this standardised position it means that a radiograph taken at one point in time can reliably be compared with one taken at another point in time.

Most radiographs are taken to look at bones; however, the cephalostat is specially adapted with an aluminium filter towards the front of the face so that the amount of x-rays reaching the x-ray film is reduced and therefore a picture of the soft-tissue contour (nose, lips and chin) is obtained. To prevent x-rays dosing the brain the beam is restricted mainly to the face; this restriction of the beam is called collimation.

Lateral cephs allow the A-P (antero-posterior; front-to-back) and vertical relationships of the teeth, jaws and soft tissues to be assessed. They will not, however, allow the analysis of the transverse (width/side-to-side) relationships as one side is superimposed on another.

To assess transverse relationships a standardised view of the patient from the front can be taken. This is called a PA ceph (postero-anterior cephalogram). These are used less frequently than lateral cephs but can be useful for looking at transverse relationships such as jaw asymmetries, e.g. after a young patient has damaged one of their mandibular condyles.

The lateral cephalogram has several uses:

- diagnosis
  - □ hard tissues
  - □ soft tissues
  - □ pathology
- growth prediction/changes
- treatment planning
- treatment progress
- research.

Diagnosis: Lateral cephalograms (cephs) are used to aid diagnosis and treatment planning and provide a baseline for monitoring treatment progress. They also provide a medico-legal record, and together with photographs they allow the soft tissues to be assessed.

Points

Po	Porion
S	Sella
N	Nasion
Or	Orbitale
PNS	Posterior nasal spine
ANS	Anterior nasal spine
A	A point
B	B point
Pog	Pogonion
Gn	Gnathion
Me	Menton
Go	Gonion

Figure 5.14 Cephalometric points.

Hard tissues: These include the underlying bones as well as the teeth. The method of assessing the relationship of the different bony structures and teeth is called cephalometric analysis (Figures 5.14 and 5.15; Table 5.4). **Cephalometrics** is the measurement of the head and allows objective assessment of the relationships, both angular and linear, of the teeth, jaws and soft tissues.

To analyse a lateral ceph requires a tracing of different points and outlines on the radiograph. The simplest way to do this is to use a piece of tracing paper secured over the top of the radiograph. To ensure the detail is easy to see, it is important to trace the ceph on a light box in a darkened room. It is best to trace the ceph using a fine, hard pencil (≤0.5 mm, 2H). Alternatively, a digitiser can be used to electronically register where all the landmarks are. Various computer programs exist that will then calculate all the relevant lengths, distances and angles.

There are many different landmarks that can be located and lines that can be drawn to give useful diagnostic information (see case example in Figure 5.15 and Table 5.4). However, the key things to identify include:

Lines

Fr Pl   Frankfort plane
Mx Pl   Maxillary plane
Md Pl   Mandibular plane
UFH   Upper face height
LFH   Lower face height
UFH + LFH = Total face height

Angles

1   SNB
2   SNA
3   ANB
4   UIMx (Upper incisor to maxillary plane)
5   UILI   Interincisal angle
6   LIMd   (Lower incisor to mandibular plane)

Figure 5.15 Cephalometric lines and angles.

Table 5.4 Cephalometric analysis.

Measurement	Case	Average (Eastman standard for Caucasians)
SNA (2)	86°	81° ± 3°
SNB (1)	80°	78° ± 3°
ANB (3)	6°	3° ± 2°
Maxillary/mandibular planes angle (MMPA)	17°	27° ± 4°
UI to Maxillary plane (4)	124°	109° ± 6°
LI to Mandibular plane (6)	93°	93° ± 6° or 120°– MMPA
Inter-incisal angle (5)	126°	135° ± 10°
LI to APog line	−4 mm	+1 ± 2 mm
LFH as % of total face height	52%	55 ± 2%

See Figure 5.15 for explanation of the planes and angles.

■ the relative size and position of the maxilla and mandible (Class 1, 2 or 3)
■ the steepness of the angle between the jaws (MMPA)
■ the angles of the upper and lower incisors to each other and their skeletal base.

Lateral cephalograms can be used in isolation, e.g. for treatment planning or to compare changes occurring over time that may be related to treatment effects with or without growth changes. If used as a comparison, the individual radiographs are traced/digitised and then the individual tracings are superimposed on each other so that the comparative changes can be visualised and measured. Superimpositions can be used to compare an individual radiograph to the average or norm (e.g. Bolton Standards) and to determine changes occurring due to growth, treatment and/or relapse. Superimpositions can be made on **De Coster's line** (base of skull), the sella-nasion line, maxillary or mandibular plane, **Bjork's structures** (lingual plate of the mandibular symphysis; crypt of the mandibular third molar; inferior dental nerve canal and anterior chin point) and/or implants. Superimposition on each of these structures will alter the perception of the changes that have occurred.

The difficulty with tracing cephs is that, even for an experienced person, identification of some of the landmarks can be very difficult so that measurements taken from them are inaccurate. Errors in cephalometric analysis can occur at all stages of obtaining the radiograph and tracing. These include problems when positioning the patient, especially rotations and then identifying the landmarks, operator reliability and the analysis used. This means that the values obtained from ceph analysis are used as a guide in context with other information gathered from the history and examination.

Soft tissues: If a ceph is taken properly the soft-tissue outline ought to be clearly visible. The lengths, thickness and relative prominence of the nose, lips and chin and how they relate to the underlying skeleton and teeth can then be measured.

Pathology: Cephs, like other radiographs, can also be used to identify pathology. It is unlikely that caries can be identified, but rarer things such as jaw cysts and tumours may be seen. More importantly, from an orthodontic point of view, it is possible to look at the position of impacted teeth, such as canines, and root length as the roots of anterior teeth can be well visualised.

Growth prediction/changes: By taking views at different times it is possible to compare the difference between the two or more dates by superimposing one tracing on top of another. If no orthodontic treatment has been undertaken then these changes will be due solely to growth. This technique is particularly useful for patients with a Class 3 jaw relationship to see if they have finished growing before orthodontic treatment is carried out in preparation for orthognathic (jaw) surgery to correct an underlying skeletal discrepancy.

Some investigators have looked at large groups of normally growing patients and produced a ceph tracing that shows the average shape and size of males and females at different ages. By superimposing a patient's ceph on top of the average tracing it may be possible to see how a patient differs from this 'normal'. This technique is known as using a proportional template.

Some analyses attempt to predict how a patient may grow in the future by looking at their current growth trend. This technique can work well if a patient is already growing fairly normally, but if a patient is not following a normal growth trend it is difficult to predict how the patient will grow in the future.

Treatment planning: It is possible to move the teeth on the tracing into the ideal positions and angles, and plan goals of where to move teeth to.

Cephs are essential in planning orthognathic surgery. Computer programmes (e.g. Opal, Quick ceph, Dolphin) can be used to simulate the repositioning of the teeth and jaws so that the distance and direction of movement required can be quantified.

Treatment progress: By taking views during treatment, movement of the teeth and jaws can be measured and treatment can be modified accordingly. Common times to take a progress ceph include:

- after using a functional appliance
- when undertaking orthodontic treatment prior to orthognathic surgery
- when assessing the position of the lower incisors, e.g. during Tip-Edge (see p. 296) or non-extraction treatment
- near the end of treatment – this can be useful to evaluate the changes caused by treatment and in the auditing of cases.

In growing patients, changes taking place during treatment are actually due to a combination of treatment effect and growth. However, in non-growing adults, any changes will be due to treatment alone.

Research tool: The technique of ceph taking and analysis is simple, relatively reproducible and internationally recognised. All of these factors make the ceph a valuable tool to use in research.

Several growth studies were conducted in the past where the growth of normal children, who had not received orthodontic treatment, was monitored every year with a ceph to establish normal growth patterns. However, such studies would not be undertaken today because of ethical considerations.

Most of what is known about how appliances work and how they move teeth has come from studies that have compared the cephalometric changes brought about by different treatments.

It is very important to realise that cephs form only part of the diagnostic information available and that data obtained from them must be integrated with findings from the clinical examination, study models and other diagnostic records. It is very easy to make errors when measuring angles and lines on the ceph, particularly if those lines and angles are formed from points that were difficult to see. Unfortunately most of the measurements or templates that patients can be compared to are averages of a small number of the population. With regard to estimating future growth changes, if a patient is growing normally it is likely that they will continue to do so. However, if they are growing abnormally then it is difficult to predict how they will grow in the future, i.e. we can predict the predictable but we can't predict the unpredictable.

Intra-oral radiographs

Periapical radiographs of 3–|–3 or an SMO can be used to assess the root length and morphology of the teeth in the upper labial segment. These radiographs are often requested to supplement information that can be obtained from an OPG. This is because the definition on an OPG in this area is often poor. They can also be used, in conjunction with an OPG or another intra-oral radiograph taken at a different angle, to assess the position of unerupted teeth, e.g. canines, relative to the line of the arch. The principle of parallax can be used to determine whether the unerupted tooth lies buccal or palatal to the line of the arch. If the tooth is lying buccal to the line of the arch it will appear to move in the opposite direction from the way the radiographic tube moved between taking the two images. If the tooth is lying palatal to the line of the arch it will appear to move in the same direction as the radiographic tube moved. NB: This can easily be checked by closing one eye and aligning your two index fingers and then moving your head to see what effect it has on the relative position of your fingers. The finger furthest away (palatal) from your eye (radiographic tube) will move in the same direction that your head moved (Figure 5.16). Comparison of the OPG (Figure 5.16a) with the periapi-

(a)

(b)　　　　　**(c)**

Figure 5.16 Unerupted maxillary canines: (a) OPG showing unerupted 3/3 overlying the pulp of 1/, mesial aspect /1 and apical third of the 1/1 roots; (b, c) peri-apical radiographs of 3/3 lying between 21/12 and near the apex of 1/1 roots.

cals (Figure 5.16b and Figure 5.16c) demonstrates parallax. Compared with the x-ray beam for the OPG, the beam has moved apically and distally to take the periapicals. This is in the same direction as the superimposition of the canine on the underlying incisors, which suggests that the unerupted 3|3 are lying palatal (lingual) to 21|12, i.e. **S**ame **L**ingual, **O**pposite **P**alatal or SLOB.

Recent advances in radiography include the introduction of **digital radiographs** that use either a charge coupled device (CCD) or phosphorus screen to produce them. The main advantage of digital images is that they expose the patient to up to 90% less radiation. It is also possible to alter the contrast of digital radiographs, which can help in obtaining a more accurate tracing. As they are digital images, they can be stored and transmitted electronically, which can aid communication between clinicians by making it easier for the images to be shared.

Photographs

Photographic records are taken before treatment commences, during treatment and post-treatment. They record the severity of malocclusion and enable the patient to judge the improvements that have been made. They are a useful record of any pre-existing pathology, decalcification or trauma to the teeth.

A complete photographic record is obtained as follows.

Initial visit
At a patient's first visit four or five standard extra-oral and intra-oral views are usually taken.

- The standard extra-oral views are (Figure 5.17a):
  - full face
  - full face smiling (this shows the lip line)
  - profile
  - three-quarters view on each side
- The standard intra-oral views are (Figure 5.17b):
  - anterior in occlusion
  - buccal – left and right sides in occlusion
  - occlusal – upper and lower.

A close-up of any areas of concern (e.g. fractures, hypoplasia, hypomineralisation, non-vital teeth, site of premature contact, fraenal attachment) can also be taken.

Mid-treatment
A selection of appropriate photographs can be taken to monitor the progress of treatment. These may include any of the standard intra-oral or extra-oral views, a close-up of any areas of unusual or noteworthy mechanics or any problem areas.

Figure 5.17 A set of clinical photographs: (a) extra-oral; and (b) intra-oral.

Post-treatment

At the end of treatment it is usual to repeat the pre-treatment views so that a direct comparison and an assessment of the changes brought about by treatment can be made.

Recommended tasks

(1) What information can be gained from a lateral cephalogram and how does it help in the management of a patient undergoing orthodontic treatment?

(2) Complete the following sentence by comparing the values for the case in Table 5.4 with the average values.

This case has a Class _____ incisor relationship on a Class _____ skeletal base with _____ vertical proportions, _____ upper incisors and _____ lower incisors.

Orthodontic appliances and treatment options

Extractions only

Occasionally the situation exists when a malocclusion can be managed by extracting teeth only. This is rarely an ideal line of treatment, but if a patient's ability or willingness to cope with orthodontic appliances, e.g. oral hygiene level or a mental or physical disability, is not suitable, it may be the best option for that patient.

Another situation where extractions only may be a suitable option is when there is severe crowding and a tooth is completely excluded from the arch and the adjacent teeth are contacting and in an acceptable relationship, e.g. a buccally or palatally excluded upper canine where the lateral incisor and first premolar are contacting.

Fixed appliances

Fixed appliances are mainly used to achieve tooth movements that are not possible with removable appliances. These appliances are fixed to the teeth and forces are applied by archwires or auxiliaries through these attachments. These appliances can:

- tip – change the mesiodistal angle of teeth
- torque – change the buccolingual inclination of teeth
- rotate
- bodily move teeth.

A fixed appliance has attachments (brackets, tubes, bands), which are attached to the teeth by composite resins (brackets, tubes) or cement (bands).

Bands

Bands are made from stainless steel and come in a variety of sizes. The band size is either etched or painted on the outside of the band. Tubes may be connected to the bands, and the sizes are 0.018″ or 0.022″. These tubes match the slot size of the bracket. There are single, double or triple tube attachments. They are made to accommodate the archwire and headgear.

Choosing and fitting bands

The bands chosen need to fit the tooth snugly and are held in place by a combination of correct fit and cement. The band needs to be clean and dry before the application of the cement. It is essential that the entire surface of the band is coated with cement to prevent any voids, which may allow plaque to accumulate and in turn result in demineralisation or caries. The band is placed into position with a band seater or bite stick. Any excess cement can be removed with a cotton wool roll or instrument before it is set.

Brackets

Brackets are fixed directly onto the teeth, usually with a composite material (either chemically or light cured). Brackets have:

- tie wings – around which the modules and ligatures are tied
- slot – into which the arch wire is placed
- base – that is curved horizontally and vertically to ensure a good fit against the tooth
- identification marks – on the distogingival tie wings of most brackets.

The angle of the slot, both mesiodistally (tip) and buccolingually (torque), and the depth of the base vary for each tooth. This is known as the **prescription** of the bracket, the best known of which are Andrews', Roth and MBT (McLaughlin, Bennett and Trevesi). See below for more details.

Brackets are usually made from stainless steel, but plastic and ceramic brackets are also available. Plastic brackets can stain and distort during treatment. Ceramic brackets do not stain but they:

- are brittle and can fracture
- are extremely hard and may cause wear of opposing enamel
- may increase the risk of enamel damage at debond
- have increased friction, which makes it harder for the teeth to slide along the archwire. To overcome this, brackets have been developed (e.g. Clarity) that have a metal insert into the bracket slot
- are more expensive.

Types of brackets

Edgewise brackets were introduced by Edward Angle in 1928 and had a rectangular archwire channel with the largest dimension horizontally. They accepted both round and rectangular wires into which bends were placed to bring the teeth into the correct position.

Begg brackets were developed by Raymond Begg in the 1950s and have a narrow vertical slot for the archwire to lie in, which allows the tooth to tip freely in all directions. Begg brackets are only used with round wires and are held in place with brass pins or auxiliaries (see Figure 5.18).

Pre-adjusted edgewise brackets (Straight Wire Appliance) were developed from the original edgewise brackets and introduced by Lawrence Andrews in the 1970s. They have tip and torque adjustments built into the slot of the brackets and the depth of the base of the brackets gives them their in/out control. This allows the teeth to be moved into their correct positions on straight wires, thus minimising the need for complicated wire bending. The amount of tip, torque and in/out control in the brackets is known as the **bracket prescription**. There are several bracket prescriptions (e.g. Andrews', Roth, MBT), each of which have advantages or disadvantages in specific situations (see Table 5.5). The Andrews prescription was the original pre-adjusted prescription and was based on the

Figure 5.18 Begg bracket. Reproduced with permission of TP Orthodontics Europe.

Table 5.5 Comparison of Andrews, Roth and MBT bracket prescriptions.

		Final crown tip			Final root torque		
		Andrews	**Roth**	**MBT**	**Andrews**	**Roth**	**MBT**
Maxillary	Central incisor	5	5	4	7	12	17
	Lateral incisor	9	9	8	3	8	10
	Canine	11	13	8	−7	−2	−7
	1st premolar	2	0	0	−7	−7	−7
	2nd premolar	2	0	0	−7	−7	−7
	1st molar	5	0	0	−9	−14	−14
Mandibular	Central incisor	2	2	0	−1	−1	−1
	Lateral incisor	2	2	0	−1	−1	−1
	Canine	5	7	3	−11	−11	−11
	1st premolar	2	−1	2	−17	−17	−17
	2nd premolar	2	−1	2	−22	−22	−22
	1st molar	2	−1	0	−30	−30	−30

finding of the average values for tip, torque and in/out control of 120 untreated subjects with ideal occlusions. Following this Roth changed the prescription slightly to give more torque in the upper incisors because he thought that they tended to be left a little upright at the end of treatment when using the Andrews prescription brackets. Roth also changed the torque in the canines and the tip in the canines, premolars and molars to be less anchorage demanding. The MBT prescription is the most recent development and has increased torque in the lower incisors to increase their anchorage potential, and upper incisors to help prevent them from being too upright at the end of treatment. There is reduced lingual crown torque in the lower molars to prevent them from rolling but increased buccal root torque in the upper molars to lift the palatal cups and help prevent the introduction of occlusal interferences.

Figure 5.19 Tipp-Edge plus bracket. Reproduced with permission of TP Orthodontics Europe.

Tip-Edge brackets were designed by Peter Kesling and introduced in 1986 (see Figure 5.19). They are a combination of a Begg bracket, to allow free tipping of teeth on a round wire in the early stages of treatment, and pre-adjusted edgewise brackets that give precision in the later stages of treatment when a rectangular wire is in place allowing the in-built prescription to be expressed. More recently the Tip-Edge Plus bracket has been introduced. As well as having a rectangular slot has a 'deep tunnel' through which a second archwire passes. There are three distinct stages during treatment with the Tip-Edge system. In **Stage I**, the teeth are aligned, the overjet and overbite reduced and any rotations and crossbites corrected and in **Stage II**, any residual extraction space is closed. In the final stage, **Stage III**, the final tip, torque and in/out control are achieved. Round archwires are used in the first two stages of treatment. Rectangular archwires are then used in the final stage of treatment, in combination with flexible nickel titanium arch wires in the deep tunnels, to allow all the in-built tip and torque of the bracket prescription to be expressed.

A more recent development of the pre-adjusted edgewise brackets are **self-ligating brackets**, e.g. Damon, SmartClip, Activa, Speed (see Figure 5.20). These brackets have the in-built tip, torque and in/out features of conventional pre-adjusted edgewise brackets but, rather than using elastomeric or wire ligatures to hold the archwires in place, they have an inbuilt clip that either holds on to the wire, e.g. SmartClip, or closes over the wire to prevent it from coming out of the slot, e.g. Damon, Activa, Speed. Their alleged advantages are that it takes less chairside time to change or re-ligate an archwire, the clinician is less reliant on their dental nurse at this stage and there is less friction between the archwire and the bracket, allowing the teeth to move more freely and, hopefully, treatment to be shorter. The evidence for these advantages is weak, but larger randomised clinical trials are being carried out to test these claims.

(a)   (b)

Figure 5.20 Self-ligating brackets. (a) Damon 3mx-340. Reproduced with permission of Ormco Europe. Copyright © Ormco Corporation. (b) Smart-Clip™ brace. Reproduced with permission of 3M Unitek. © 2010 3M Unitek. All rights reserved.

Archwires

The choice of archwire depends on the stage of treatment it is being used in and the properties needed to bring about the tooth movements that are required. At the **initial alignment** stage an archwire is used that provides gentle forces, is flexible enough to engage the brackets on the malaligned teeth and is resistant to breakage. Nickel titanium (NiTi) wires, e.g. Sentalloy, are most commonly used at this stage as they have the ability to return to their original shape after they are distorted, i.e. they have **shape memory**, which in turn moves the teeth. Stainless steel wires can also be used at this stage but as stainless steel needs to have a very small diameter to be flexible enough to tie into irregular teeth, individual strands are twisted into a larger diameter wire to prevent breakage, e.g. Twist-Flex. After the initial alignment has occurred, a transition archwire is needed that is midway in size and stiffness between the aligning and working archwires. This wire can be larger diameter nickel titanium, e.g. 0.018″ × 0.025″, or stainless steel, e.g. 0.018″ or 0.020″. During the **mid-treatment** stage, archwires are used to reduce the overbite and move individual or groups of teeth to reduce the overjet and close residual space as required. Most of the tooth movement at this stage is done on 0.019″ × 0.025″ stainless steel working archwires when using an 0.022″ × 0.028″ pre-adjusted edgewise appliance. **Finishing** archwires are usually flexible to allow final adjustments to tooth position to be made. Braided stainless steel archwires can be used that are made up of many fine strands that are woven into a rectangular arch wire, e.g. 0.018″ × 0.025″. Alternatively, beta-titanium can be used as it can be deformed easily, unlike normal nickel titanium that is used earlier in treatment. The finishing tooth movements can be brought about using bends in the archwire or by using elastics to seat the teeth.

Table 5.6 Effect of thickness on the stiffness of round stainless steel wire.

Diameter (")	Relative stiffness
0.014	1.00
0.016	1.71
0.018	2.73
0.020	4.16

Table 5.7 Effect of interbracket span on stiffness.

Span (mm)	Relative stiffness
6.0	1.0
5.0	1.7
4.0	3.4
3.0	8.0
2.0	27.0

Force applied by archwires

Ideally, archwires exert the lowest force necessary to achieve the desired tooth movement. The amount of force that an archwire exerts depends on its **stiffness**, which in turn is related to the **thickness** of the wire, its **length** and the type of **material** the archwire is made of. The stiffness of a round wire is proportional to its **diameter** to the power of four, i.e. stiffness $\propto$ (diameter)^4. This means that small increases in size lead to large increments in the stiffness and in turn the force delivered (see Table 5.6). For rectangular wires the stiffness is proportional to the width of the wire multiplied by the cube of the height, i.e. for a 0.019" × 0.022" archwire the vertical stiffness $\propto$ (0.019) x (0.022)^3. However, the horizontal stiffness increases even more for small changes in size, which means that it is very difficult to correct rotated teeth on a rectangular archwire.

The stiffness of a wire is inversely proportional to its **length** cubed, i.e. stiffness $\propto 1/$ (length)^3. This means that as the distance between two brackets decreases, e.g. between the lower incisors compared to the upper incisors, the stiffness increases dramatically (see Table 5.7).

The stiffness of wires made from different materials is dependent on its Young's modulus, which determines how far it will bend under any given force.

Archwire materials

The main archwire materials used in orthodontics include stainless steel, nickel titanium (e.g. nitinol, sentalloy, titanol) and beta-titanium (titanium molybdenum alloy- TMA).

Stainless steel is made from chromium and nickel, in an 18:8 ratio, together with some iron. Stainless steel:

- is relatively stiff but can be made more flexible by twisting several very thin lengths of wire together, e.g. three strands of 0.0075″ to give an 0.016″ multistrand archwire that has similar flexibility to a similar sized nickel titanium archwire
- is easily adjusted allowing bends and curves to be placed in the wires as required
- has low friction so that the brackets move along the wire more easily
- can be welded and soldered allowing it to be joined to other components, e.g. ball hooks
- is relatively cheap, thus making it a near ideal archwire.

Nickel titanium archwires come in many forms and their structure determines their mechanical properties. Changes in the structure of the NiTi wires can be brought about by deflecting the archwire, e.g. when tying it into a displaced tooth (Chinese NiTi, Nitinol SE, Sentinol, Titanol), or a change in temperature, e.g. when placing the wire into the mouth (Thermal NiTi, Neo-Sentalloy). The heat-activated NiTi wires are flexible at room temperature; they become even more flexible if cooled but stiffer when warmed up, e.g. in the mouth. This means that the wire can be tied into displaced teeth more easily if cooled, e.g. with ethyl chloride, and then when the wire warms up in the mouth it becomes stiffer and returns to its original shape taking the attached teeth with it.

The changes in structure that can be brought about by deflecting the wire or by temperature change allow NiTi wires to exhibit:

- shape memory, i.e. they return to their preformed shape having been tied into a displaced tooth in the mouth
- super elasticity, i.e. the ability of the wire to exert the same force over a wide range of deflection.

More recently NiTi wires have been developed with added copper (Copper NiTi) and they have the added benefit of:

- tolerating repeated loading and unloading better, which is good in cases with severely displaced or rotated teeth where the archwire will stay in place for several visits during the alignment phase
- increasing its strength
- allowing the temperature at which it changes its structure to be changed.

Stabilised beta (β) titanium (TMA) is made from 80% titanium, 10% molybdenum and 6% zirconium. Its stiffness for any given wire size lies between stainless steel and nickel titanium archwires. It is formable, allowing curves and bends to be put into the archwire. It is also weldable allowing it to be joined to other wire or auxiliaries if necessary. These properties mean that it can bring about precise tooth movements making it a good archwire for the finishing stages of treatment.

Auxiliaries

These are:

- ligatures
- elastics
- springs
- separators.

Advantages and disadvantages of fixed appliances

Advantages

- They can be used for multiple tooth movement.
- Precise control over force distribution to individual teeth is possible.

Disadvantages

- They are complex to make and use.
- The components are usually costly.
- Oral hygiene is more difficult to maintain.

Removable appliances

Removable appliances are orthodontic appliances that can be removed from the mouth by the patient for cleaning. They can be used as active appliances where springs, wires, bows, screws, elastics or the acrylic baseplate are designed to achieve tooth movement. Their main **advantages** are that it is easy for patients to maintain good oral hygiene, they are simple, relatively cheap to make, easy to adjust and they can be a useful addition to fixed appliances. However, these features can be a **disadvantage** in that patients can take them out and leave them out; removable appliances can only tilt the teeth, are inefficient at moving multiple teeth, can affect patients' speech and lower ones are difficult to tolerate. The **indications** for removable appliances include being used to guide the eruption of teeth, tip teeth, reduce overbites, maintain space and act as appliances to apply headgear to and retainers.

When designing a removable appliance it needs to have components that are active, provide retention and anchorage that are joined together by a baseplate. Active components include springs, bows and screws. Clasps and bows can provide retention and anchorage while the baseplate joins the components together and can help provide retention and anchorage.

Active components

Springs are made from 0.5–0.7mm diameter stainless steel wire. The force delivered by a spring depends on how far it is deflected together with the length, radius (½ diameter) and stiffness of the wire. The force is inversely proportional to the cube of the length and proportional to the radius to the power of four, i.e. $\text{Force} \propto \dfrac{\text{Deflection} \times \text{Radius}^4}{\text{Length}^3}$.

This means that if the length of the wire is doubled the force applied is reduced to an eighth of the original, but if the radius is doubled the force increases by a factor of 16. To increase the length of the wire in a spring, coils or loops are often incorporated into their design, and to keep the force applied low, as thin a wire as possible (that won't fracture or be distorted easily) is used, which in practice is 0.5 mm diameter, but even so they will need some protection either from acrylic (e.g. palatal finger spring) or an outer casing of wider diameter tubing along part of its length (e.g. buccal canine retractor).

Springs can apply their force from the palatal or buccal side. Straight **palatal springs** are used to move a tooth along the line of the arch e.g. a premolar or canine. The force needs to be applied at a point that is at right angles to the direction the tooth needs to move. The spring is activated to provide about 40 g of force. The amount of deflection required to deliver this force will depend on the diameter of the wire but is in the region of 2–3 mm for a 0.5 mm diameter wire but only 1–1½ mm for a 0.7 mm diameter wire. Springs should be activated as close to the coil or loop as possible using spring former pliers (no. 65). **Z-springs** (double cantilever) can be used to procline incisors, e.g. to correct an anterior crossbite, whereas **T-springs** can move canines, premolars or molars buccally. Z-springs are activated by pulling the labial arm forward parallel to the direction of the tooth movement required. T-springs are activated by lifting the 'T' away from the baseplate. **Buccal retractors** are used on teeth, usually canines, which have been displaced buccally and need to be moved palatally as well as distally; they can be made of 0.5 mm diameter wire but tend to be very vulnerable to distortion or breakage, so the ascending arm tends to be protected by a 0.7 mm diameter tube. If they are made out of only 0.7 mm diameter wire they have a limited range of action due to the increased force for any deflection that is produced by the larger diameter wire (see above).

Bows join two loops (e.g. U-loops in a labial bow) or springs (e.g. buccal retractors in a Roberts' retractor) together across the labial segment and can be used to tip teeth palatally or lingually. A labial bow can be used to bring about a small reduction in overjet or provide retention in combination with other active or retentive components. A Roberts' retractor, usually in combination with a flat anterior bite plane, can be used to reduce a larger overjet that is amenable to being reduced by tipping the teeth.

Screws can be incorporated into the baseplate to deliver a force to several teeth. They can be used in the midline to produce buccal expansion, anteriorly to procline incisors, e.g. to correct a crossbite, or at right angles to buccal teeth to move them distally. They are usually activated by a quarter turn (0.25 mm) once or twice a week until the necessary tooth movements have been achieved after which they can be stabilised, e.g. by placing composite over the screw, to retain the changes produced.

Retention

The retention of a removable appliance is its resistance to being displaced, i.e. what keeps it in. An appliance usually needs anterior and posterior retention and this can be provided by several designs of clasps and bows. **Adams'** clasps or cribs are used on buccal teeth and are made out of 0.7 mm diameter wire. They are designed so that the arrowheads engage the mesio- and distobuccal undercuts, usually, of the first permanent molars, but they can also be used on premolars, incisors and second molars. Adams' clasps can be adapted to support tubes for extra-oral traction and to span two teeth. They can be adjusted at the arrowhead or on the flyover to improve retention. **Southend** clasps are used anteriorly to engage the undercuts between the contact points between two incisors and are made out of 0.7 mm diameter wire. **Bows** can be used labially in the anterior segment and can be plain or fitted. They are most effective when the incisors are proclined. **Ball-ended** clasps are made from 0.7 mm diameter wire with either blobs of solder on the ends of the wire or a tightly wound loop to engage individual undercuts between adjacent teeth. They can be used anteriorly or posteriorly. **Plint** clasps are designed with a loop that engages the undercut gingival to the tube on a molar band and are useful when a patient is wearing the removable appliance in conjunction with a fixed appliance.

Anchorage

Anchorage is the resistance to unwanted tooth movements, e.g. when retracting a canine the molar and premolar will move forward according to Newton's third law of motion that for every action there is an equal and opposite reaction. In the situation of retracting a canine, the molar and premolar together have a greater root surface area than the canine so will not move forward as much as the canine will move back. The unwanted movements can be reduced further by making it harder for the molar and premolar to move and easier for the canine to move, e.g. by clasping the molar and extending the baseplate up to the molar and premolar and into the inter-proximal areas while trimming the baseplate away from the canine. The baseplate has a large surface area in contact with the vault of the palate and can provide a considerable amount of anchorage, but sometimes headgear will need to be added when the anchorage demands are high. The facebow of the headgear can be inserted into tubes that are soldered to the bridge of the Adams' cribs.

Baseplate

The main function of the baseplate is to hold the individual components together to form a rigid and robust appliance. The baseplate also provides a considerable amount of anchorage through its contact with the vault of the palate or lower alveolus. The baseplate is made from acrylic (polymethylmethacrylate) that can be cold or heat cured. In most situations the acrylic is cold (self) cured but in situations where it needs to be stronger, e.g. bite-blocks, it can be heat cured. A baseplate can be passive or built up to provide an active component, e.g. anterior bite plane, buccal capping. An **anterior bite plane** is used to reduce an overbite and is made by increasing the thickness of the acrylic behind the upper incisors so that when the patient bites together, the lower incisors bite onto the bite plane and the buccal teeth are out of contact. Over time, the buccal teeth erupt to regain contact so that when the patient bites together without the bite plane in, the buccal teeth are in occlusion but there is a vertical gap between the upper and lower incisors into which the upper incisors can be moved. If necessary, a bite plane can be reactivated by adding more acrylic to it. Bite planes are usually flat but can be inclined, e.g. a 'steep and deep' appliance that is used to maintain the overjet reduction during the transition phase between treatment with a functional and fixed appliance (see below). **Buccal capping** is usually used to disclude the occlusion when a crossbite (anterior or posterior) is being corrected. This is necessary because when normal occlusal contacts are maintained during crossbite correction, movement of teeth in the one arch (usually maxillary) can result in movement of the opposing teeth and the crossbite not being corrected. The buccal capping causes the bite to open and the incisors to be out of contact so that they can be moved labially, without interference from the lower incisors, and out of the crossbite. Similarly, when correcting a buccal crossbite, the buccal capping prevents the buccal cusps of the lower molars from interfering with the upper molars as they are moved buccally out of crossbite.

Some appliance designs

A **Nudger** or **Ten Hove** appliance is used in combination with headgear and often a lower fixed appliance to reduce an overbite and maintain the position of the first permanent molars during the day that have been moved by the headgear during the night. This appliance typically has:

- Adams' clasps 4 | 4
- Southend clasp 1 | 1
- palatal finger springs 6 | 6
- flat anterior bite plane
- baseplate extending to the mesial of 6 | 6.

A **Roberts' retractor** appliance is used to reduce an overbite and overjet and is made of:

- Adams' clasps 6 | 6
- Roberts' retractor 321 | 123
- flat anterior bite plane
- baseplate extending to the distal of 6 | 6.

An appliance to correct an **anterior crossbite** involving two or more teeth (e.g. 1 | 1 2) may have:

- Adams' clasps 6 | 6
- Southend clasp 1 | 1 2
- buccal capping 654 | 456
- split baseplate and anterior screw.

An appliance to correct an **anterior crossbite** involving one tooth (e.g. 1⌊) may have:

- Adams' clasps 6 ⌊ 6
- Southend clasp ⌊ 1 2
- Z-spring 1 ⌊
- buccal capping 654 ⌊ 456
- baseplate extending to the distal of 6 ⌊ 6.

An appliance to correct **posterior crossbite** involving may have:

- Adams' clasps 6 4 ⌊ 4 6
- buccal capping 654 ⌊ 456
- split baseplate and midline screw.

A **Steep and Deep** appliance can be used to maintain the overjet and overbite reduction during the transition phase between treatment with a functional appliance and fixed appliance. It may have:

- Adams' clasps 6 ⌊ 6
- labial bow 321 ⌊12 3
- inclined anterior bite plane
- baseplate extending to the distal of 6 ⌊ 6.

An appliance to **retract buccal canines** may have:

- Adams' clasps 6 ⌊ 6
- Southend clasp 1 ⌊ 1
- buccal canine retractors 3 ⌊ 3
- stops mesial to 5 ⌊ 5
- baseplate extending to the distal of 6 ⌊ 6 and trimmed in 43 ⌊ 34 region.

A **space maintainer** appliance may be used to hold space, e.g. for unerupted canines to erupt into following the extraction of first premolars. It may have:

- Adams' clasps 6 ⌊ 6
- labial bow 21 ⌊ 12
- stops mesial to 5 ⌊ 5
- baseplate extending to the distal of 6 ⌊ 6.

Headgear

Uses of headgear

Headgear can be used to:

- maintain the position of the maxillary buccal segments (extra-oral anchorage, EOA)
- move the maxillary buccal segments distally (extra-oral traction, EOT)
- modify facial growth by restricting maxillary growth in Class II cases or to protract the maxilla in patients with a Class III malocclusion.

The effect that headgear has on the teeth and maxilla depends on the level and direction of force applied and the duration or wear.

- EOA – 200–250 g per side for 10–12 hours per day applied just above the occlusal plane and through the furcation of the first molars, which is the centre of resistance of the teeth.
- EOT – 400–500 g per side for 14–16 hours per day applied through the centre of resistance of the teeth.
- Growth modification requires >500 g per side for 14–16 hours per day applied above the occlusal plane and through a point between the premolars, which is the centre of resistance of the maxilla.

The direction of the pull of the headgear needs to be considered because it can have rotational effect on the molars and even the whole arch if it is worn enough. If the force is directed below the occlusal plane, i.e. **cervical** headgear using a neck strap only, it will have an extrusive effect on the upper molars which will tend to open the bite and rotate the maxillary arch in an anti-clockwise direction. These movements are often wanted in patients with an increased overbite but can cause problems for patients with a reduced overbite, so cervical headgear is best avoided in patients with increased vertical proportions or reduced overbite. On the other hand, with **high pull** headgear using a headcap only, the force is directed above the occlusal plane which will tend to intrude the upper molars and rotate the maxilla in a clockwise direction. This helps to control the vertical dimension and prevent the loss of an overbite so it is best to use high pull headgear in patients with an increased maxillary-mandibular plane angle and/or reduced overbite. **Combination pull** or **straight pull** headgear uses the headcap and neckstrap at the same time and is ideal for patients with average vertical dimensions.

Components of headgear

Headgear usually involves the use of the following.

- **Facebow** – the inner bow fits into the headgear tubes on molar bands and the outer bow is attached to the headcap and/or neckstrap via a plastic tag (see below).

- **Headcap** and/or **neckstrap** – these are adjusted to apply the required amount of force to the teeth/maxilla via the facebow. They are often used together (combination headgear) to apply a straight distal force but can be used on their own. The headcap will produce a distal and intrusive force to the molars/maxilla. It is often used for patients with increased vertical dimensions. A neckstrap will exert a distal and extrusive force on the molars/maxilla and can be used in patients with reduced vertical dimensions.

■ **Force mechanism** – the force is usually generated by a spring that is attached to the headcap or neckstrap and then to the outer arm of the facebow via a plastic tag with holes in it so that the force can be varied as necessary. For safety reasons (see below) the spring usually has a 'snap-away' feature so that if undue force is applied to the headgear it will become disengaged rather than causing a recall injury.

Reverse headgear (facemask)

When posterior teeth are required to move forwards and there is inadequate resistance to this from the anterior teeth, e.g. in a Class III case, then a force is required to resist the unwanted distal movement of the anterior teeth and encourage the posterior teeth to move forwards. In this situation a reverse headgear can be applied. This consists of an external frame that rests on the forehead and chin that is attached, via elastics, to hooks on an upper fixed appliance. Reverse headgear can be used to increase anterior anchorage or modify maxillary growth in a similar, but opposite, way to conventional headgear.

Headgear safety

Although, in the vast majority of cases, headgear can be used without causing any damage to the teeth, mouth or face, there have been a few cases reported where severe injuries have occurred. The most devastating injuries have involved damage to the eyes caused when the facebow has become dislodged from the headgear tubes and then the distal ends of the inner bow have recoiled into the patient's eye. The physical damage has often been complicated by infection due to oral flora being introduced into the eye. In the most serious cases the patient has lost the sight in the affected eye.

For this reason, the British Orthodontic Society has issued an advice sheet on the use of headgear and facebows. The advice is that 'where possible, all headgear has two safety mechanisms: one to prevent accidental disengagement and the second to prevent recoil injuries'. Safety mechanisms to prevent accidental disengagement include the following.

■ A **rigid neck strap** which prevents the face bow from being pulled forwards and the bow from being disengaged. However, to be effective the strap has to be adjusted correctly and this may be too tight for some patients to tolerate.

■ **Locking mechanisms**: these ensure that the face bow cannot be removed from the buccal tubes, e.g. NiTom^2 facebow, but they can be fiddly and the patients may find them difficult to fit and remove.

■ **Locating elastics:** short, strong elastics may be used between hooks on the inner bow and the buccal tubes to reduce the likelihood of the facebow becoming dislodged. However, the elastics may be variable in effect, and may present difficulties for the patent to fit and remove.

Safety mechanisms to prevent recoil injuries include the following.

- Anti-recoil devices designed to 'snap-away' when excessive force is applied to the headgear. However, there is considerable variation in the amount of force required to activate the snap-away mechanism and they do not always prevent enough force to displace the facebow from the headgear tubes.
- A rigid neck strap which prevents the forward displacement of the face bow (see above).

Other safety mechanisms include **'safety ends'** that do not actually prevent the accidental removal of the face bow from the buccal tubes, but provide a blunt end to the inner bow which may reduce the incidence of penetrating injuries.

Functional appliances

Functional appliances are a group of orthodontic appliances that aim to modify the growth of the jaws by using the forces generated within the masticatory and facial muscles.

Types of functional appliance

Most functional appliances are removable but some, e.g. Herbst appliance, are fixed to the teeth for the duration of active treatment. The majority of functional appliances have been designed to correct Class II malocclusions, although some have been modified to correct Class III malocclusion, e.g. the Frankel FR3 appliance. Functional appliances to correct a Class II discrepancy are designed to hold the mandible forward often to an edge-to-edge position. For a Class III discrepancy only minimal posterior positioning of the mandible is possible so the mandible is held open. Most functional appliances, e.g. Andresen, Harvold and medium opening activators, the bionator and Frankel appliances, are made in one block of acrylic, which is designed not only to hold the mandible forwards but also to open the bite. The Twin Block appliance is the most commonly used functional appliance in the UK and is unusual in that it is made in two parts. It has buccal bite blocks with inclined planes that encourage forward posturing of the mandible into an edge-to-edge relationship. Additional components, e.g. labial bow, expansion screw, clasps and Adams cribs, can be incorporated into the appliance to bring about tooth movement or aid retention of the appliance.

Mode of action

Most functional appliances are worn full time and work in a similar way. For Class II cases, the appliances hold the mandible forward so that the teeth are not in occlusion, the condyles of the mandible are displaced from the glenoid fossa and the muscles of mastication are stretched. For Class III cases, the appliances hold the mandible in a posterior position and open in an attempt to redirect mandibular growth in a downward and backwards direction. In each case the repositioning of the mandible generates forces that are directed primarily to the teeth but can also have an effect on the growth of the maxilla and/or mandible. There are several theories on how functional appliances bring about the changes they do. These include the following.

Dentoalveolar changes: Evidence on the effects of functional appliances suggests that most of the changes (70–80%) that they bring about are due to changes in the dentoalveolar complex. In Class II cases the maxillary incisors retrocline and the eruption of teeth in the maxillary buccal segments is directed distally during treatment. In the mandibular arch the lower incisors tend to procline and the teeth in the buccal segments erupt in a more mesial direction. The reverse occurs in Class III cases.

Skeletal changes: Evidence on the effects of functional appliances suggests that only 20–30% of the changes that they bring about are due to alterations in the growth of the maxilla or mandible. In Class II cases there is minimal restriction of maxillary growth and about 1–3 mm increase in mandibular growth over what would be expected in the same time if patients had not worn an appliance. In Class III cases studies show that there is 1–2 mm increase in maxillary growth and 1–2 mm restriction of mandibular growth. Whether this *extra growth* is sustained after active treatment and is clinically worthwhile is debatable. Functional appliances also have the effect of redirecting mandibular growth downwards and backwards which may not be beneficial in Class II cases but gives the appearance of improving a Class III relationship.

Changes in the glenoid fossa: Animal studies have shown that when the condyle of the mandible is displaced from the glenoid fossa, it remodels causing the temporomandibular joint and mandible to move forwards. However, the evidence that this also happens in humans is weak and if it does occur the changes it causes are minimal.

Indications for using functional appliances

There are some general criteria that patients need to fulfil before considering treatment with a functional appliance as part of their orthodontic treatment.

■ In Class II cases, functional appliances are most successful when patients are undergoing maximum growth. Patients therefore need still to be growing and preferably be in their most rapid phase of growth. This is between 10 and 12 years of age for girls and between 11 and 13 years of age for boys.

■ In Class III cases, patients need to be treated before the maxillary sutures fuse if any enhancement of maxillary growth is to be obtained. These patients therefore need to be treated between 8 and 10 years of age.

■ The aim of functional appliances is to correct a mild/moderate skeletal discrepancy and improve the occlusion. It is therefore important that patients have a skeletal discrepancy, which can either be Class 2 or Class 3. This usually corresponds to the overjet, which is increased in Class II cases and reduced or reversed in Class III cases.

■ Detailed tooth movements are not possible with functional appliances, so ideally patients having functional appliance treatment will have well-aligned upper and lower arches. However, functional appliances are often used as the first phase of treatment to correct the incisor relationship. Patients will then go on to have a phase of fixed appliance therapy when detailed tooth movements can be undertaken in the second phase of treatment.

Interdisciplinary treatment

Interdisciplinary treatment can be defined as orthodontic treatment combined with minor oral surgery, or orthognathic surgery, or restorative treatment.

Minor oral surgery

Unerupted teeth

The teeth most commonly found to be unerupted or impacted beyond the normal time of eruption are maxillary canines and incisors. The aim of treatment for an impacted tooth is either to align the tooth if it is in reasonable position, the patient is prepared to wear fixed appliances and has good oral hygiene; or to remove the tooth if it is in a poor position, the patient is not prepared to wear fixed appliances or has poor oral hygiene.

Canines: Upper canines usually erupt at about 11–12 years of age and lower canines at about 9–10 years. The upper canines are usually palpable in the buccal sulcus by the age of 10 years. If they are not palpable they may be missing, but this is rare (0.08%), or displaced palatally and impacted (1–3%). Girls are more commonly affected then boys (70% and 30% respectively). Impacted canines may cause damage (resorption) to the adjacent teeth (lateral or central incisors). This occurs in about 12% of patients with impacted canines, in girls more then boys, and, if it occurs, has usually started by the age of 12 and rarely after the age of 14 years. Impacted canines are associated with peg or missing lateral incisors and Class II division 2 malocclusions. Impacted canines are usually displaced palatally but occasionally can become impacted buccally (a ratio of 6 to 1).

Buccally impacted teeth usually erupt and are displaced from the line of the arch thus needing alignment or removal. If they don't erupt, surgery may be needed to expose the canine. They can be exposed by simply cutting a window of overlying mucosa away to uncover them, using an apically repositioned flap or bracket, with a gold chain attached, and closed exposure followed by orthodontic traction. However, the bracket/gold chain may perforate the buccal gingivae as the tooth is pulled into the line of the arch.

Palatally impacted canines usually need active intervention as they rarely erupt on their own. Unerupted palatal canines need to be checked for at the age of 10 years. At this stage either the deciduous canine is mobile or the permanent canine should be palpable in the buccal sulcus. If it is not palpable, radiographs need to be taken to locate the tooth. To locate the tooth the **rules of parallax** are applied to two radiographs (see p. 290). These can be an OPG and SMO or periapical or two periapical views taken from different positions.

If, at the age of 10 years, the permanent canine is found to be lying palatally then evidence suggests that if the deciduous canine is extracted, the permanent canine may improve its position sufficiently to allow normal eruption to occur. The amount of improvement seen will depend on how displaced the permanent canine is. If the canine is only overlapping the distal half of the lateral incisor root up to 91% will erupt into a reasonable position, whereas if the canine is overlapping the pulp of the central incisor, only 64% will erupt into a near normal position.

Unfortunately, unerupted palatal canines often present in the mid-teens with the deciduous canine retained and firm and the permanent tooth palpable palatally. They may be associated with small or missing upper lateral incisors and often (60%) have few other problems.

The treatment options for palatally impacted canines include the following.

■ Leave and monitor – however, the dental follicle may undergo cystic change or the canine causes resorption of the lateral incisor. Both these repercussions are uncommon, occur more frequently in girls and have often started by the age of 12 years. For these reasons this option is acceptable for patients who are not willing to undergo active treatment as they can be monitored with radiographs every 1–2 years.

■ Remove the unerupted tooth and replace the deciduous canine when it is lost, or close any residual space with a fixed appliance so that the first premolar acts as the canine. This can be a reasonable option if there is less than 3–4 mm space between the first premolar and lateral incisor and/or the canine is in a poor position.

■ Align the unerupted tooth using a fixed appliance having either surgically exposed the tooth or attached a gold chain to it to allow orthodontic traction to be applied. The prognosis for alignment of an impacted canine depends on the position of the canine in terms of its height, angulation and mesiodistal position. If the crown of the canine is overlying the incisal third of the root of the lateral incisor, at an angle of less than 45° and only overlapping the distal part of the root of the lateral, the prognosis for alignment is good. However, if the crown of the canine is overlying the apical third of the root of the incisors, at nearly right angles to the incisor roots and only overlapping the pulp of the central incisor, the prognosis for alignment is very poor and consideration should be given to other treatment options.

In the end, the option taken will depend on the position of the unerupted tooth and the adjacent teeth, any associated pathology (e.g. resorption, cyst formation) and the patient's compliance.

Canines can either be exposed by an open or closed procedure. In an **open** exposure, a palatal flap of mucosa is raised to allow the bone overlying the canine to be removed. Once the crown of the canine has been uncovered, the palatal flap is replaced and a window of mucosa is cut out to allow the canine to be seen. The palatal flap is then replaced and the area is covered with a surgical pack or dressing plate for 7–10 days to prevent the mucosa from healing over the canine again. Following this the dressing is removed and the canine is allowed to erupt on its own before orthodontic traction is applied and the canine gradually moved into the line of the arch. With a **closed** exposure, a palatal flap is raised and the bone cleared over the canine in the same way as for the open exposure, but rather than make a window in the mucosa to pull the tooth through, a bracket with a gold chain attached to it is bonded to the canine. The flap is then replaced intact with the gold chain emerging through the suture line in the canine region. Orthodontic traction is then applied, via a NiTi piggy-back wire or elastomeric thread/chain, to move the canine into the line of the arch. It is common to fit a transpalatal arch to the maxillary molars to increase the anchorage.

Incisors: Contra-lateral incisors rarely erupt at the same time but if one is still unerupted six months after eruption of the contralateral tooth, suspicions should be raised and investigations instigated to determine why the tooth has not erupted. The incidence of unerupted incisors is less than 1% of the population and in 30–60% of cases is related to a supernumerary tooth although there are other causes that include the following.

- **The root being dilacerated** (crown and root are at different angles) – this can occur following trauma to the deciduous teeth that causes the developing permanent tooth to become deformed. These teeth can be aligned but is dependent on the degree and position of the dilacerations.

- **Obstruction** – this can be due to **supernumerary** (extra tooth that is of abnormal shape or form, e.g. conical) or **supplemental** (extra tooth that resembles a normal tooth, e.g. extra lateral incisor) teeth in the area that block the path of eruption of the permanent incisor.

- **Crowding** – this may be due to a tooth tissue discrepancy or premature loss of the deciduous teeth that has allowed the others to drift into the space required for the permanent successors.

The treatment options for impacted incisors largely depend on the cause. If the tooth is unerupted because it has a dilacerated root, it can be aligned or removed depending on the degree of dilaceration and position of the dilacerations together with the ability and willingness of the patient to undergo treatment with a fixed appliance. If there is an obstruction, then that (e.g. supernumerary or supplemental tooth) has to be removed. At this stage some clinicians leave the unerupted incisor to erupt on its own, and 50–75% of them will erupt. However, if there is inadequate space for the tooth, or even though the obstruction has been removed and there is adequate space, it can fail to erupt. It is for these reasons that some clinicians place an attachment and gold chain on the tooth at the time of surgery to remove the obstruction, thus avoiding the need for another surgical intervention and general anaesthetic if the tooth doesn't erupt. Once the obstruction has been removed a fixed appliance can be placed to create adequate space, if necessary, or apply traction, via a fixed appliance attached to a gold chain, to the unerupted tooth to bring it into the line of the arch. If there is crowding, then adequate space needs to be created and then the unerupted tooth can be pulled into the line of the arch.

Orthognathic surgery

If a patient has a significant skeletal discrepancy then orthodontic treatment alone may not be sufficient to correct all aspects of the malocclusion and facial disproportion. In such cases it may be necessary to consider orthodontic treatment combined with orthognathic surgery. Orthognathic surgery is that branch of surgery concerned with the correction of dentofacial deformity, and particularly with disproportions of the tooth-bearing segments of the jaws, and associated facial skeleton. Therefore, the aims of orthognathic surgery are to correct the functional and aesthetic consequences of severe dentofacial deformity through a combination of orthodontic and surgical treatment.

History

Orthognathic surgery, to correct Class III malocclusions with mandibular prognathism, was originally developed late in the 19th century, but it was not until the 1960s that Obwegeser popularised the sagittal split mandibular osteotomy. Later, in the 1970s, Bell introduced the one-part maxillary osteotomy which allowed the maxilla to be impacted to correct vertical dento-skeletal discrepancies. Subsequently, segmental osteotomies have been devised, which give the maxillofacial surgeons the ability to correct transverse discrepancies surgically. Surgically assisted rapid maxillary expansion (SARME) has been developed to correct transverse discrepancies gradually over a period of 10–14 days. Most recently, distraction osteogenesis, originally used to distract the long bones of the arms and legs, has been adapted for use in the craniofacial region.

Mandibular surgery

The **sagittal split osteotomy** allows the mandible to be advanced or set back up to about 10 mm and/or rotated to correct mild asymmetries. The versatility of this operation has meant that it has become widely accepted as a predictable and effective orthognathic surgical procedure for the correction of both mandibular prognathism (Class III) and retrognathism (Class II) malocclusions. The incisions for this operation are made intra-orally, from behind the terminal molar into the buccal sulcus, and the bony cuts obliquely across the angle of the mandible. The biggest risk of this operation is damage to the inferior dental nerve which can lead to numbness or altered sensation in the distribution of the mental nerve (lip and chin).

An alternative to this operation for patients needing a mandibular setback is the **vertical sub-sigmoid osteotomy**. The incisions for this procedure are usually made extra-orally, thus leading to scars on the face; they may also be made intra-orally, but special instruments are then required to make the bony cuts which run from the sub-sigmoid notch to the lower border of the mandible. The risk of nerve damage is much less with this technique.

A **genioplasty** may be used as a supplemental operation, e.g. in a patient with a Class II division 2 malocclusion with a prominent chin button who has had a mandibular advancement to correct the dental discrepancy. A genioplasty can also be used occasionally to simplify surgical procedures if the dentition can be corrected orthodontically or is acceptable as it stands, e.g. a mild asymmetry or well-compensated Class II or Class III malocclusion.

Maxillary surgery

The bony cuts for maxillary surgery follow the fracture lines described by Le Fort in 1901 and can be made on three levels. The **Le Fort I** osteotomy is the most commonly used maxillary osteotomy and involves an incision made high in the buccal sulcus from 6 | 6 and the bony cut being made from one maxillary tuberosity to the other, above the roots of the maxillary teeth, via the pyriform fossa and through the nasal septum and maxillary sinus. The dento-alveolar part of the maxilla can then be freed from the remaining parts of the maxilla and advanced, impacted or moved down to correct maxillary discrepancies of up to 7–10mm depending on which direction it is moved. Once the Le Fort I osteotomy cuts have been carried out, the maxilla can also be sectioned to allow transverse discrepancies to be corrected. However, it is extremely difficult to move the whole maxilla posteriorly, due to the anatomy and structures contained in the pterygomaxillary fissure so, if the maxilla is protrusive, a **segmental osteotomy** can be performed where a section of bone is removed, usually from the first premolar region, and the anterior segment (3 | 3) is moved posteriorly. If the maxillary deficiency lies higher in the face than the dentoalveolar complex, a higher level osteotomy can be performed. The biggest risk of this operation is damage to the inferior-orbital nerve which can lead to numbness or altered sensation of the cheek, upper lip and nose on the effected side.

The **Le Fort II** osteotomy allows the mid-face to be advanced by involving the nasal bones and zygomatic process. Incisions for this operation have to be made intra-orally, as for the Le Fort I osteotomy, and extra-orally in the infra-orbital region. For patients with severe craniofacial abnormalities a **Le Fort III osteotomy** can be carried out, which allows the whole of the maxilla, including the nasal bones, floor of the orbit and zygoma to be moved forward. Access, to make the necessary bony cuts, is usually gained through a bi-coronal flap.

Correcting transverse discrepancies of the maxilla with a sectional Le Fort I osteotomy carries the risk that the blood flow to the segments may be reduced and the segments may undergo necrosis and be lost. Also, the stability of these operations is unpredictable. It is thought that the relapse occurs because the associated soft tissues are stretched suddenly and do not have time to adapt. In an attempt to overcome these problems **surgically assisted rapid maxillary expansion (SARME)** was developed to remove the need for segmental cuts of the maxilla and allow the maxilla to be expanded gradually. There are variations on where the bony cuts are made but, in general, the cuts are made at the Le Fort I level and a rapid maxillary expansion device, attached to the maxillary molars and premolars, is fitted and then activated twice a day (2 × 0.25mm). This opens the mid-palatal suture steadily until the desired expansion is achieved, after which the transverse dimensions are stabilised to allow bony healing. The theory is that because the soft tissues are expanded slowly they can stretch and adapt better, thus reducing the risk of relapse, and because the maxilla is not sectioned its blood supply remains intact and the risk of bone necrosis is reduced.

A similar process is used in **distraction osteogenesis** where much larger movements of the position of the maxilla and/or mandible are required to correct severe discrepancies, usually in growing children thus, hopefully, reducing the number of operations that they will need and increasing the stability of the correction. In this situation bone cuts are made and then, after a few days, a force is applied across the healing bone (callus) that causes new bone to be laid down between the bone ends thus producing an increase in length and/or height of the bone.

Fixation

In the past, bony segments were held into position with wires and stabilised by inter-maxillary fixation. However, these days, the maxilla is usually stabilised with mini-bone plates and if necessary bones grafts, while the mandibular segments are secured using bicortical screws and/or mini-bone plates. The use of plates and screws has meant that intermaxillary fixation is rarely required these days. This has considerably reduced the risks and morbidity of the orthognathic surgery, as well as the hospital stay needed, and allows patients to start moving their jaws, allowing them to eat and speak, within a day or two of surgery.

Skeletal discrepancy

Skeletal discrepancies can occur in all three planes of space.

- Antero-posterior:
  - Class 2, where the mandible lies significantly posterior to the maxilla usually due to the mandible being smaller than normal
  - Class 3, where the mandible lies significantly anterior to the maxilla. This is occasionally due to the mandible being larger than normal or the maxilla smaller than normal, but usually patients have a combination of the large mandible and small maxilla.

- Vertical:
  - AOB, where there is no vertical overlap of the anterior teeth. In severe cases this can extend to include the premolars and first molars. This can be due to excessive vertical growth of the posterior part of the maxilla, a short mandibular ramus and/or growth that tends to be in a downward and backward direction
  - vertical maxillary excess (VME), where there is excessive gingival show either at rest and/or when smiling. This is due to excessive vertical growth of the maxilla and should not be confused with patients who have a short upper lip and appear to have increased maxillary growth.

- Transverse:
  - crossbite, where the buccal cusps of the upper buccal teeth occlude lingual to the buccal cusps of the lower buccal teeth. Crossbites that exist before treatment can be true or apparent crossbites. A true crossbite occurs when the maxilla is physi-

cally narrower than the mandible, but an apparent crossbite can exist due to the relative anterior-posterior position of the maxilla and mandible. Apparent cross-bites can often be seen pre-treatment in Class III cases where the maxilla is set back relative to the mandible so that a narrower part of the maxilla is occluding with a broader part of the mandible. However, if the study models are reposi-tioned so as to simulate the surgery, the crossbite almost always reduces and often disappears. On the other hand, in Class II cases that appear to have a normal transverse relationship pre-treatment, the patients often develop a crossbite as the mandible is brought forwards to correct the skeletal discrepancy

☐ asymmetry occurs when there has been asymmetrical growth of one or both jaws. This can be the result of excessive or reduced growth on one side of the mandible and/or maxilla. This abnormal growth pattern may be the result of a congenital deformity (e.g. hemifacial microsomia), trauma that caused damage to the growth centre (e.g. condyle) or may occur spontaneously.

A patient may present with a skeletal discrepancy in one or more of the three planes of space.

Stages of treatment

There are several stages of treatment for patients undergoing a combined orthodontic/orthognathic treatment plan. They include the following.

- **History and examination** – When initially seeing the patient it is important to estab-lish the patient's motivations for treatment. These may include aesthetic concerns regarding their teeth and/or face or functional problems that may give rise to difficul-ties eating certain foods, signs and/or symptoms of temporomandibular joint dys-function or a speech impediment. It is also important to determine whether there are any external pressures on the patient to have their teeth/jaws corrected or whether they are self-motivated towards treatment. Patients vary in how much they focus on their teeth and/or jaws and their expectations about what treatment will do for them. If there is a discrepancy between the patient's malocclusion, their perception of how severe it is and/or how their life will be changed by having it corrected, then it is usually advisable to have a psychological opinion on the patient's suitability for treat-ment as they may have body dysmorphic disorder. The extra- and intra-oral examina-tions are carried out in the normal way (see p. 276).

- **Preliminary planning** – The preliminary planning is carried out away from the clinic by the orthodontist and surgeon using the study modes, cephalometric analysis and photographs together with the findings from the history and examination. At this stage an assessment is made of where the skeletal discrepancy lies in all three planes of space to establish what surgery will be required to correct it. The surgery may involve the maxilla, mandible or both jaws and occasionally other procedures, e.g. genioplasty. From an orthodontic point of view the expected tooth movements needed to be undertaken pre-surgically and extractions necessary are planned.

■ **Pre-surgical orthodontics** – The aims of pre-surgical orthodontics are to maximise the benefit of the surgery. In order to do this it is usually necessary to:

☐ *relieve crowding* – just like in conventional orthodontics, any crowded teeth are straightened during the pre-surgical phase of combined orthodontic/orthognathic treatment. Extractions may or may not be needed to gain the space to straighten the teeth. The need for extractions will depend on whether the incisors need to be maintained in their anterior-posterior position, retroclined or proclined and whether any arch expansion is required. In turn, the need for these tooth movements is determined by the need to decompensate the incisors and co-ordinate the arches (see below)

☐ *correct centre-lines* – the centre-lines need to be corrected relative to the facial centre-line and those of the individual jaws. The dental centre-lines may not be coincident with each other, depending on whether the patient has an asymmetry (usually mandibular) or not. Again, extractions may or may not be needed to gain the space required

☐ *decompensation* – during the development of a malocclusion the upper and lower incisors tend to compensate for the underlying skeletal discrepancy. This means that for a Class II malocclusion, the upper incisors tend to be more upright and the lower incisors more proclined than normal in an attempt to reduced the overjet and hide the difference between the relative sizes of the maxilla and mandible. In Class III malocclusions the upper incisors procline and the lowers retrocline to minimise the reverse overjet. The implication of compensation on orthognathic surgery is that the amount the jaws can be moved is limited so, in order to maximise the movement of the jaws the surgeon can undertake, the incisors usually have to be moved so that they are at the correct angle to their respective jaw. In a Class II case this means that the upper incisors may need to be proclined and the lower incisors usually have to be retroclined which often means that extractions are needed in the lower arch. Conversely, in a Class III case, the upper incisors often need to be retroclined and the lower incisors usually have to be proclined which typically requires extraction in the upper arch but not the lower. These tooth movements are the absolute opposite of what are needed during conventional orthodontic treatment

☐ *arch co-ordination* – as mentioned earlier, the dental arches may be in cross-bite pre-treatment that then improves during surgery, i.e. in Class III cases, or go into a cross-bite relationship once the mandible is moved forward in a Class II case. In both situations the width of the arches needs to be adjusted so that it fits in a normal buccolingual relationship when the jaws are in their new position after surgery. Any changes (usually expansion) in the transverse dimensions are mainly carried out in the maxilla because it is much harder to change the width of the mandibular arch

☐ *levelling or maintaining the curve of Spee* – the need for this is determined by the presenting malocclusion. In patients with reduced vertical proportions and increased overbite, the **curve of Spee** is often maintained preoperatively, and only levelled in the postoperative phase, so that the vertical increase obtained during surgery can be maximised. On the other hand in cases with increased vertical proportions and a reduced overbite or anterior open bite, the curve of Spee is levelled preoperatively to minimise the amount of vertical tooth movement that occurs postoperatively, which may result in some reduction of the overbite. However, if an anterior open bite has a bowed occlusal plane, e.g. resulting from a digit sucking habit, then the different sections (right buccal, anterior and left buccal) are levelled independently and their levels are then corrected surgically by moving the buccal segments up or the anterior segment down.

- **Final planning** – At this stage full records of the patient are taken so that a check can be made that the planned orthodontic tooth movements have been achieved. Special attention is paid to the centre-lines, incisor angulation and fit of the arches. It is only at this point that the amount of skeletal movement required to correct the malocclusion, in all three planes of space, can be determined. If the inclination, position and fit of the teeth appear to be good, then the working archwires are made passive, so that no further tooth movement takes place, and several ball hooks are attached to the archwires. Working study models are made and mounted on an articulator so that the anticipated jaw movements can be simulated and the planned occlusion achieved. From these models acrylic wafers are made that the surgeon uses to guide the teeth and jaws into position during the surgery.

- **Surgery** – In theory it is possible to move the jaws in three planes of space; however, some movements are harder to do or not as stable as others. The most frequently carried out surgical movements and their limits are:
  in the **maxilla**:
  □ advancement of 7–10 mm in cases with a Class 3 discrepancy
  □ expansion in cases with a transverse discrepancy
  □ impaction of 7–8 mm in cases with an AOB or VME
  □ down fracture (and bone grafting) of 5–6 mm to correct vertical deficiencies
  in the **mandible**:
  □ advancement of 7–10 mm in cases with a Class 2 discrepancy
  □ set back of 7–10 mm in cases with a Class 3 discrepancy.

All these procedures can be carried out in isolation or in combination with one or more other surgical corrections. Most procedures are carried out from within the mouth so that it is rare for patients to be left with any external scars following surgery. The jaws are usually held in their new position by small titanium plates or screws. These usually remain *in situ* for life but occasionally may need removing if they become infected or if they bother the patient.

The main **complications** of these specific procedures are nerve damage, swelling and bruising. **Nerve damage** can involve the infra-orbital nerves in patients who have undergone maxillary surgery, which leads to numbness or altered sensation over the affected cheek and side of the nose. In the mandible it is the inferior dental nerve that can be damaged, which leads to numbness or altered sensation over the affected side of the chin or lip. Immediately following surgery most patients have a degree of altered sensation or numbness over the affected areas. This usually subsides over the following weeks or months but about 10% of patients will be left with a small area of numbness or altered sensation overlying the exit of the nerve from the respective jaw. This does not affect the way the patients move their facial muscles as the nerves concerned are sensory.

Patients are very **swollen** immediately after the operation but the swelling usually goes down rapidly during the first 2–3 weeks and then continues to reduce more slowly over the next 6–9 months. They are also quite **bruised** but this has usually gone by four weeks after the operation. After the operation, patients are only able to eat a soft **diet**. For the first few days this will need to be liquid only and then they gradually build up to soft then normal foods over a period of 4–6 weeks. Patients are usually in hospital for 3–5 days coming into hospital the day before and then leaving 2–3 days after the operation. Orthognathic surgery is a major operation so patients need to take it easy for the 2–3 weeks after the operation and be away from education or off work for about four weeks.

- **Post-surgical orthodontics** – Immediately after surgery it is common for patients to have a limited number of teeth in occlusion, i.e. incisors and terminal molars (three-point landing), so that there are lateral open bites between the teeth that then need closing down with the aid of inter-arch elastics and flexible archwires. The aims of post-surgical orthodontics are therefore to:
  - □ maintain the surgical correction achieved
  - □ level the curve of Spee if necessary
  - □ close down the lateral open bites
  - □ finish and detail the occlusion to achieve maximal intercuspation.

These tooth movements can be brought about using small, appropriately positioned inter-arch elastics on flexible archwires. Once the best possible occlusion has been achieved the fixed appliances can be removed and a period of retention commenced.

Restorative treatment

If patients have missing or malformed teeth or have had severe periodontal disease they may require a combination of orthodontic and restorative treatment to achieve the best possible occlusion.

Missing teeth (hypodontia)

Teeth may be congenitally missing or missing due to trauma or pathology. The most commonly congenitally missing teeth are upper lateral incisors, upper and lower second premolars and lower central incisors. The treatment options for patients with missing teeth are to either open space and replace the missing teeth or close space and modify the adjacent teeth to resemble those that they are replacing. The aim of orthodontic treatment in such cases is to move the existing teeth into positions that make it easier or eliminate the need for the restorative dentist to replace the teeth that the patient is missing.

Space closure and modification of the adjacent teeth is most frequently chosen in cases where there is another feature of the malocclusion that requires space to correct it. This includes an overjet in a Class II division 1 case, crowding or an increased overbite. The teeth adjacent to the missing teeth can then be modified to resemble those they are replacing, e.g. modifying upper canines to look like lateral incisors or upper lateral incisors to resemble central incisors. This can be achieved by enamel grinding, composite additions, veneers or crowns.

Space can be maintained or recreated and the missing teeth replaced in cases where there is excessive space or it cannot be used to correct another aspect of the malocclusion. These cases include those with a Class I or III incisor relationship, spacing and/or an average or reduced overbite. The missing teeth can be replaced by a denture, bridges, implants or occasionally other teeth that can be auto-transplanted into the site of the missing teeth.

Malformed teeth

The crown or the root of a tooth can be malformed and need restorative treatment to modify it to improve its appearance or allow a good occlusion to be achieved following orthodontic treatment.

The crown of a tooth may be smaller (**microdontia**) or larger than normal (**macrodontia**). Microdontia most commonly affects upper lateral incisors that may be anything from slightly smaller than usual but of the correct shape through to a very diminutive tooth that is conical in shape (peg shaped). Such teeth can be modified to restore normal proportions using composite additions, veneers or crowns.

Macrodontia most commonly affects upper central incisors, which may be fused with the adjacent lateral incisor or a supplemental tooth. It is often difficult to modify such teeth due to the size of the pulp and the likelihood of pulpal damage if the tooth is reduced in size. It may, therefore, be necessary to extract very unaesthetic macrodonts and either replace them or move the upper lateral incisor into their place.

The roots of teeth may be malformed as a result of abnormal development or trauma. A dilacerated root may arise as the result of abnormal development or trauma to the deciduous teeth that affected the development of their permanent successor(s). It is difficult to align these teeth so it may be necessary to extract them and either replace them or move the adjacent teeth into their place.

A root may become **ankylosed** (fused to the bone) either spontaneously, e.g. deciduous molars, or as a result of trauma, e.g. upper central incisors. Ankylosis may result in the tooth becoming infra-occluded (**submerged**) and it is impossible to move these teeth. Occasionally an infra-occluded tooth may be restored with a veneer or an onlay to re-establish occlusal contacts. However, it may be necessary to extract these teeth and either replace them or close the residual space and modify the adjacent teeth as necessary.

Teeth of poor prognosis

Teeth may have a limited prognosis if they have been affected by caries or trauma. Caries most frequently affects the first permanent molars, in which case their extraction may be built into the overall orthodontic treatment plan and the remaining space closed. This would be the treatment of choice if extractions were required to correct another feature of the malocclusion, e.g. to relieve crowding or reduce an overjet. Occasionally incisors may become carious to such an extent that the longevity of the tooth is questionable, e.g. lateral incisors with a dens-in-dente, in which case it may be necessary to extract the tooth and either replace it or close the space and modify the adjacent teeth to resemble it.

Trauma most commonly affects the upper central incisors and if the prognosis of the tooth is poor, such as a tooth with a root fracture or resorption, it may be necessary to extract the tooth and either replace it or close the space and modify the adjacent teeth to resemble it.

Periodontal disease

When a patient has suffered from advanced periodontal disease there is reduced bony support for the teeth. This means that the resistance of the teeth to the normal pressures of the tongue and lips is reduced and the teeth may move into a new position of balance. Frequently this results in proclination and spacing of the teeth in the upper labial segment that may move out of the control of the lower lip. Many patients find this unaesthetic and request orthodontic treatment to improve the situation. In these cases it is very important that the periodontal disease is controlled because orthodontic treatment in patients with uncontrolled periodontal disease can hasten the periodontal breakdown. The aims of treatment in these cases are to reduce the spacing of teeth and bring them under the control of the lower lip again. Treatment may be carried out with a URA but it is probably more efficient to use a fixed appliance. Whichever way the tooth movements are carried out it is likely that this group of patients will require some form of permanent retention either with a bonded or removable retainer.

Timing of orthodontic treatment

In most cases the timing of orthodontic treatment is related to the stage of dental development.

Deciduous dentition

Treatment is rarely indicated in the deciduous dentition, but in the case of severe skeletal discrepancy an exception may be made.

Mixed dentition

Treatment in the mixed dentition can involve the extraction of deciduous teeth, the correction of an anterior or posterior crossbite and/or growth modification.

Early permanent dentition

The majority of fixed orthodontic treatment is carried out at the early permanent dentition stage.

Adult dentition

Many forms of treatment can be undertaken later on. Orthognathic surgery is delayed until late teens.

Orthodontic treatment for many people is optional rather than essential.

Cleft lip and palate

Aetiology

The aetiology of clefts of the lip or palate (CL/P) is multifactorial and debatable. It is likely to be a combination of genetic and environmental factors. For some cases the cleft is part of a syndrome and in others it may occur on its own. In some families there is a strong family history of clefting and it appears that these families have a pre-disposition to clefting. However, for most cases there is no family history and no single cause. Clefts may be related to environmental factors that affect the foetus at critical embryonic stages. Some drugs are known to increase the incidence of clefting, e.g. vitamin A, heroin.

Incidence

Clefts of the lip and/or palate are one of the most common congenital abnormalities. In the UK they occur in about 1:700 live births. This means that about 1,000 babies are born in the UK every year with a cleft of the lip and/or palate. The incidence varies with racial origin. It is slightly higher in Indian Asian races (3.6/1,000) but lower for Negroid races (0.5/1,000). In Caucasians the incidence is higher in boys (3:2) and unilateral clefts occur more commonly on the left.

Development

Facial development is very complex and not fully understood. The tip of the nose, upper lip and primary palate develop from three processes. These normally fuse from the incisive foramen anteriorly in about the seventh to eighth week of pregnancy (fifth to sixth week of intra-uterine life (IUL)). Failure to fuse leads to a cleft of the lip and/or alveolus that may be unilateral or bilateral. The secondary palate (hard and soft palates) develops from two shelves that initially lie vertically either side of the tongue. At a critical time the tongue lowers and the shelves elevate and join in the midline. This occurs during the ninth to tenth week of pregnancy (seventh to eighth week of IUL). Failure of the tongue to drop, fusion to take place or a breakdown of the joint will result in a cleft of the palate. The cleft can vary in size from a cleft of the soft palate to one extending and possibly joining with a cleft of the alveolus and lip to form a complete cleft of the lip and palate (Figure 5.21).

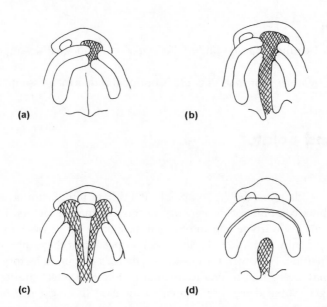

Figure 5.21 Types of cleft lip and/or palate: (a) unilateral cleft of the left lip and alveolus; (b) complete unilateral cleft of the lip and palate; (c) complete bilateral cleft of the lip and palate; and (d) cleft of the soft palate.

Diagnosis

Some clefts are hard to diagnose, e.g. submucous cleft, and may not be detected until the baby or child is older and the defect causes problems with feeding or speech.

Classification

Clefts of the lip and palate can range from very small defects, e.g. bifid uvula or small notch of the upper lip, to a complete bilateral cleft of the lip and palate. For this reason several classification systems have been suggested. However, many clinicians simply prefer to give an exact description of the cleft rather than classify it to a specific type.

Management

Antenatal care

With recent developments in ultrasonic scanning, defects can be detected from about the nineteenth week of pregnancy (seventeenth week of IUL). However, such diagnosis is difficult and even experienced scanners may miss these defects and false positives have been reported. When an antenatal diagnosis of a CL/P is made the parents are informed and referred to the local cleft team for further counselling.

Postnatal care

Diagnosis of a CL/P usually occurs at birth. It is usually a paediatrician who makes the initial diagnosis and informs the parents. This has to be handled sensitively. Ideally, the parents need to be informed as soon after birth as possible and put in touch with the local cleft team within 24 hours of birth so that specialist advice and counselling can be given and any necessary treatment started.

Each type of cleft can give rise to different functional or aesthetic problems. Immediately after birth the priorities are breathing and feeding. Clefts of the lip and/or palate rarely give problems with breathing unless associated with a retrognathic (small) mandible. This is most commonly associated with **Pierre-Robin syndrome**, which usually consists of a small mandible, a cleft of the hard and soft palate, and a small tongue that is positioned too far posteriorly. The small mandible and the posteriorly positioned tongue may cause the airway to become partially or fully obstructed if the baby is placed on their back. This results in the baby becoming cyanosed or having periods of not being able to breathe. For this reason such a baby needs to be nursed on their side and may need a nasopharyngeal airway or, rarely, a tracheostomy to allow them to breathe.

About a quarter of babies with a CL/P have problems in feeding and have poor weight gain for the first two to three months. Problems with feeding arise due to the inability of the baby to achieve an adequate seal around the breast or bottle teat or to produce the negative intra-oral pressure that is required to breast-feed successfully. However, with appropriate support successful feeding is usually achieved and babies rarely need to be fed via a naso-gastric tube. This can vary from simple advice on how to position the baby to using specially designed teats or bottles or the baby being provided with a feeding plate.

The use of intra-oral plates in babies with CL/P is controversial. Some clinicians advocate their use to help with feeding (feeding plates). Others suggest that the plates can mould the segments of the maxilla (pre-surgical orthopaedics). The aim in this situation is to make later surgery easier and possibly less traumatic, with the hope that this produces less scarring and growth restriction. However, there is very little evidence either supporting or refuting the use of such plates and clinicians remain divided as to whether or not to advocate their use.

Pre-school care

The priorities during the pre-school years are speech and language development, hearing, general growth and social development, and general dental care.

Most children with a cleft palate develop speech disorders. Many will require several interventions throughout their childhood and adolescence to achieve some cases surgery. The main problems that a child with a cleft palate has with speech are those of hyper-nasality and difficulty in pronouncing consonants. These can be due to physical problems, e.g. oro-nasal fistulae, velopharyngeal insufficiency where the soft palate is unable to make a seal against the anterior wall of the pharynx, poor hearing, neurological, social and psychological reasons. Hyper-nasality occurs because air can escape from the mouth to the nose due to a fistula or from the pharynx to the mouth or nose due to velopharyngeal insufficiency.

Patients with a cleft palate are prone to middle ear infections that can cause loss of hearing. This is because the attachments of the eustachian tube are abnormal which means that secretions in the middle ear do not drain properly so infection is more likely. It is therefore important that a child with a cleft palate has their hearing checked regularly so that any hearing impairment can be detected early and appropriate intervention carried out, e.g. placement of grommets.

The impact of early problems with feeding usually resolve and babies have caught up their growth by six months of age. However, older children with a cleft palate are frequently shorter than their peers. Although growth hormone deficiency is more common in children with a CL/P, it cannot fully account for the frequency of short stature in children with a cleft palate.

Social development of pre-school children is important if they are to adjust well to the school environment. However, children with a CL/P often fail to mix well. This can be due to a combination of factors, including hearing problems, speech disorders and lack of previous social contact with peers due to multiple hospitalisations or parents being overprotective thus limiting social interaction and nursery school attendance. Although orthodontic treatment is not required in the pre-school period it is important for children with a CL/P to attend their dentist regularly for routine dental care. The importance of good oral hygiene and a well-balanced diet with a minimum exposure to sugary foods and drinks needs to be stressed. Where tap water is not fluoridated then appropriate fluoride supplements can be prescribed.

Care of the child at infant/junior school

This period is very important for the child with a CL/P. It is the time when peer groups are established and children who do not conform to the norm may well be excluded or be the subject of bullying. This may lead to poor self-esteem and depression in later years. It is therefore very important that the child is fully supported by their family, teachers and healthcare professionals. From a dental point of view it is the time that the permanent dentition starts to erupt and significant facial growth occurs. Orthodontically, treatment centres around trying to establish a positive overjet and overbite and preparing the maxillary dentition for secondary alveolar bone grafting where appropriate.

Secondary alveolar bone grafting has, in many ways, revolutionised the treatment of patients with alveolar clefts and allows the alveolar process to be fully restored so that teeth adjacent to the cleft can erupt or be moved into the grafted bone. This minimises the need for a prosthesis to replace missing bone or teeth. In addition, oronasal fistulae can be closed, the gingival contour and health of the teeth adjacent to the cleft can be improved and the additional bone often gives increased support to the nasal tip. Expansion of the maxillary arch is often required prior to alveolar bone grafting. This can be achieved relatively quickly (six months) with a quad-helix appliance. Bone grafting is usually undertaken at around 10–11 years of age, prior to the eruption of the canine(s) so that they can erupt through the grafted alveolar bone. Bone is usually taken from the iliac crest of the pelvis and within about three months the grafted bone is indistinguish-able radiographically from normal alveolar bone.

Care of the adolescent at secondary school

Psychosocial aspects of development are important and poor self-esteem can lead to depression and even suicide in older age groups. Psychological counselling can play an important role in enabling adolescents to cope better with their facial disfigurement. **Changing Faces** is a charity established to help those with facial disfigurement and can be contacted at 27 Cowper Street, London EC2A 4AP or via its website (www.changing-faces.co.uk)

It is during adolescence that the effects of differential growth of the maxilla and mandible become apparent. Scarring of the maxillary soft tissues resulting from the primary surgery often means that growth of the maxilla becomes restricted and a Class III malocclusion and skeletal discrepancy results. It may be possible to camouflage any resulting skeletal discrepancy with orthodontic treatment by proclining the upper labial segment and retroclining the lower labial segment to create a Class I incisal relationship. However, a proportion of patients will require orthognathic surgery to correct the underlying skeletal discrepancy. This usually involves advancement of the maxilla with or without a mandibular setback. Prior to surgery, patients will require orthodontic treatment to decompensate the upper and lower labial segments and co-ordinate the arches.

Infection control

As with every other aspect of clinical dentistry, infection control procedures when under-taking orthodontic treatment are essential to ensure the safety of both patients and staff in the workplace. All members of the dental team must be adequately trained in the procedures necessary to implement appropriate infection control. Impressions and ortho-dontic appliances must be cleaned and disinfected before being dispatched to the laboratory.

After an impression is removed from the mouth it must be rinsed under cold running water (to remove any debris, blood or saliva) until visibly clean and then immersed in a disinfection solution according to the manufacturer's recommendations. The impression is then removed and rinsed under running water again and dispatched to the laboratory with the appropriate paperwork, including details of the disinfection procedure. Appliances that have been removed from the mouth must follow the same procedure before being sent to the laboratory.

Clinical waste must only be disposed of by a registered waste carrier and it is essential that it does not contain any sharps (needles, scalpels, orthodontic wires, brackets or bands, debonding burs). All sharps must be disposed of in approved, puncture-proof containers, which must not be more than two-thirds full when sealed. All clinical waste should be stored securely until collection for disposal.

Recommended task

(1) As a member of the orthodontic dental team, what are your responsibilities in relation to cross-infection control?

Laboratory skills

Materials

The material used to make all orthodontic models is **gypsum** (calcium sulphate). Gypsum is a rock, which, during the manufacturing process, is crushed into a fine powder and has chemicals added to improve the strength and control the setting time. A colouring agent is also added. A fine powder is produced, which, when mixed with water forms a material that can be vibrated into the impression, producing a strong model when set. The basic plaster of Paris is white in colour, porous, weak and expands on setting. **Kaffir D** dental stone has the advantage of controlled expansion and a slower setting time, producing a stronger model that is yellowish in colour.

A fine (plaster of Paris) orthodontic model material is available for casting presentation models. This is more expensive but has the advantage of being very strong and very accurate, with a slow setting time, resulting in a model which, when trimmed, has an exceptionally white appearance. Some presentation models are soaked in a soap solution (pure soap flakes) for a few minutes and then polished with a paper towel to give a high gloss shine to them.

Preparation of models

Study models are an important diagnostic aid and should be prepared with the utmost care. The impressions should be cast as soon as possible and a model made which has a base of about half the depth of the anatomical area.

The impressions should be removed from the models as soon as the stone has fully set. If the cast is left with the alginate material in place after the final set of the stone material the alginate will dry out (**syneresis**). This leads to shrinkage of the alginate material and hardening. If this should happen there will be a danger of damage to the study cast during the removal of the hard alginate. Although it is necessary to keep the alginate impression moist during transit to the laboratory to reduce the risk of shrinkage, if the impression is submerged in water for a length of time it may swell and render the cast inaccurate (**imbibition**). To stabilise alginate impressions on a temporary basis they should be covered with a damp dental napkin and placed in a polythene bag and sealed.

Study models are constructed from the initial impressions (normally in alginate) and poured in dental stone (Kaffir D) with a base of 50/50 stone/plaster. The study models are then trimmed so that they can be articulated in any position that may be required for observation purposes. The base of the upper model is first trimmed parallel to the occlusal plane. The model is then placed on its base and the sides are trimmed at least 7 mm away from the buccal surfaces of the teeth (see Figure 5.13). The two models are placed in the correct occlusion (ICP), and the base of the lower model trimmed parallel to the upper base. The sides are then trimmed so that they are in the same planes as the upper (see Figure 5.13).

Orthodontic appliance materials

Acrylic resin is used for orthodontic appliances and over the past 25 years a self-curing resin has been used as the baseplate material for appliances. The technique for the use of this material allows the appliance to be built up freehand on the model, without any damage to the fine springs and clasps. The acrylic is built up in layers by applying first the powder (polymer) and then the liquid (monomer), which is applied to the powder. When the required thickness is reached the model is immersed in a curing vessel of water at 45–50°C at a pressure of 2 bar (approximately 30psi) for 10 minutes. After curing the model is removed from the vessel and the acrylic trimmed and polished in the usual way. The use of this self-curing resin is ideal for the range of functional appliances that are currently being used.

Before the use of the self-cure acrylic resin, appliances were made using heat-cured acrylic resin; the disadvantage with this method was the distortion of the fine spring components of the appliances. These could be damaged during the curing process.

Stainless steel is used to make springs, labial bows and expansion screws. The various types of stainless steel were first discovered in Sheffield by Brearley in 1913. There are essentially three types:

- austenitic
- martensitic
- ferritic.

The stainless steel used in orthodontic appliances is the austenitic hard drawn steel known as 18/8. This is composed of 71% ferrite, 18% chromium, 8% nickel and 0.15% carbon. The main advantages of austenitic stainless steel are that it:

- has excellent corrosive resistance in the mouth
- is very strong even when used in thin sections
- is comparatively easy to manipulate
- is inexpensive
- can be spot welded or soldered using silver solder.

These materials are used in functional appliances, active and passive retainers, and transpalatal arches.

Recommended task

(1) Describe why study models are an important tool for use in orthodontic treatment.

Oral health and care of appliances

The patient's oral health is a major consideration before any orthodontic treatment is carried out. The obvious risks associated with orthodontic treatment, and the patient's responsibility in maintaining a good level of oral hygiene and taking care of the appliances so that the risks are minimised, are discussed at the initial appointment stage. In some instances the patient will have to improve their oral health before treatment can begin.

The dental nurse has an important role in discussing diet, toothbrushing and appliance care with the patient.

Dental health education

Diet

The general aspects of diet and its influence on caries are covered in Chapter 2 and the aspects specific to orthodontic treatment only will be covered in this section. In some cases, a patient's diet will have to be modified so that some of the risks of treatment are minimised.

Patients need to be given advice regarding the types of food and drink that should be reduced or eliminated from their diet. It is also important to discuss with patients the effect that the frequency of sugar intake (in food and drinks) can have on the tooth enamel (e.g. demineralisation and caries).

Patients are also advised to eliminate chewy, sticky and hard foods (chewing gum, toffees, boiled sweets, crusty bread, apples, etc.) from their diet as these can contribute to appliance breakage. It is helpful for patients to be given advice in terms that they can relate to on the level of stickiness or hardness that can be eaten, e.g. to eat nothing harder or chewier than a Twix bar without taking special care such as cutting it up. This advice is important because eating hard foods can damage the appliance; brackets can debond or bands loosen and chewy foods can get tangled in the appliance and damage it. Archwires can become distorted so that they exert the wrong level or direction of force.

Oral hygiene

The correct toothbrushing technique should be demonstrated to patients prior to them starting treatment in order to show them how to effectively remove plaque and food debris from the teeth and appliance. Patients should then be allowed to demonstrate their understanding of the technique shown by competently using the aids available, which include:

- specially designed orthodontic toothbrushes
- interdental brushes (bottle brushes)
- interspace brushes (single tufted).

These brushes are designed to fit in and around the various structures of a fixed appliance. The teeth and gingival tissues should be brushed at least twice a day with a fluoride toothpaste, and especially after eating. If a removable appliance is worn, this should be removed first. Plaque disclosing tablets may be used on a regular basis to perfect toothbrushing technique or to monitor plaque control. Asking patients to floss with a fixed appliance on is rather impractical and a good level of oral hygiene can be maintained by other means.

Fluoride mouth rinses can be recommended for patients who have fixed appliances and are particularly valuable when used just before the patient goes to bed. The use of these is described in Chapter 2.

The importance of keeping regular appointments with the patient's dentist for routine dental check-ups and any follow-up treatment should be stressed. Patients need to be monitored regularly to ensure that their oral hygiene is maintained to a high standard.

Appliance maintenance

Patients who have removable appliances are advised to take them out after eating and clean the appliance, removing food debris and plaque from around the clasps. A removable appliance should be brushed and rinsed outside the mouth over a basin half full of water to prevent damage to the appliance if it is accidentally dropped.

Should an appliance be lost, broken, damaged or causing trauma, the patient should be told to contact the surgery or clinic at the earliest opportunity. Failure to do so could result in permanent damage to the patient or be detrimental to the success of the treatment. Until help can be obtained it is possible to apply orthodontic wax to an offending wire or bracket of a fixed appliance. This will reduce the amount of discomfort and trauma suffered by the patient.

Patients need to be advised to wear removable or functional appliances if at all possible, even if they are broken or causing some trauma. Again wax can be applied to relieve pressure areas. If the appliance is not worn the teeth will move quickly so that, within a day or two, the appliance will not fit and will need remaking rather than simply repairing.

Patients should be told that if there is a problem with headgear coming detached or dislodged from the headgear tubes it should not be worn until it has been adjusted. This is because the major risk of trauma from headgear is when it comes apart.

A removable appliance should be removed if the patient is participating in contact sports and placed in a suitable container to prevent loss or damage.

Fixed appliances need careful cleaning and particular attention needs to be paid to the areas around the brackets and bands. If debris and plaque are not removed from these areas decalcification of the enamel can occur in as little as six weeks, i.e. between two appointments.

Headgear

Patients who wear a headgear appliance can be given a chart on which to record the amount of time spent wearing this appliance. Patients will have been advised by the orthodontist about how many hours a day the headgear should be worn (normally 14 hours per day). Some patients may find that they have problems sleeping when wearing the appliance, but they need to be encouraged to persevere with the treatment and the problems may soon resolve. It is usual to ask the patient to build up their hours with the headgear so that for the first few days they only wear the appliance in the evenings to get used to wearing something around their head. This means that when they sleep with the headgear on for the first time it is not a completely new experience. It is also wise to suggest that the first night they try sleeping with the headgear on is at the weekend, so that if they do have a disturbed night they are not too tired for school the following morning.

The patient must be made aware of the importance of bringing the headgear with them to every appointment, as it will need to be checked by the orthodontist. If any problems do arise from wearing the appliance then the patient should be asked to contact the surgery as soon as possible. It is important to stress to the patient that the headgear will only work while they are wearing it. The dental nurse should be able to show the patient how to fit and remove the headgear. It is important that the headgear is fitted in the correct way so as to avoid accidental damage when the headgear is not fully assembled.

The facebow is fitted first, followed by the head/neck strap(s) and safety strap (if one is being used). The inner bow of the facebow fits into the headgear tubes on the maxillary molar bands. Most facebows have a U loop along the inner bow and the patient must be told which way up the loops face so that they insert it the correct way up. Usually the patient has to insert one side of the inner bow first and then the other. At first the patient will need to use a mirror to see where to insert the ends of the inner bow, but with practice patients are often able to insert the facebow by feel alone. For younger patients, help from their parent/guardian may also be required initially. Some facebows have additional safely catches which need to be demonstrated. These are usually clips that fit over the back of the inner bow once it is in place. The importance of these in preventing accidental dislodgement of the bow should be stressed.

Once the facebow has been inserted the head/neck strap(s) can be attached to the outer bow. It is important to stress at this stage that some pressure is maintained on the facebow to stop the inner bow from being dislodged from the headgear tubes when unilateral force from the head/neck strap(s) is applied when fitting them. Finger pressure applied in the midline will be adequate to prevent this from happening. Again the straps have to be applied one side at a time. To help the patient know which hole to attach the straps by, it is advisable to mark the correct hole on the tags with a marker pen. The hole tags can be cut to length to help prevent them catching the cheek or eye if they are excessively long. Patients are sometimes advised to wear an additional safety strap fitted around the back of the neck to prevent the facebow from becoming dislodged during sleep.

Cases have been reported where the facebow has become dislodged during sleep or while playing. In such circumstances severe damage can result. This includes blinding and trauma to the face or soft tissues of the mouth due to the recoil of the facebow, and trauma from the ends of the inner bow. It is therefore important to stress the safety precautions that need to be taken when wearing headgear. Patients need to be advised not to mess around when wearing their headgear and only wear it while doing quiet activities (e.g. homework or watching television) and using all the additional safety features (e.g. safety clip or strap) that have been provided.

Recommended tasks

(1) Ask a colleague or friend to pretend to be the patient so that you may rehearse your response and answers to the following tasks using role-play.
   (a) A patient asks you to explain what a fixed appliance feels like to wear and how it will affect his lifestyle.
   (b) You have been asked to provide a patient, who has just had a fixed appliance placed, with information on how to care for her brace.
   (c) The orthodontist you work with has asked you to explain to a patient how to fit headgear and how it should be worn.
(2) Develop an oral health education aid that you can use to support the information given to a patient who requires dietary and toothbrushing advice. Discuss with a colleague ways in which a patient can be motivated into acting on this advice.

Orthodontic stock control

The ordering and organisation of equipment and materials is usually the responsibility of the dental nurse. The nurse assigned to this task needs to have good organisational and inter-personal skills. To run an efficient ordering system it is important to:

- know what needs to be purchased
- have prices and codes for the items
- decide on the quantity required related to usage
- have a contact list of the supply companies.

It is also necessary to ensure that stock is used on a rotational basis and stored correctly, according to the manufacturer's instructions. Expiry dates should be checked regularly. Forward planning (ordering weekly or monthly) is vital in making sure that stock levels are maintained and shortages do not occur. Stock information may be recorded in a book or on computer disk.

When ordering products such as fluoride, etchant gels, fixatives or adhesives and acrylics it is important to note that these need to be stored in a cool, dark cupboard which should be kept locked (Health and Safety and COSHH regulations apply). Some items, such as certain types of archwire, have special storage instructions (Neo sentalloy must be stored in a fridge); it is therefore important to adhere to the manufacturer's instructions on storage.

Single-use items (e.g. brushes for etchant, disposable impression trays, etc.) help to reduce cross-infection in the surgery. Most single-use items are marked as such on their packaging. Auxiliary items, such as modules, will perish over a period of time so it is important not to over-stock. If these items are stored in a fridge they become brittle; if cold sterilised they lose their elasticity.

All labels and packaging have a **CE mark** on them. This is useful if the product proves to be faulty as it allows the product to be traced back to its origin. It is useful to either record these numbers/letters or keep the packaging for reference.

Maintenance of instruments

The following points are particularly important.

- Always keep cutters sharp and oil regularly.
- Use only cutters for cutting.
- Do not put cutters in an ultrasonic bath as it will damage them. Place them in a non-ionic solution.
- Always follow the manufacturer's instructions on how to look after instruments to maximise their life.

Recommended tasks

(1) Check the COSHH assessment sheets in your workplace to find out if they are complete and up to date.
(2) What information would you expect to see on a stock record/control sheet? How would this information influence your decision when ordering items?

Medico-legal aspects

Confidentiality

Every aspect of a patient's dental care must be considered confidential. The duty of confidentiality is a responsibility of all staff. Breaches of confidentiality on the part of staff are usually a disciplinary matter, which may warrant a dismissal. All staff should be made aware of the need for strict confidentiality. This includes inside and outside the surgery. The duty of confidentiality is emphasised in many documents such as:

- Hippocratic Oath (500BC)
- FDI (International Dental Federation) Principles (1947 and 1986)
- General Dental Council (*Maintaining Standards*, 1997)
- European Convention on Human Rights (article 8 – the right to privacy)
- Human Rights Act 1998.

Patients may sue dentists who breach confidentiality. They may complain to the GDC, who will decide if such a breach constitutes serious professional misconduct. Dentists may face the GDC to account for the actions of their staff.

Confidentiality can be breached in many ways, some not always apparent. For example:

- being overheard in the workplace and elsewhere
- on video display screens
- via intercoms
- on answer-phones
- via emails
- through the internet
- in professional publications.

Orthodontic records

High-quality patient care cannot be delivered without the maintenance of good dental records (radiographs, study models, photographs and correspondence). It should be remembered that dental records may be required in the context of litigation which may arise long after the event that has given rise to the action, therefore retaining orthodontic records for some considerable time after treatment has been completed is advisable. This in itself can prove a problem because of storage.

Dental records

Dental records should be:

- clear
- concise
- comprehensive
- accurate
- constrained
- signed and dated.

In addition, any records that are computerised should be:

- secure
- functional
- tamper-proof
- virus protected
- compatible with other systems
- serviceable
- have defined user access.

Referral letters

Patient referral letters should also be retained. The relevant information required on a referral letter includes:

- patient details (including date of referral)
- relevant medical and dental history
- specification as to whether advice or treatment is required
- level of urgency
- name of consultant/specialist
- source of referral
- name and signature of writer
- relevant radiographs and/or models.

When records are no longer required they should be disposed of in a way that will ensure no breach of confidentiality.

Data protection

The contents of dental records must not be disclosed to a third party without the patient's permission. The **Data Protection Act 1998** requires a patient to be given access to their dental records within a period of 40 days from their written application. However, some situations may arise where it might be considered appropriate to disclose records without the consent of the patient; professional advice should be sought before disclosure. Acceptable disclosure, beyond the immediate healthcare needs of the patient, may include:

- reporting an adverse drug reaction
- reporting a notifiable disease
- assisting the police to:
  - □ identify a body
  - □ identify the driver in a road traffic accident
  - □ prevent terrorism

    ☐ prevent or detect a serious crime
    ☐ help the coroner investigate a suspicious death
    ☐ prevent serious risk to others
■ disclosure of records to a third party (this is acceptable with the patient's consent).

Maintenance and storage

Day-to-day management of records

It is very important that a patient's records are readily available for each visit. This will mean that notes, radiographs and study models are accessible and cross-linked to allow them to be traced and retrieved easily. It is desirable to have all the necessary records before the clinic starts. This will mean retrieving the notes from file and radiographs and study models from store in preparation for the clinic.

Patients' clinical notes have conventionally been recorded in paper files; however, electronic storage of patient records is increasing. In a paper-based system records are usually stored alphabetically. They may be separated into groups according to the stage of a patient's treatment, e.g. under pre-treatment review, under treatment or discharged. If such a system is in operation it may be helpful to keep track of where patients are in the system, e.g. a card index. Increasingly, patient records, including radiographs and photographs, are stored and accessed electronically. There are several commercially available patient administration systems that have been designed specifically for orthodontic practices.

Radiographs are often stored in a patient's case notes or file, so are retrieved with the notes. Where this is not possible the radiographs will need to be stored separately. It is common to store them alphabetically in large envelopes. All radiographs need to have the patient's name and the date the radiograph was taken on them, either written directly or on a label.

The storage of study models is more of a problem and a system needs to be established to link the notes with the models. Study models are usually stored in boxes. Unlike radiographs that are usually stored alphabetically, study model boxes are usually numbered and stored in numerical order. The boxes have to be linked to case notes – by writing the relevant number on a patient's case notes in a prominent position – and also to an independent system, e.g. card index, so that a patient's box can be identified independently of the case notes.

Long-term management of records

Records not only have to be retained to monitor the progress of treatment but also for medico-legal reasons. Compared with other branches of dentistry the litigation rate is low for orthodontics; however, systems need to be in place to ensure that relevant records are stored for an appropriate length of time in case litigation arises. Although most dental claims are brought within four years of a causative event, the Department of Health has suggested that medical records held in NHS trusts and health authorities need to be kept for 10 years *after* treatment has been completed. However, records relating to patients who were children when treated should be kept until the patient's twenty-fifth birthday or twenty-sixth birthday if there was an entry made when the patient was 17 years old. In the General Dental Services there is a legal requirement to keep the records for two years after treatment.

This obviously presents a huge problem for orthodontic practices and departments to retain clinical records for such a length of time. It is therefore necessary to have systems in place to ensure that records are moved and tracked through the different stages before they are destroyed.

Once a patient has been discharged, the models and notes can be removed from the main system and put into long-term storage. It is common for discharged records to be stored according to the *year of discharge*. The **British Orthodontic Society** (BOS) has suggested that records should be graded and marked as *low risk/short-term storage* or *high risk/long-term storage* at the end of treatment and that this is marked clearly on the records. If this system is used it would then be possible to separate the records that can be destroyed after 10 years or the patient's twenty-fifth or twenty-sixth birthday from those that need to be kept for longer. The BOS suggests that *high-risk* cases would include multidisciplinary cases, those with high levels of treatment difficulty or those where there was a complication or dispute.

Whichever system is used it is necessary to keep a record of which patients have been discharged in any one year and into which larger box or holding area the records have been placed, so they can be retrieved again if necessary. For ease of use and tracking it is preferable that this record is kept alphabetically.

Over the working lifetime of an orthodontist, tens of thousands of models could potentially accumulate. It is therefore necessary to cull records regularly. However, it is important that no records are destroyed without being reviewed and that the timing of the destruction takes into account the 10-year and birthday guidance. The BOS has suggested that for *high-risk* cases:

- records should be retained for 10 years after treatment or until the patient's twenty-fifth or twenty-sixth birthday in their original form
- clinical notes need to be retained by the clinician
- secondary records may be held by the patient, thus placing the onus on the patient to produce them in case of litigation.

For *low-risk* cases:

- clinical notes should be retained by the clinician for 10 years after treatment or until the patient's twenty-fifth or twenty-sixth birthday
- secondary records may be destroyed after six years
- electronic storage of all records may be considered after six years provided there are appropriate audit trails, safety and security guarantees to allow the destruction of the original records.

System for management of records.

- Alphabetical notes ± radiograph storage.
- Numerical box storage.
- Methods to:
  - ☐ link box to patient, e.g. written on case notes, computer database
  - ☐ link patient to box, e.g. card index, computer database
  - ☐ link main store box with discharge box, e.g. card index, computer database.
- Record of the:
  - ☐ year of discharge, e.g. alphabetical list within a diary, computer database
  - ☐ whether case *high* or *low* risk
  - ☐ year of record destruction or transfer to another, e.g. electronic, medium.

Regulation of orthodontics

Registration

Orthodontics is a branch of dentistry and as such is regulated by the GDC. The GDC also keeps lists of dental specialists. Any registered dentist can work in a particular branch of dentistry, such as orthodontics, if they have the necessary competence. However, only those on a Specialist List can call themselves specialists in that discipline. To join a Specialist List, dentists have to show how they are qualified to use the title *specialist*. Usually they will have undertaken an approved period of training that leads to the attainment of a relevant qualification. However, when the lists were first established dentists who were able to show that they had enough experience or training to be called a specialist were also included on the lists (transitional arrangements). The orthodontic Specialist List was established in July 1998 and the relevant qualifications for entry on to the list are the Membership in Orthodontics (MOrth) or Diploma in Orthodontics (DOrth) from one of the royal colleges, although some dentists will be included on the list if they have a masters degree in orthodontics (e.g. MSc or MDentSci) that was awarded by a university. Specialist Lists are published annually in paper and electronic formats.

Education and training

As well as having responsibility for setting up and maintaining specialist lists, the GDC has overall responsibility for standards of education and training for the dental specialities. The GDC fulfils this responsibility in partnership with the faculties of dental surgery, the universities, the postgraduate dental deans and directors and the Joint Committee for Specialist Training in Dentistry.

Scope of practice

The Specialist Lists include registered dentists who are entitled to use a specialist title, e.g. specialist orthodontist, but do not restrict the right of any registered dentist to practise in any particular field of dentistry or the right of any specialist to practise in other fields of dentistry.

Informed consent

The orthodontist needs to inform patients and their parent (if appropriate) about any risks that may be involved during the course of orthodontic treatment. It is important that the orthodontist obtains valid (informed) consent before treatment commences. For consent to be valid the following points need be considered:

- the information needs to be up to date and current
- the person agreeing to the procedure needs to be able to understand and retain the information being given
- the person needs to be able to come to a reasoned decision.

Some of the main points that patients need to be made aware of before making a decision about treatment are:

- what type of appliance/s will be needed
- the need for retainers after the active treatment stage
- whether any teeth will need to be removed
- how long treatment will take, and the fact that it will be increased if they don't wear the appliance as advised, break their appliance or miss any appointments
- how often they will need to attend for appointments
- the need for excellent oral hygiene and the implications of not keeping appliances clean – also a change in dietary habits may be required
- the treatment may be stopped early if oral hygiene, attendance, care or wear of their appliance is poor
- the need to continue to have regular dental check-ups with their dentist throughout orthodontic treatment
- the risks associated with their treatment
- the limitations of the treatment.

Ideally written consent for orthodontic treatment should be obtained from the patient or parent/guardian if the patient is under 16 years of age. However, many orthodontists use implied consent – the patient attends regularly for treatment and allows the appliances to be fitted and adjusted – in view of the fact that most orthodontic procedures are reversible. This practice is likely to change in the future, as all parties are becoming more aware of the issues surrounding informed consent and the possibility of litigation.

Occlusal indices

Uses of occlusal indices

Occlusal indices have been developed for several reasons. They can be used for the following.

- **Diagnostic classification**, e.g. incisor (British Standards Institute) and molar (Angle's) classifications. Diagnostic classification aids communication and allows a quick description of a case in general terms without reference to any records.

- **Epidemiological purposes**: indices used for the collection of epidemiological data include data on all features of a malocclusion and are used for estimating the prevalence of occlusal traits within a population. Indices for such purposes include those developed by the FDI and World Health Organization (WHO).

- **Treatment need/priority**: several indices have been developed to assess patients' need for treatment and priority for care under public and private healthcare systems throughout the world. In the UK, the Index of Orthodontic Treatment Need (IOTN) was developed in response to the report of the Inquiry into Unnecessary Dental Treatment. It is based on the index developed for the Swedish Health Board and was originally developed to determine whether or not to give prior approval to an orthodontic assessment. In practice it is now used to determine which patients are accepted for hospital/NHS treatment in the UK.

- **Treatment standards**, e.g. Peer Assessment Rating (PAR). Some indices have been developed to assess standards of treatment that can then be used for audit or research purposes (see later).

- **Treatment complexity**, e.g. Index of Complexity Outcome and Need (**ICON**). This is the only index that has been developed specifically to assess treatment complexity. It is based on IOTN and PAR and gives a summary score based on the severity of the malocclusion and the difficulty of the proposed treatment.

- **Aesthetics**, e.g. IOTN aesthetic component. The expectation that orthodontic treatment will improve appearance is a strong motivating factor for seeking and complying with orthodontic care. To objectively rate dental attractiveness *in vivo* and from photographs or study models several indices that grade the aesthetic impact of a malocclusion have been developed.

- **Specific features** of a malocclusion, e.g. Little's index. Several indices have been developed to measure dental irregularities. The irregularity of the labial segments has been a characteristic of malocclusion that has been singled out for quantification because of the arbitrary descriptions of mild, moderate and severe crowding or spacing that have frequently been applied.

For an index to be useful it must be:

- **valid**, i.e. it measures what it intends to measure
- **reproducible**, i.e. it is probable that the same score/rating is given to an individual's malocclusion when the patient is re-examined by the same or different examiner
- **quick and simple** to use, ideally not needing specialist personnel or equipment.

Treatment need

The IOTN was developed from the Index of Treatment Priority used by the Swedish Dental Board for use in the UK. It grades malocclusion in terms of the significance of various occlusal traits on a patient's dental health and aesthetics. It aims to identify individuals who are in most need of and are likely to benefit most from orthodontic treatment.

Dental health component

The dental health component (DHC) of the IOTN was determined by considering the potential harm that a particular occlusal trait can have on the longevity of the dentition. Each occlusal trait is defined and categorised into five grades with clearly defined cut-off points. The grades are:

Grade 1 no need for treatment
Grade 2 little need for treatment
Grade 3 moderate need for treatment
Grade 4 great need for treatment
Grade 5 very great need for treatment.

When allocating a grade for the DHC, only the worst feature of the malocclusion is scored. The grade is made up of two components: the first, a grade (1–5), which defines the need for treatment; and the second, a suffix, which denotes which feature of the malocclusion was the reason for the classification. The features are looked at in the following order of priority (MOCDOB):

Missing teeth
Overjet
Crossbites ± displacements
Displaced teeth
Overbite
Buccal segment occlusion.

For example, if a malocclusion has an overjet of 12 mm and a canine that is missing and assumed to be impacted, both features put the malocclusion into grade 5, but it is the canine that determines the suffix, not the overjet. The suffix is primarily used for research to allow the clinician to see the relative frequencies of the different features of a malocclusion that need treatment (Table 5.8).

Aesthetic component

The aesthetic component was developed by Evans and Shaw (1987) by showing 1000 orthodontic photographs to a panel of six non-dental personnel who graded them on a

Table 5.8 Index of Orthodontic Treatment Need (IOTN) – Dental Health Component.

Grade	Description
Grade 1	**(None)**
1	Extremely minor malocclusions including displacements less than 1 mm
Grade 2	**(Little)**
2a	Increased overjet greater than 3.5 mm but less than or equal to 6 mm with competent lips
2b	Reverse overjet greater than 0 mm but less than or equal to 1 mm
2c	Anterior or posterior crossbite with less than or equal to 1 mm discrepancy between retruded contact position and intercuspal position
2d	Displacement of teeth greater than 1 mm but less than or equal to 2 mm
2e	Anterior or posterior open bite greater than 1 mm but less than or equal to 2 mm
2f	Increased overbite greater than or equal to 3.5 mm without gingival contact
2g	Pre-normal or post-normal buccal occlusions with no other anomalies. Includes up to half unit discrepancy
Grade 3	**(Moderate)**
3a	Increased overjet greater than 3.5 mm but less than or equal to 6 mm with incompetent lips
3b	Reverse overjet greater than 1 mm but less than or equal to 3.5 mm
3c	Anterior or posterior crossbite with greater than 1 mm but less than or equal to 2 mm discrepancy between retruded contact position and intercuspal position
3d	Displacement of teeth greater than 2 mm but less than or equal to 4 mm
3e	Anterior or posterior openbite greater than 2 mm but less than or equal to 4 mm
3f	Increased and complete overbite without gingival or palatal trauma
Grade 4	**(Great)**
4a	Increased overjet greater than 6 mm but less than or equal to 9 mm
4b	Reverse overjet greater than 3.5 mm with no masticatory or speech difficulties
4c	Anterior or posterior crossbite with greater than 2 mm discrepancy between retruded contact position and intercuspal position
4d	Severe displacements of teeth greater than 4 mm
4e	Extreme anterior or posterior open bite greater than 4 mm
4f	Increased and complete overbite with gingival or palatal trauma
4h	Less extensive hypodontia requiring pre-restorative orthodontics or orthodontic space closure to obviate the need for a prosthesis
4l	Posterior lingual crossbite with no functional occlusal contact in one or both buccal segments
4m	Reverse overjet greater than 1 mm but less than 3.5 mm with masticatory or speech difficulties
4t	Partially erupted teeth, tipped and impacted against adjacent teeth
Grade 5	**(Very great)**
5a	Increased overjet greater than 9 mm
5h	Extensive hypodontia with restorative implications (i.e. more than one tooth missing in any quadrant) requiring pre-restorative orthodontics
5i	Impeded eruption of teeth (with the exception of third molars) due to crowding, displacement, the presence of supernumerary teeth, retained deciduous teeth and any pathological cause
5m	Reverse overjet greater than 3.5 mm with masticatory or speech difficulties
5p	Cleft lip and/or palate
5s	Submerged deciduous teeth

Note: **MOCDOB M**issing teeth, **O**verjet, **C**rossbites ± displacement, **D**isplacement of contact points, **O**verbite and then **B**uccal occlusion.

Figure 5.22 Index of orthodontic treatment need: aesthetic component.

linear scale of attractiveness. Ten photographs were then selected to represent malocclusions at points equidistant along the scale (Figure 5.22). The photographs were selected on aesthetic grounds only and not on specific occlusal traits, e.g. spacing or buccally placed canines. The grade given indicates the need for treatment on aesthetic grounds and implies the psycho-social impairment that patient may suffer from.

The grades of the aesthetic component can be categorised to define the need for treatment on aesthetic grounds:

Grades 1/2	no need for treatment
Grades 3/4	slight need for treatment
Grades 5/6/7	moderate need for treatment
Grades 8/9/10	definite need for treatment.

The IOTN index can be used during clinical examination or on study models. This index is relatively quick to learn and with the specially designed measuring/prompt ruler it is quick to use.

It is purely an index of treatment need and makes no allowance for the complexity of treatment required to treat a particular malocclusion. For example, a canine that is displaced 4 mm from the line of the arch palatally may need 18 months of fixed appliance therapy to treat but it will score the same as one that is displaced the same distance buccally but may only require extraction therapy.

Treatment standards

The concept of audit is not new but very little work has been done to objectively evaluate the results of orthodontic treatment. The PAR index was developed to assess the outcome of orthodontic treatment from pre- and post-treatment study models. It has been found to be valid and reproducible and is quick to apply.

The concept of the PAR index is to assign a score to various occlusal traits that make up a malocclusion. The individual scores are then weighted and summed to obtain an overall total that represents the degree a case deviates from normal alignment and occlusion. A score of zero indicates good alignment and higher scores (rarely above 50) indicate increasing levels of irregularity. The overall score is recorded from pre- and post-treatment study models. The difference between these scores represents the degree of improvement as a result of orthodontic intervention and active treatment. There are five components to the PAR score and each is weighted according to the importance placed on it by the validation panel (Table 5.9).

Assessment of improvement

Treatment success can be determined by comparing the pre- and post-treatment PAR scores and can be expressed by:

- the percentage reduction in PAR score; and/or
- a reduction in PAR score plotted on a nomogram (Figure 5.23) to show the category change, e.g. a case with a pre-treatment score of 30 and post-treatment score of 5 will be greatly improved, but a case with a pre-treatment score of 20 and post-treatment score of 5 will only be improved.

Table 5.9 Peer Assessment Rating (PAR) weightings.

Component	Weighting
Upper anterior segments	1
Lower anterior segments	1
Right and left buccal segments	1
Overjet	6
Overbite/open bite	2
Centre-line	4

Figure 5.23 Peer assessment rating (PAR) index nomogram.

Category change in PAR score

Worse/no different   A change in weighted PAR Score of less than 30%
Improved   A change in weighted PAR Score of greater or equal to 30%
Greatly improved   A change of 22 weighted PAR points

Disadvantages of PAR

The PAR index has no weighting as to the difficulty of achieving the end result. However, a recently developed index – ICON – incorporates aspects of IOTN and the PAR index to develop a score that represents how complex a case will be to treat. The weightings of the PAR index put very little emphasis on the buccal occlusion compared with the overjet. Also, no account is taken of the inclination, angulation or rotation of the teeth and residual spacing in the buccal segments is not scored.

Treatment complexity

Index of Complexity, Outcome and Need (ICON) was developed by Daniels and Richmond in 2000. It is based on a combination of IOTN and PAR and was developed in collaboration with an international panel of 97 orthodontists using 240 initial and 98 treated study models. Each of the occlusal traits was scored according to a defined numerical protocol and statistical tests were used to determine the traits that were deemed to be predictive of the complexity of orthodontic treatment required. Five highly predictive occlusal traits were identified:

- IOTN Aesthetic Component
- crossbite
- upper arch crowding/spacing
- buccal segment antero-posterior relationships
- anterior vertical relationship.

Each occlusal trait contributing to a malocclusion is assigned a score. These are then summated and divided into five grades of complexity and improvement.

Provision of orthodontic treatment

Complexity

When considering who is the most appropriate person to undertake treatment for a patient the complexity of the likely treatment needs to be taken into account. There are several factors that determine how complex treatment is likely to be. When thinking about the complexity of the likely treatment for a patient the following points need to be considered.

■ What the problem is from a professional point of view and from the patient's point of view.
■ Whether the most appropriate treatment for the individual patient is the ideal, text-book treatment or some degree of compromise.

These two factors will largely determine what treatment is considered and are closely related to a patient's willingness/ability to cope with appliances, commitment to treatment and mouth care. Cases that are considered complex are those with (IOTN):

■ severe hypodontia   (5h)
■ overjet of 9 mm or more   (5a)
■ traumatic overbites   (4f)
■ CL/P   (5p)
■ anchorage demanding cases that will require treatment with fixed appliances and headgear
■ interdisciplinary cases that will require orthodontic treatment in combination with surgery or restorative treatment.

Orthodontic providers

There are several possibilities as to who can legally provide orthodontic treatment in the UK. These include:

■ general dental practitioner with clinical assistant training
■ specialist practitioner
■ Senior Dental Officer (SDO Ortho.)
■ hospital consultant.

Sometimes there is no choice in an area, but how the decision is made depends on the reason for referral. Patients may be referred for:

■ advice on the need for orthodontic treatment
■ a diagnosis and treatment plan
■ diagnosis and provision of treatment
■ a second opinion.

The different providers have different levels of training and can therefore only provide the level of service for which they are appropriately trained.

General dental practitioner with clinical assistant training

They cannot provide specialist advice but can provide treatment for patients with mild/ moderate malocclusions who need simple treatment with single-arch fixed appliances or removable appliances. However, whether those patients who are likely to have relatively mild problems need treatment and will benefit from having treatment needs to be considered.

Specialist practitioner/orthodontic SDO

They can provide specialist advice on the need for orthodontic treatment, developing malocclusions and any intervention required in a developing malocclusion. They can provide treatment for patients with moderate/severe malocclusions who need more complicated treatment with upper and lower fixed appliances with/without anchorage support, removable appliances or functional appliances.

Hospital consultants

They can provide specialist advice on the need for orthodontic treatment, developing malocclusions, any intervention required in a developing malocclusion and treatment planning for treatment carried out by general dental practitioners.

The hospital service can provide treatment for patients in greatest need who have severe malocclusions or need complex treatment with fixed appliances with or without anchorage support, removable appliances or functional appliances. It is also best equipped to provide treatment for those patients that require interdisciplinary treatment, e.g. combined with orthognathic surgery or restorative treatment.

In general, patients with severe malocclusions needing complex treatment are best treated within a hospital department. These include cases with (IOTN):

- impacted teeth   (5i)
- severe hypodontia   (5h)
- severe skeletal discrepancies   (4/5a, 4/5b, m or 3/4e)
- crossbites with slide   (>2 mm, 4c)
- Severe tooth irregularities   (4d)
- traumatic overbites   (4f)
- patients who fulfil the training needs of undergraduates, specialist registrars or clinical assistant training programmes.

When a patient is referred for an orthodontic opinion the malocclusion needs to be assessed systematically; the IOTN and the likely complexity of the treatment required needs to be determined. A decision about who is the most suitable person to carry out the treatment can then be made.

Quality measurement and improvement

A range of institutions and processes contribute to ensuring as far as possible that standards for patient care can be clearly identified and improved upon. These are:

- clinical effectiveness guidelines
- National Service Frameworks
- evidence-based practice
- clinical audit
- National Institute for Clinical Excellence (NICE)
- Commission for Health Improvement (CHI).

These are discussed in Chapter 6.

Risk management

This includes:

- identification of risks
- risk assessment
- risk reduction, elimination and transfer
- reporting and recording adverse events
- complaints procedures.

References and further reading

Egermark I, Magnusson T and Carlsson GE (2003) A 20-year follow-up of signs and symptoms of temporomandibular disorders and malocclusions in subjects with and without orthodontic treatment in childhood. *Angle Orthod* **73**: 109–115.

Ellis PE and Benson PE (2002) Potential hazards of orthodontic treatment – what your patient should know. *Dent Update* **29**: 492–496.

Evans R and Shaw W (1987) Preliminary evaluation of an illustrated scale for rating dental attractiveness. *Eur J Orthod* **9**: 314–318.

General Dental Council (1997) *Maintaining Standards*. London: GDC.

Helm S and Petersen PE (1989a) Causal relation between malocclusion and caries. *Acta Odontol Scand* **47**: 217–221.

Helm S and Petersen PE (1989b) Causal relation between malocclusion and periodontal health. *Acta Odontol Scand* **47**: 223–228.

Isaacson KG, Thom AR, Hormer K and Whaites E (2008) *Guidelines for the Use of Radiographs in Clinical Orthodontics*. London: British Orthodontic Society,.

Kim MR, Grabe TM and Viana MA (2002) Orthodontics and temporomandibular disorder: a meta-analysis. *Am J Orthod Dentofacial Orthop* **121**: 438–446.

Luther F (1998a) Orthodontics and the temporomandibular joint: where are we now? Part 1. Orthodontic treatment and temporomandibular disorders. [Review] *Angle Orthod* **68**: 295–304.

Luther F (1998) Orthodontics and the temporomandibular joint: where are we now? Part 2. Functional occlusion, malocclusion, and TMD. [Review] *Angle Orthod* **68**: 305–318.

Mitchell L (2001) *An Introduction to Orthodontics* (2e) Oxford: Oxford University Press. (This is an excellent textbook that is well written with an abundance of clear illustrations covering all aspects of orthodontics.)

Nightingale C (2001) Belle Maudsley Lecture 2001. Risk management in orthodontics – making clinical practice safer. *Dent Update* **28**: 437–441.

Pilley JR, Mohlin B, Shaw WC and Kingdon A (1997) A survey of craniomandibular disorders in 500 19-year-olds. *Eur J Orthod* **19**: 57–70.

Shaw WC, O'Brien KD, Richmond S and Brook P (1991) Quality control in orthodontics: risk/benefit considerations. *Br Dent J* **170**: 33–37.

6 Dental Implantology

Ulpee Darbar

Introduction

Dental implantology has undergone a significant revolution in the past 20 years with dental implants having become a more predictable tooth replacement option. The ongoing change has been triggered by two key factors, namely the improved technology relating to how implants integrate into the jaw bone and the increasing demands from patients wanting teeth like their own. While at present the field of implantology is not recognised as a separate speciality, to ensure protection for patients the General Dental Council (GDC) has enlisted training requirements for all those involved in implant dentistry. The successful outcome of implant treatment embraces the close working of the whole team, which includes the patient, the clinician, the dental nurse and the technician, not forgetting the hygienist and the radiologists who may have a more remote input but one that is equally important. To this end the dental nurse has a vital and crucial role in ensuring the smooth provision of implant treatment to the patient, as they will be the person to whom the patient is most likely to address questions. It is therefore important that the dental nurse has the necessary knowledge and understanding to be able to communicate effectively with the patient and the clinician. They should also be able to anticipate potential problems and appreciate the importance of patient aftercare, thus offering the support that is integral to a successful outcome. This chapter provides an overview of some of these aspects and guides the reader through the basic concepts of dental implantology.

Management of the missing tooth

Replacement options for missing teeth

Missing teeth are a problem for all groups of patients and can significantly compromise a patient's psychosocial well-being, with loss of confidence one of the most important aspects. Different types of device have been used for the replacement of missing teeth and the choice is primarily dependent on the number of teeth missing. Other factors that need to be assessed when making this choice are both patient related and site related and include the following:

- number of missing teeth
- amount of soft tissue (including the gingivae) lost
- underlying bone support
- condition of the remaining teeth and the gingival tissues in the mouth
- patient's smile line
- patient's expectations.
- patient's general health.

As the patient demands have grown over the years, a number of these factors pose challenges and the choice of replacement should be carefully evaluated against the objective of the tooth replacement. Tooth replacement options fall into two main categories: those that are supported by teeth and those that are supported by external devices, called **implants**, inserted into the jaw bone to anchor/support the replacement teeth. Within each category the replacement options fall into two groups:

- Removable prostheses (dentures): these are removed by the patient for cleaning and are usually considered when there has been a significant degree of soft tissue loss that needs replacing. The dentures can be **complete** (full) when the patient has lost all their teeth or **partial** when only some of the teeth are missing.
- Fixed prostheses: these are secured into the patient's mouth and can only be removed by the clinician. These can either be single crowns or multiple linked crowns, called **bridges,** supporting the missing teeth.

Most patients are not keen on wearing dentures and prefer to have something fixed in the mouth. The feasibility for a fixed prosthesis is determined by the degree of soft tissue lost and the amount of facial support required to restore aesthetics. Currently dental implants have become a predictable, albeit costly, alternative treatment option which many patients are seeking. However, implant treatment predictability is dependent on careful patient and site assessment as well as treatment planning, which is an essential and integral part of the decision-making process for the implant patient.

Dental implants

A dental implant is a device made from a biocompatible material that is placed within, or on, the bone of the jaws (maxilla or mandible) to provide support for a prosthetic reconstruction, which could be a single tooth, multiple teeth or all the teeth (e.g. a denture). **Endosseous** (also called **endosteal**) **implants** have been available for a number of years, with **ramus implants** used for edentulous patients with atrophic ridges (Figure 6.1b) and **blade implants**, the first-generation implants, being used widely in the past (Figure 6.1a). The second-generation implants, also called **root form implants** because their shape resembles that of a root, first gained acceptance in the early 1980s and have currently largely replaced all other types of implant device. These implants are rigid and will remain the focus of this chapter. These implants help to maintain and stimulate the alveolar bone, as well as providing an anchor for the prosthetic device.

(a)

(b)

Figure 6.1 (a) A blade vent implant; (b) a ramus implant.

Denture

Clips that insert
into denture

Bar retainer

Fixture (implant)

(a)

(b)

Figure 6.2 (a) A denture retained on an implant; (b) a crown retained in an implant.

Components of dental implants

An implant retained construction is made up of two components (Figure 6.2).

- The **fixture** (also referred to as the implant or screw). This is surgically placed into the jawbone using a series of specialised cooled drills under controlled conditions.
- The **teeth** (also called the prosthesis). This is usually initiated after a period of healing following placement of the fixture. Today with improved understanding about the way in which implants work, the prosthesis can be connected onto the fixture at the same time as it is placed in the jawbone. However, the latter is only feasible if certain conditions are met.

Treatment with dental implants occurs in two phases:

■ The **surgical phase**, which involves all the procedures that are necessary to place the fixture into the jawbone to facilitate the prosthetic tooth replacement.
■ The **prosthetic phase**, which includes all the procedures required to construct a restoration that is connected into the fixture.

Each phase requires specialised equipment to ensure predictable outcomes. Depending on the treatment plan, once the fixture is placed in the jawbone it is allowed to integrate for a period of time before the prosthetic phase during which the prosthesis is constructed. Today, with the correct environment, implant restorations can be constructed on the same day as implants being placed surgically.

Biology of implantology

The success of the second-generation endosseous dental implants is dependent on the close connection between the surface of the fixture and the bone. This phenomenon is called **osseointegration** and was originally defined on a histological basis as a direct structural and functional connection between ordered and living bone and the surface of a load-carrying implant (Brånemark *et al.*, 1969). Today this concept has been redefined using clinical parameters as 'a process whereby clinically asymptomatic and rigid fixation of an alloplastic (non-biologic) material is achieved, and maintained, in bone during functional loading'.

Osseointegration is a time-related phenomenon and its predictability is dependent on:

■ the surface of the fixture
■ the host bed (environment in which the fixture is placed i.e. the bone)
■ the patient.

The fixtures are made of commercially pure titanium which is biocompatible with the host tissues. The surface of the fixture forms an oxide layer when it is exposed to the environment. Once the fixture is surgically secured into the bone, the site will heal with a blood clot forming around the fixture. This blood clot carries the bone cells (**osteoblasts**) which play a role in determining the rate at which osseointegration occurs. It is therefore crucial that the host environment is protected during and immediately after the surgery to ensure that any trauma to the site is minimised. Any factor that affects this, e.g. poor surgical technique, trauma caused by the suction, excessive loading immediately after the surgery or smoking, will compromise the healing response and contribute to failure of the fixture to integrate into the bone.

The surface of the fixture also plays a key role in determining the rate of integration and the healing time period as it attracts the bone cells that are important for osseointegration to occur. While machined surface fixtures were the first type of fixtures introduced to the market, today most companies provide fixtures with surfaces that are treated and modified by etching and/or grit blasting the surface to increase the surface area onto which the bone cells adhere. This enhances healing thereby reducing the time it takes for the fixture to integrate into the jawbone. This enables the fixture to be restored either on the same day as the fixture placement or within eight weeks of placement as opposed to the six months that was traditionally quoted when the second-generation implants were first introduced. The fourth-generation fixtures are the latest development and have surfaces that are chemically modified to further increase the rate at which bone cells bond to the fixture surface, hence hastening the osseointegration process and enabling restoration to take place in shorter time frames (the same day or within four weeks) in high-risk patients.

It is essential that during the planning phases all these factors are taken into consideration and the host factors, including the site-specific factors, e.g. bone quality and quantity, as well as the patient-related factors are carefully evaluated such that the treatment outcome is predictably defined. Details of these and other parameters are covered later in this chapter.

Healing around implants

Healing around the implants occurs at two levels: the bone interface and the soft tissue interface. The predictability of the bone healing and osseointegration (discussed earlier) is dependent on strict protocols that must be followed to ensure a favourable outcome. The following key features must be observed during the healing phase.

- **Aseptic sterile technique**. This minimises the risk of infection and contamination.

- **Strict drilling protocol**. This protocol ensures that the site preparation is undertaken sequentially with incremental enlargement of the site in which the fixture is to be placed with adequate cooling. The drills used must be sharp to ensure that there is minimal trauma to the bone during the preparation, and the drilling should be undertaken intermittently to ensure not only efficiency in the bone cutting but also to enable any debris collected during the preparation to be removed. The drills used are all marked to the required length of the fixture and also come in different sizes in line with the final width. To ensure that the drills remain sharp a number of companies produce one-use only drills. Multiple-use drills must be closely monitored and changed regularly. The nurse plays a key role in ensuring that the drills are sharp and replacements are available if needed.

- **Adequate cooling**. The cooling is an essential aspect of the drilling protocol as any overheating of the bone will lead to death of the bone cells (**necrosis**) that are needed for osseointegration to occur.

The healing around the fixture once placed is dependent on the vascularity (blood supply) to the site. This has a key role in the osteogenic (bone forming) process which is the precursor to ensuring integration of the fixture into the alveolar bone. To ensure that the precursors of the bone cells within the blood clot have the optimum opportunity to develop into osteoblasts, it is crucial that there is no trauma or movement of the blood clot during the immediate postsurgical period. During the surgical placement, this movement is minimised by ensuring that the fixture has stability when it is placed in the jawbone. This initial stability is referred to as the **primary stability**. Following the sequential drilling, the final drill used is usually a size smaller than the fixture, thus ensuring maximum adaptation to the bone walls thereby providing the primary stability of the fixture which is crucial during the immediate postsurgical healing period. The threaded nature of the fixture and the design of the threads further enhance the primary stability, which is also dependent on the bone quality. Soft bone will need specific techniques to help ensure that this stability is achieved, and in bone that is very soft the final preparation may be undertaken using special instruments called '**bone condensers**'. Many implant systems have fixtures with different thread configurations for use in sites of soft bone to help ensure that good primary stability is achieved. After the surgical placement, the stability of the blood clot immediately afterwards is crucial to ensure that healing occurs with bone formation as opposed to fibrous tissue formation. Any pressure or trauma to the site at this time can lead to fibrous healing, thus leading to failure of the fixture to integrate into the jawbone. Hence patients are often advised not to wear their prosthesis for at least one week immediately after the surgery. Tooth-supported prosthetic devices can be used providing they do not traumatise the underlying surgical site and the patient is careful. This also helps minimise the risk of abnormal loading during eating and chewing on the fixture in the immediate postoperative period as any excessive overload on the site can also lead to fibrous union of the fixture during this critical time period thus leading to failure.

Sites that need augmentation (see p. 365) at the time of fixture placement also need to be managed carefully. It is usual to leave the fixture to integrate for a period of 4–6 months depending on the material used for augmentation and the extent of augmentation needed, e.g. repair of a dehiscence (fissure) or fenestration (hole). The rationale for augmentation is covered later in this chapter. Studies have shown that the osseointegration that occurs in augmented sites is similar to that which occurs in sites that have not had augmentation, and the success rate of the implants in such sites has also been shown to be equivalent to those not requiring augmentation.

The soft tissue healing around implants differs by virtue of the phenomenon of osseointegration. Unlike teeth, the fixture does not have a **periodontal ligament** when it integrates into the jawbone, as described earlier. Additionally the soft tissue/gingival tissue anatomy at a microscopic level around implants differs from a tooth in that the connective tissue fibres run parallel to the surface of the abutment (Figure 6.3). The vascularity is also reduced as the bulk of the blood supply in the region is derived from the basal tissues; as a result, implant-retained restorations are at a higher risk of failure if the cleaning is not maintained at an optimal level. Bacterial contamination can cause catastrophic failure with severe bone loss and ultimately loss of the implant, especially if there is occlusal overload, e.g. bruxists.

Types of dental implant

Implant fixtures are available in different lengths and sizes to match the teeth and the sites in which placement is being planned. The first fixtures were of a standard size;

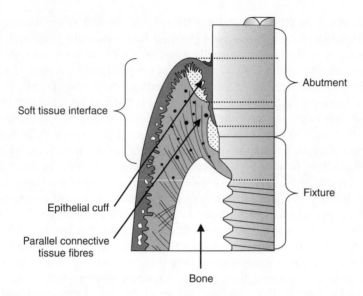

Figure 6.3 Soft tissue implant interface showing the parallel configuration of the connective tissue fibres.

however, today, with the aesthetic demands and restorative driven planning, different widths to accommodate the different sizes of teeth are now available with narrow fixtures (diameter of 3.3 mm and less) and regular fixtures (diameters of 3.75 mm to 4.1 mm) being most commonly used, followed by the wide diameters (greater than 5 mm), which are predominantly used for molar teeth and occasionally upper canine teeth.

Design of implants

The fixtures come in two main designs.

■ **Cylindrical**: these do not have a screw thread on the outside and are inserted into the site as a press fit. These fixtures are seldom used today

■ **Screw**: these are also called threaded parallel-sided fixtures and are screwed into the jawbone, offering better primary stability. These fixtures are the most commonly used today.

Tapered fixtures are available in both configurations and are designed with a narrower apical end resembling the shape of the root of the tooth. They were developed primarily to facilitate implant placement into the socket of a tooth as soon as it was extracted. The intention was to achieve better primary stability and also minimise the loss of bone that would normally occur after extraction. There is evidence to show that the latter does not happen and the remodelling changes in the bone are still seen post extraction. As a result their predictability remains variable and the use of tapered implants remains highly technique sensitive. These fixtures have special tapered drills that must be used to prepare the site and while still available are seldom used today.

Newer designs incorporating a combination of the taper coronally and screw form apically are also available especially for use in extraction sockets such that primary stability coronally is enhanced.

Other newer concepts such as **platform switching**, which focus on the preservation of the bone coronally once the fixture-retained restorations have been placed, have emerged in the past 3–5 years. The standard success criteria used for assessing outcome of implant treatment measure the bone levels around the fixture/restoration interface, with the accepted annual bone loss at this interface being around 0.1 mm or up to the first thread during the first year, depending on the system used. The concept of platform switching is aimed at eliminating this type of bone loss such that the bone levels at the coronal end of the fixture remain stable throughout the life of the implant-retained restoration. This occurs by switching the position of the abutment connection on the fixture platform, thus moving it inwards (Figure 6.4a). The tissues do not recognise this change and thereby remodel around this, allowing the bone to be preserved at the coronal height of the fixture (Figure 6.4b).

Connection of the implants

Two types of connection are used (Figure 6.5).

- **External connection**: this is where the connection via which the prosthesis is joined to the fixture sits above the coronal level of the fixture. The external connection fixtures are based on a hexagon design and the term **external hex** is often used to describe them.

- **Internal connection**: this is where the connection into which the prosthesis fits is inside the fixture itself. To improve the stability and anti-rotation (stops the prosthesis from moving around), different configurations are used, with some having a morse taper and others using double configured hexagons.

The majority of fixtures today adopt the internal connection as this offers the best stress distribution once the prosthesis is connected.

Type of placement

The fixtures are designed to be placed in one or two stages.

- **Two stage**: the fixture once placed is protected with a cover or closure screw and buried under the gingival tissue (Figure 6.6a). This type of fixture will need to be exposed to the mouth following a minor surgical procedure. At the end of the second surgical procedure a healing abutment is connected to allow the healing of the soft tissues before the impression can be taken for the prosthetic phase.

Figure 6.4 (a) The platform-switching concept aimed at bone preservation; (b) radiograph showing the platform-switch concept versus standard abutment.

Figure 6.5 Components of fixture (implant) retained prosthesis.

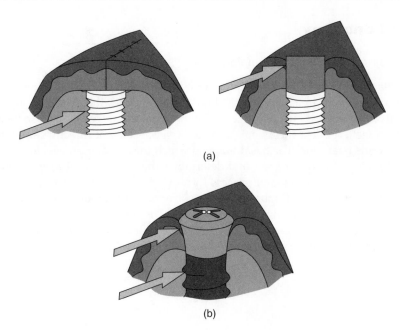

(a)

(b)

Figure 6.6 The two-stage (a) versus the one-stage (b) surgical techniques used for implant placement.

- **One stage**: the implant is inserted surgically into the jawbone and a protective cap called the **healing cap** or in some cases the **healing abutment** is connected to protect the top surface of the fixture (Figure 6.6b). At the end of the process the top of the protective cap is visible in the mouth. The key advantages of this type of placement are that the patient is not subjected to another surgical procedure to expose the fixture and the placement of the abutment will allow the soft tissues to remodel around the fixture thus providing a better soft tissue contour during the prosthetic phase.

Recommended tasks

(1) List the different tooth replacement options that are used for the replacement of missing teeth.

(2) List the factors affecting osseointegration and the criteria used to assess success.

(3) List the different types of implant fixture and their connections, including your understanding of primary stability.

(4) Access the Association of Implantology (ADI) website and download the patient information leaflet. List the information that should be given to a patient considering implant treatment.

Applied anatomy

Maxillary structures relevant to implantology

The maxilla or the upper jaw consists of a body and four processes. The areas of key importance in implant treatment are the body, which houses the **maxillary air sinuses**, and the **alveolar process**, which projects downwards and develops in response to the teeth. When teeth are lost the alveolar process remodels if not directly stimulated and bone loss occurs over time. The **basal bone** on which the alveolar process forms remains stable and undergoes little change, and determines the basic skeletal relationship of the teeth (Figure 6.7a). The **horizontal process** forms part of the hard palate and houses the incisive canal and foramen (Figure 6.7b). The structures of importance during implant placement are the incisive canal and the sinus floor. The **sinus** has a complicated anatomy and an awareness of this is essential if implant placement in the posterior maxilla is being planned especially if the bone height is minimal (Figure 6.7c).

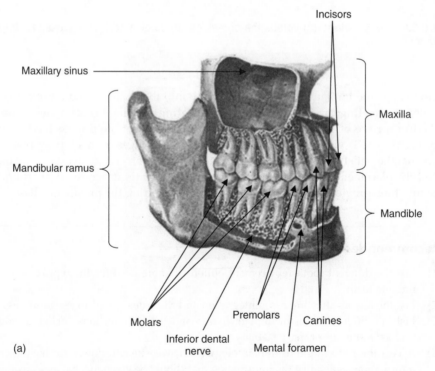

Figure 6.7 (a) Lateral view of the maxilla and mandible showing the key structures; (b) palatal view of maxilla; (c) lateral view of the maxillary sinus; (d) posterior view of the maxillary sinus.

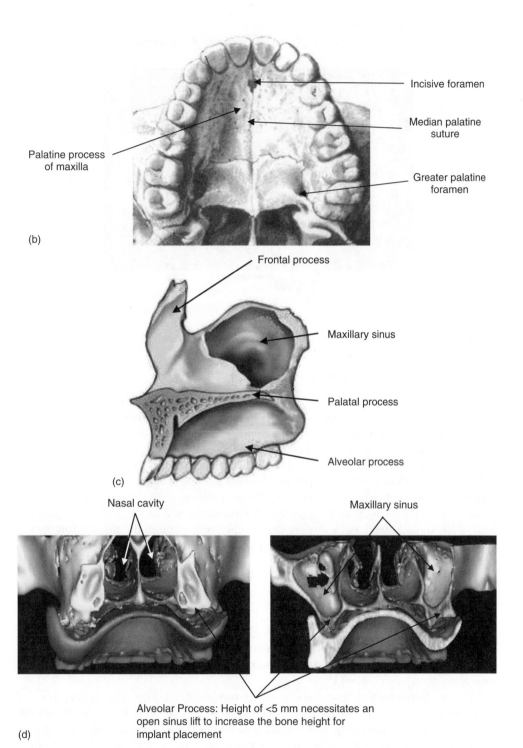

(b)

Incisive foramen

Median palatine suture

Greater palatine foramen

Palatine process of maxilla

Frontal process

Maxillary sinus

Palatal process

Alveolar process

(c)

Nasal cavity

Maxillary sinus

Alveolar Process: Height of <5 mm necessitates an open sinus lift to increase the bone height for implant placement

(d)

Figure 6.7 *Continued*

Mental foramen   Inferior dental canal

Figure 6.8 Anatomy of the mandible.

Mandibular structures relevant to implantology

The mandible consists of two halves that join in the middle. Each half is made up of the **ramus** and the **body**. The **alveolar process** forms on the body when the teeth develop. The **inferior dental nerve canal** in which the inferior dental bundle (nerves and vessels) lies traverses through the body and exits it at the mental foramen, where the vessels and nerves also exit (Figure 6.8). The ramus contains the opening of the inferior nerve canal called the **mandibular foramen**. The lingual nerve sits in the soft tissue lingual to the region where the ramus joins the body. As the bone resorbs in the mandible, the alveolus is lost and the bone height moves closer to the inferior dental canal. A knowledge of the path of the canal as well as the exit of the mental nerve through the **mental foramen** is crucial, especially if the bone height in the mandible is compromised.

Bone quality and quantity

Bone quality

Bone consists of cortical and cancellous bone. The **cortical plate** forms the outer surface of the bone and the **cancellous bone** lies within this cortical plate. Bone quality is determined by the distribution of the cortical and cancellous bone and four types (types I–IV) have been described (Table 6.1).

Type I is mainly cortical bone and is very dense and hard. This type of bone has the least vascularity. Type IV is mainly cancellous bone and remains very soft. It has the highest amount of vascularity. The maxilla usually has bone of type II/III with the posterior regions being type III/IV, whereas the mandible usually has type I/II. More often, the quality of bone will vary across the four types within the same site with a predomi-

Table 6.1 Types of bone quality.

Type	Description	
I	Mainly cortical bone. Comparable to oak wood	Cortical bone / Cancellous bone
II	Softer than type I, comparable to pine wood	
III	Less dense than type II comparable to balsa wood	
IV	Mainly cancellous bone. Least dense and comparable to polystyrene	

nance of one type. An awareness of the bone quality helps to ascertain the need for different equipment to ensure that the implants can be placed with predictability. Type IV bone, which is soft, may provide the biggest challenge in achieving primary stability when fixtures are placed in such bone. Equally, hard dense bone, e.g. type I, may need special screw taps to prepare the site prior to the placement of the fixture to minimise the heat that could be generated. While type I bone is the best type for primary stability it is the worst type for vascularity and may compromise the treatment outcome; patients should be made aware of this at the outset. An awareness of the bone quality is also important if the area needs to have any augmentation undertaken, especially in hard type I bone where the vascularity is compromised.

Bone height and width

A minimum height of bone is needed to ensure successful outcomes to implant treatment. In the past, fixtures of 7 mm were used; however, the failure rate with these when used alone remains high, and if used, they should only be used with other longer fixtures.

The minimum height of bone needed to place fixtures is 7 mm. Most systems have varying lengths of fixtures; the most common lengths used are the 10–13 mm lengths. The length of the fixture, depending on the site of placement, will help determine the primary stability. In the posterior maxilla, where more patients are asking for dental implants, the compromised bone height can be enhanced by raising the floor of the sinus, a method called **sinus lift**. Sinus lift procedures can be undertaken in two ways depending on how much bone height is present. If there is 4–5 mm bone height present then the sinus lift (raising the floor of the sinus by lifting the membrane) can be undertaken through the osteotomy site prepared for the fixture placement. The site is drilled to a length that is 1 mm short of the bone height. Special instruments called osteotomes are used to tap the floor of the sinus, lifting the membrane up. If grafting material is to be placed then this is done maintaining the prepared length, which is determined by special markers on the osteotomes. If, however, the bone height is less than 4–5 mm then a window of bone is removed laterally and the sinus membrane is exposed and raised using special instruments. The grafting material is placed and the sinus closed, and the site is allowed to heal for a period of 4–6 months prior to being prepared for fixture placement (Figure 6.9). However, it is important that in partially dentate patients the position of the natural teeth in relation to the bone level is ascertained such that any degree of soft tissue loss is also accounted for and the correct fixture to crown ratio is obtained. When a fixture is placed, there must be a minimum of 1 mm bone surrounding the fixture in all four directions. Today, with the use of augmentation, as long as primary stability is achieved the site can be augmented at the time of fixture placement to achieve these dimensions.

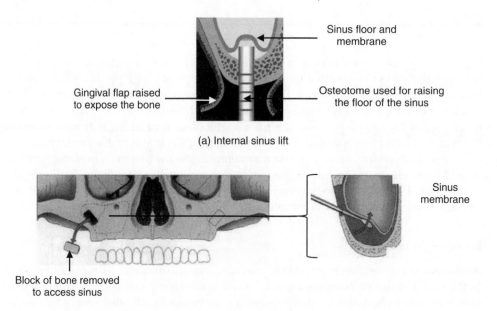

(a) Internal sinus lift

(b) External sinus lift (for alveolar bone < 5mm in height)

Figure 6.9 (a) The internal sinus lift procedure using an osteotome; (b) the external sinus lift procedure.

Augmentation of hard and soft tissue

Hard tissue augmentation

Hard tissue **augmentation** either during fixture placement or prior to fixture placement has become the norm, as placement of the fixture is usually driven by the prosthetic (restorative) treatment needs. This invariably means that bone volume has to be recreated to ensure that the fixture can be placed such that the proper aesthetic profile can be achieved. The materials available for hard tissue augmentation fall into the following categories.

- **Autografts** – bone obtained from the same human. Autogenous bone remains the gold standard; however, problems with morbidity and quantity lead to a need for the material to be mixed with other materials.
- **Allografts** – bone obtained from another human. This bone is usually freeze-dried or decalcified and freeze-dried.
- **Xenografts** – bone from an animal, e.g. cows, pigs. Cow bone is the most widely used material for augmentation today.
- **Alloplasts** – synthetic derivatives, e.g. bioactive glass and calcium sulphate derivatives. These have limited predictability in bone regeneration but have been used widely as alternatives with varying results of success.

Hard tissue augmentation can be undertaken:

- at the time of fixture placement, called **simultaneous augmentation**. If the fixture can be placed with good primary stability within the restorative envelope but there are local dehiscences or fenestrations, then the site can be augmented at the time of fixture placement. Healing is usually allowed for a period of at least four months, depending on the nature of the augmentation, prior to the prosthetic treatment phase starting

- prior to placing the fixture, called **staged augmentation**. If there is inadequate bone to achieve primary stability of the fixture the site must be augmented first to build up the bone such that future fixture placement can be achieved to meet the restorative treatment needs. The days of placing the fixture into the sites where the bone was present without considering the final position of the prosthetic teeth is no longer appropriate because of the prosthetic complications that occur, compromising the end result. Once augmented, the site is usually allowed to heal for up to six months subsequent to which the planning of the implant-retained prosthesis is commenced. The length of time for healing is also dependent on the type of grafting material being used, with autogenous bone requiring less time for healing.

Hard tissue augmentation is often undertaken using autogenous bone that has been collected during site preparation for fixture placement. The graft provides a scaffold over which the bone cells can migrate, thus enabling bone formation. Often, the bone is mixed with one of the other bone grafts because of the limited amount that can be collected. Currently, due to the fast resorption rate of autogenous bone, bone is often mixed with xenografts or synthetic grafts to slow the resorption rate. The grafting material may be protected with a barrier membrane. The nurse has to be aware of the materials and the equipment that is going to be used so that these are prepared and made available for the surgery. Additionally, the patient must be informed of the origin of the material, which should be recorded to provide the tracking information needed for the device in the event of a potential problem.

Soft tissue augmentation

Currently the awareness and need for aesthetically driven treatment has increased. As a result, there has been a rising interest in soft tissue augmentation around implants. There are two types of augmentation techniques that can be used.

- **Free gingival graft**: this is used to increase the band of keratinised tissue to facilitate cleaning and maintenance. The graft is normally taken from the roof of the mouth or other edentulous sites in the mouth. The main disadvantage with this is the difference in colour that is often visible.

- **Connective tissue graft**: this is normally taken from the roof of the mouth to provide a thicker band of tissue. This graft helps to change the biotype of the gingival tissue from a thin type to a thick type with more predictable outcomes. It gives excellent results providing patients with improved outcomes.

Soft tissue grafting can be undertaken prior to implant placement, at second stage surgery or after the prosthetic connection. With the latter, often the problem needs to be carefully evaluated to ensure the best outcome to the treatment. The appropriate type of sutures with the correct needle size should be used for soft tissue grafting. The needle sizes recommended are, usually 5.0 and 6.0 due to the delicate nature of the tissues that are being handled.

Recommended tasks

(1) Detail the key anatomical landmarks that are important during implant placement in the maxilla and mandible.
(2) Why is bone quality important in implant placement and what types are you aware of?
(3) Why do you need to augment bone? List the materials used for this. At what stage would bone augmentation be considered?
(4) Soft tissue grafts are being used increasingly in implant surgery. What types of soft tissue grafts do you know of and when are they used?

Patient assessment

The patient assessment is an essential part of the process when implant treatment is planned. This assessment is undertaken in two phases:

- **The preparative phase**: during this phase the expectations and the patient's primary dental problems are addressed and any medical problems identified. Treatment is initiated so that the patient can be assessed with a view to progressing into the definitive phase, when planning for the implant retained prosthesis takes place.

- **The definitive planning phase**: this phase usually occurs after the preparative phase, during which the primary problems have been dealt with. A full assessment and evaluation for planning the replacement of the missing teeth with an implant-retained prosthesis is undertaken and includes an assessment of the site where the fixtures are going to be placed with the bone height, width and the soft tissues being evaluated.

The assessment phase enables the dental team to obtain a full evaluation of the patient, including their concerns, expectations and medical history. The patient's attitude to treatment can be ascertained and the rapport established during this time is essential to build up the patient's confidence for the planned treatment. The patient's needs must be closely evaluated so that a clear understanding of their expectations is achieved. The treatment can then be planned such that the patient's intended treatment outcome is fulfilled. Equally this also enables the patient to be alerted to when it is not possible to meet their expectations.

Complaint and patient history

This is the first step in the assessment phase. It will help ascertain what the patient's main concerns are and their expectations of treatment. The latter is a fundamental aspect of the process as it helps to understand where the patient sees the treatment going. It will also help identify patients who have unrealistic expectations of the treatment outcomes. The history the patient gives will help identify the cause of the tooth loss and gives some indication about the level of patient compliance and motivation for treatment. It also gives an opportunity to identify whether the patient is wearing a prosthesis to replace the missing teeth and how they are coping with this. The patient's suitability for surgery and their ability to cope with lengthy procedures is also determined during this phase. It is important that the nurse assisting the operator listens closely to the discussion as the patient will often share confidences with the nurse and ask the nurse questions about things they may not have understood at the consultation.

Medical history

A thorough medical history is mandatory for all patients and should be taken and updated regularly by the clinician. It is essential that any concerns are raised and to help ensure that a through history has been undertaken, the use of medical history proformas can be considered. It is essential that the patient's drug history, including a list of the medications they are taking, is noted. The medical history should be updated at every visit and while there are no absolute contraindications to implant treatment, patients who have bleeding disorders or on certain medications, e.g. warfarin, may need to be handled differently. It is important that patients with complicated medical histories are planned such that the treatment is organised around the medical history. In situations where there is ambiguity of the medical history, clarification should be sought from the patient's doctor.

Examination

The examination phase is undertaken in two sections, the extra-oral and the intra-oral assessment. The **extra-oral assessment** includes an assessment of the patient's smile line, the facial height and facial profile, as well as the asymmetry and the patient's mouth opening.

The **intra-oral assessment** should be undertaken sequentially as follows.

■ **Soft tissue assessment:** an assessment of the soft tissues, including the sulcus depth and the contour, is undertaken and the relationship with the adjacent teeth evaluated.

■ **Periodontium:** the health of the gingival tissues is determined, including the quality of the gingival tissues called the **biotype**. The amount of keratinised tissue present is also noted in the site of the implant placement.

■ **Teeth:** the teeth present, including their condition, is assessed together with the recording of any missing teeth. The intended tooth position is determined and evaluated against the underlying soft tissue. Additionally, the presence of any drifting or over-eruption is also noted.

■ **Occlusion:** the intra- and inter-occlusal relationship of the teeth is assessed and an analysis undertaken of any interferences.

■ **Other investigations:** orthopantomograms and periapical radiographs are taken. These give an overview of the dental structures and also an indication of the anatomical structures in relation to the site of the missing teeth, as well as the alveolar bone height and the condition of the teeth. Issues relating to magnification remain a concern and ball bearings incorporated into radiographic stents are often used to help calculate the magnification factor. While easily accessible, neither of these radiographs gives an indication of the bone quality or density. Lateral cephalometric radiographs have been used; however, these are mainly beneficial for ascertaining the bone height in edentulous patients.

The basic assessment undertaken will enable the clinician to judge the patient's suitability for implant treatment. Depending on the case complexity, supplementary diagnostic information relating to the bone height and width as well as the type of prosthetic replacement will have to be obtained prior to finalising the treatment plan. The patient at this stage is usually given an overview of the feasibility of implant treatment and the need for further investigations is discussed. It is good practice to confirm the verbal information in writing and supplement it with patient information leaflets. This will help the patient to make an informed choice during the final planning stages once all the required information has been gathered.

Diagnostic aids to planning

The increasing patient demands and associated case complexity have resulted in the need for meticulous planning of implant-retained restorations as a treatment option for missing teeth. To supplement the basic assessment, additional diagnostic aids are needed to help finalise the treatment plan. These can include the following.

Photographs
These enable the clinician to have a more critical evaluation of the area being planned for fixture placement and can also be valuable to remind the patient of their appearance prior to treatment.

Study casts
These give an accurate assessment of the site of fixture placement viewed outside the mouth. The casts should ideally be mounted on an articulator so that the relationship of the upper and lower jaws is determined and an assessment of the teeth can be undertaken three dimensionally. The study casts also provide a reference of the preoperative starting point, which can be shown to the patient for comparison against the planned procedure.

Diagnostic wax-up
This is a mock-up of the intended position of the teeth to be replaced and is undertaken on the study cast. The wax-up is beneficial as it will help identify the shape and size of the teeth to be replaced and their relationship to the existing teeth, the impact of any soft tissue loss and any possible need for augmentation. It can be used as a tool for discussion with the patient, who can also see what the replacement teeth would look like, which can help the clinician to ascertain potential difficulties that may be encountered during the placement and restoration of the fixtures. In cases where multiple teeth are lost, the wax-up will help ascertain the need for soft tissue replacement and its potential impact on the facial appearance. The diagnostic-wax up is also used to obtain radiographic and surgical guides thus ensuring the intended replacement tooth position is replicated accurately.

Radiographic template
This is normally made using the diagnostic wax-up or the denture, if the patient has been wearing a denture where the tooth position is acceptable. The radiographic guide will

Radiographic template   Incisive canal   Bone width

Palatine process of maxilla

Figure 6.10 Radiographic template in situ against the alveolar bone.

contain a radiopaque material in the teeth to be replaced, so that when the radiograph is taken with the stent *in situ*, the intended tooth position is replicated onto the radiographic image thus relaying this position to the underlying bone and soft tissue (Figure 6.10). The radiographic templates help incorporate the patient's proposed treatment plan into the radiographic examination so that an indication of the need for soft and hard tissue augmentation to meet the restorative needs can be made

Bone mapping

This is usually undertaken when additional radiographic facilities are not available and is particularly useful for single tooth replacement. This can also be a cost-effective alternative to gain some information of the buccolingual dimension of the bone available for implant placement. The method involves giving local anaesthesia in the potential implant site, and a sharp probe with markers is used to assess the depth of the soft tissue at recorded intervals and transferred to a cross sectioned study cast at the intended implant site (Figure 6.11).

Specialist x-rays

In addition to the basic radiographs detailed above, the field of implantology has become more complex as the boundaries are pushed further out. A number of specialised radiographic techniques are now available that enable the clinician to have a visual understanding of the site to be operated on well before the surgical procedure is undertaken. Many of the latest inventions in digital radiography offer the advantage of lower radiation doses with three-dimensional imaging such that the bone volume and height, including the bone quality, can be obtained. The following specialised radiographs are of value in dental implantology.

(a)

(b)

Figure 6.11 (a, b) Ridge/bone mapping.

- **Lateral tomograms:** these films give an indication of the buccolingual dimension and are inexpensive. However, they can sometimes be difficult to interpret.

- **Computerised tomograms:** a number of sophisticated techniques are now available and utilise digital mathematical procedures, thus giving an outline of both the soft and hard tissues. Axial and three-dimensional images can be obtained and give a good indication of the bone volume in relation to the tooth position, especially when used with a guide. Interactive three-dimensional imaging has become more popular and can provide axial, cross-sectional and panoramic views with greater detail of the bone as well as soft tissue volume. This helps during the planning, giving visual representation of the bone prior to the surgical intervention. These images can be shown to the patient during the discussion, thus enabling them to understand more fully the risks associated with the proposed treatment.

Decision making

The decision-making process involves the assimilation and integration of all the data collected during the assessment phase, along with the additional aids, to derive a risk-assessed treatment plan that is intended to satisfy the patient's presenting complaints. The patient is shown the diagnostic wax-up and all the tooth replacement options, including dental implants, are discussed. The patient is alerted to the potential risks associated with the implant treatment and is also shown the specialist radiographs if any have been taken. The patient is also informed about the potential need for bone and/or soft tissue augmentation that may be required either during or prior to the fixture placement to improve the predictability of the treatment. The decision-making process will alert the patient to the following:

- the type of implant retained restoration that will be feasible
- the need for bone augmentation either prior to or during the fixture placement
- the need for soft tissue augmentation
- the type of surgery required and how it would be undertaken
- the healing period and the time frame within which the patient will have the final prosthesis
- the risks associated with treatment, which includes failure of the fixture to integrate into the bone, trauma or damage to any adjacent vital structures
- the short- and long-term complications associated with the treatment
- the need for long-term maintenance and support to ensure longevity of the restorations.

The patient is an integral part of this decision-making process and plays a key role in formulating the definitive plan. The information sheet given to the patient will enable them to actively participate in the decision-making process. Once the final plan has been agreed with the patient, these verbal discussions should be confirmed in writing so that the patient is able to have a clear understanding of the treatment proposed and the associated risks, as well as their compliance and commitment to the treatment proposed.

Patients will often seek advice from the dental nurse about some of the issues discussed with them, especially if they are anxious. It is therefore important that the nurse assisting in implant treatment is fully aware of the types of procedure that can be undertaken, the grafting materials available and investigations required, and also understands what the clinician has discussed with the patient to ensure that they are able to accurately and appropriately reassure the patient.

> ### Recommended tasks
>
> (1) A patient presents requesting replacement of a missing tooth with an implant. What are the steps the clinician would take to plan the replacement of the tooth?
> (2) What type of diagnostic investigations can be used to supplement the planning for implants?
> (3) What is the decision-making process and how should it be undertaken?

Implant treatment

Aims of implant treatment

The key aim of implant treatment is to provide the patient with a tooth or teeth that resemble their own, thus improving function, aesthetics and psychological well-being. While implants are the best option in the majority of patients, provision of implants in some patients could be detrimental to their well-being.

Benefits of implant treatment

The potential benefits of implant treatment include:

- replacement of missing teeth with teeth closely resembling the patient's own teeth
- improved aesthetics
- continued maintenance of oral health
- improved psychological well-being
- improved self-confidence
- retention of teeth so that the teeth feel like natural teeth.

Risks of implant treatment

Implant treatment, like any other surgical intervention, is associated with a number of risks. These risks should be evaluated during the planning phase and the patient made aware of them. The dental nurse should be aware of the risks as patients will often ask the nurse about things they are worried or unclear about. A well-informed nurse will be able to play an active role in comforting and reassuring the patient during the pre- and postoperative phases as well as during the surgical and restorative phases. The risks that can be associated with implant treatment can be assessed at three stages.

Planning phase
Teeth adjacent to the site planned for the implant placement can flare up and contribute to implant failure. Teeth that are deemed as high risk should be assessed during the planning phase to minimise this risk and if necessary planned loss should be undertaken during the implant planning.

During surgical placement and immediately afterwards

Care during the surgical stage is important to ensure that complications during the surgical placement as well as immediately afterwards are minimised. The key risks are:

- trauma during the surgery – torn flaps that can occur when the flaps are raised or trauma as a result of inappropriate use of flap retractors and the suction equipment
- excessive bleeding during the surgery – this is minimised if care is used during the raising of the flaps. Applying pressure during the surgery will help minimise the bleeding
- abnormal anatomy – during surgery the ridge shape may be noted to be unfavourable or the bone quality poor. Fixture placement should either be aborted or an alternative plan considered
- perforation during site preparation.
- fracture of the osteotomy wall
- paraesthesia – this can occur due to trauma to a nerve, e.g. the inferior dental nerve, mental nerve
- perforation of the sinus floor
- postoperative swelling and bruising beyond what would normally be expected.
- postoperative infection.

Many of these risks can be minimised if the surgical site has been planned well and the tissues and site are handled carefully. In the event that the risk is deemed severe, then the placement of the fixture should be aborted, the site closed and the patient informed.

At the prosthetic connection and after the fit of the prosthesis

- Failure of the fixture, noted by movement at the time the impression coping is connected. The fixture should be removed and the site assessed for the potential causes of the failure and re-planned if appropriate

- Loosening and/or fracture of the prosthetic screw. This usually occurs after the restoration has been inserted and connected for some time. Screw loosening was a common problem with some implant systems; this has largely been rectified, although it does still occur in some patients. The main cause is due to parafunction or occlusal overload.

- Fracture or wear of the bridge.

- Inflammation of the soft tissues.

The risks at each of these stages can be minimised or avoided with thorough planning, careful tissue handling and good patient co-operation. The patient will often phone the surgery and the nurse may be the first person the patient speaks to. It is important that the nurse is able to give the patient the correct information to reassure them and if necessary arrange for the patient to attend in an emergency.

Phases of implant treatment

Implant treatment is divided into two stages. The first involves the surgical placement of the fixture and the second is the restoration of the fixture to support a prosthesis.

Surgical placement

The surgical placement is undertaken such that an aseptic sterile technique is followed. The fixture is placed into the jawbone as directed by the surgical guide, which gives the clinician an idea of the final tooth position and helps to ensure that the fixture is placed within the desired prosthetic location. If this placement is not feasible then insertion of the fixture should be aborted. The site is prepared using a sequential drilling protocol, which is customised to the implant system that is being used. It is essential that the nurse assisting with the procedure is aware of this protocol as they will play a key role not only in supporting the process but also in the postoperative disposal of contaminated materials and sterilisation of instruments. The site preparation is undertaken systematically with optimal cooling such that trauma to the bone does not occur. The key objective of site preparation and fixture placement is to achieve primary stability of the fixture such that there is no movement of the fixture in the bony socket. The concept of **bicortical stabilisation** used in the 1980s where the fixture was placed such that the cortical plate coronally and apically was engaged is no longer followed. Following the fixture placement, the site is allowed to heal for the required period. If the fixture is buried under the gingival tissue, a second surgical procedure is needed to expose the fixture in the mouth. In this case the same aseptic surgical protocols that are used for the first stage surgery are followed. After exposure, the fixture is connected to the mouth with a healing cap/abutment and after a few weeks of healing the prosthetic phase can begin. If the fixture has been placed using the one-stage protocol, the patient will be ready to start the prosthetic phase following the healing period.

Prosthetic reconstruction

The prosthetic reconstruction starts after the healing period and can be undertaken at:

■ 4–6 months after osseointegration
■ 4–8 weeks after osseointegration
■ immediately at the time of placement of the fixture.

The choice between the above options will be dependent on the reason for the tooth loss, the degree of primary stability achieved at the end of the surgery, the need for augmentation and the planned procedure, including the type of prosthesis to be made. This would have been decided on during the planning phase, i.e. whether removable or fixed (see p. 373). Irrespective of the type of prosthesis, the prosthetic reconstruction follows the same stages.

■ **Impression taking** using specialised impression copings. These are taken either at the fixture head level or at the abutment level. For the latter an abutment has to be connected to the fixture head. The impression is sterilised, labelled and marked with the patient's details and a laboratory card with instructions of what is needed is completed and sent off to the laboratory.

- **Pouring the working cast:** the laboratory connects the replicas of the fixture or the abutment depending on type of impression taken. They will then proceed with the fabrication of the prosthesis using the customised prosthetic components. Where multiple teeth are missing the laboratory may be asked to make a bite block with which the jaw registration is carried out.

- **Jaw registration:** this is undertaken by the clinician using the special jaw registration jigs or the bite block that the laboratory has constructed. A facebow transfer is undertaken at this stage if needed. The assembly is sent to the laboratory with an indication of the shade needed. The laboratory will work on the set-up and construct the framework onto which the prosthesis is to be made.

- **Framework try in:** the framework is connected onto the fixtures in the patient's mouth and checked for fit and passivity.

- **Try in:** the prosthesis is then tried in for the patient to assess the aesthetics and comfort and to ensure that they are happy with it.

- **Fit:** this is completed as determined by the type of prosthesis.

The above stages are an overview and will vary depending on the complexity and type of prosthesis being made, and the patient's expectations. The nurse should be aware of all these stages to ensure that all the laboratory work as well as the clinic is set up for the clinician's needs. Additionally there is a need for the nurse to be able to liaise with the clinician and technician as well as the patient in the event that there is a query.

When immediate restorations are constructed a similar sequence is followed; however, the jaw registration is undertaken at the same time as the impression taking phase. The prosthesis is usually constructed as a temporary prosthesis and the site allowed to heal prior to the final prosthesis being made. These types of restorations will not necessarily be placed under load at this time. The alternative type of prosthesis is one that is fitted and loaded immediately after the fixtures are placed. These require special techniques and skills to be constructed both in the clinic and the laboratory.

Recommended tasks

(1) Discuss the benefits of implant treatment and the risks associated with this type of treatment.
(2) What are the phases of implant treatment and why should the dental nurse be aware of these phases?
(3) What type of restorations can be constructed on implants?
(4) Describe why diagnostic wax-ups are used in implant planning.

Types of surgical procedure

The types of surgical technique and procedure used have changed over the years as predictability has improved. As discussed earlier the fixture can be placed either as a two-stage procedure where the fixture is buried under the gingival tissue or as a one-stage procedure where the top of the healing abutment is visible in the mouth. Irrespective of the type of placement or technique, the surgical set-up must follow a strict protocol of sterility to ensure that the risk of infection and failure is minimised.

Aseptic technique

The predictability of implant treatment is dependent on ensuring that an aseptic technique is observed at all times. This technique helps ensure that optimum sterility is maintained and no contamination of the equipment or implants occurs during the surgery. The aseptic technique involves the concepts of asepsis and antisepsis. **Asepsis** is the absence of living pathogenic organisms and is used to minimise the risk of bacterial contamination by the use of sterile instruments and the no-glove touch technique. **Antisepsis** is the removal of microorganisms from the skin and the reduction of bacterial flora in the oral cavity. This is usually undertaken by asking the patient to rinse out with chlorhexidine mouth rinse preoperatively and also by wiping the skin around the oral cavity with an antiseptic, e.g. Tisept. During the whole surgical process sterility is maintained by using strict clinical protocols.

Types of fixture placement

Fixtures can be placed surgically at different times depending on the site that is being treated and the objective of the treatment.

Standard placement

This type of approach is used when the teeth have been lost for a number of years and the patient is now seeking replacement with an implant. Additionally those sites that need bone augmentation prior to implant placement will also fall into this type of placement as the site is allowed to heal for a period of 4–6 months following the bone graft before the implant can be placed. This type of placement gives the best outcome as the bone and soft tissues have healed and remodelled to a predictable level. The key challenges associated with this type of placement are related to the degree of bone loss that could have occurred following the loss of the teeth.

Delayed placement

This approach has become more popular and the majority of patients today are treated this way. The teeth are removed and the site allowed to heal for a period of 6–8 weeks prior to the surgical placement of the fixture. The objective behind this approach is that it enables the soft tissues to heal completely, thus improving the soft tissues available and also minimising the loss of bone that normally occurs if the site is allowed to heal for 4–6 months. In sites where major bone grafting becomes necessary due to the excessive bone loss, this type of placement would not be suitable due to the lack of bone. Depending on the reasons for the tooth loss, this type of placement may cause problems with achieving primary stability.

Immediate placement

With this approach the teeth are removed and the fixtures inserted at the same time into the socket of the tooth. This type of placement is highly unpredictable and requires a high level of skill. A number of companies have produced tapered implants to fulfil the objectives of immediate placement by producing a device that resembled the shape of a tooth root; however, currently these have been largely replaced with cylindrical implants. In patients with a thin quality gingival biotype, this type of approach is not recommended, especially in the aesthetic zone, as problems with ongoing bone loss can lead to exposure of the fixture threads and compromised aesthetics. Immediate placement does give predictable outcomes, but remains highly case sensitive. If this approach is used it is crucial that healing caps are available to protect the fixture and support the gingival tissue.

Flapless surgery

This is used to minimise the exposure of bone that occurs when a full flap is raised. The intention is that access to the bone is achieved either via the socket of the tooth if it is an immediate placement or alternatively by the use of a **punch**, which removes a collar of the keratinised tissue in the planned site of implant placement. This type of surgery works well in experienced hands but can lead to an increased risk of failure as the whole bone anatomy in the site of the fixture placement is not evident.

Teeth in a day

This approach uses specialised computerised guided stents that are made to fit the patient's mouth, and the bone is accessed using a flapless approach to place the fixtures. The restorations are connected immediately afterwards.

As technology advances, different types of high-risk procedure are being reported; however, it is important to remember the predictability of the treatment is dependent on the patient and any associated risk factors. The increasing number of surgical techniques, and therefore choices, have been driven by patient demand as well as improved technology. It is essential, albeit demanding, for the dental nurse to keep up to date, as often patients may have heard about something and will approach the nurse with questions. The crucial role that the nurse plays in the preoperative setting up of the surgery as well as the assistance provided cannot be underestimated and it is important that the nurse understands the different procedures used to ensure that the whole process works smoothly for both the patient and the clinician.

Post-operative cleaning of instruments

A systematic approach to cleaning the instruments is essential to ensure their longevity of use and to provide appropriate infection control. On completion of the operative stage used drills must be wiped and soaked in saline immediately after use to minimise contamination with blood. Drills that are multiple use must be checked for wear or damage and new drills ordered if necessary. A log should be kept of the number of times the drills are used in order to ensure that new drills are ordered well before they are needed for the next surgical procedure. Single use only drills should be discarded. At this time all manual torque wrenches and devices should be dismantled prior to sterilisation. The nurse should also check all the equipment and kit contents and arrange for replacement of any items that are either worn or damaged. To ensure that the nurse is able to provide the best support for the procedure, communication and joint team working with the clinician is of paramount importance.

Recommended tasks

(1) What types of surgical techniques are available for implant placement and when would they be used?
(2) What is the sequence that should be followed after the implant surgery?
(3) What are the sequences that are followed for prosthetic reconstructions?

Implant-retained prostheses

An implant retained prosthesis can either be screwed or cemented and falls into the falling categories:

- removable
- fixed
- a combination called a **hybrid**.

The choice of the type of prosthesis will be determined by the amount of soft tissue loss, the aesthetic needs of the patient, the amount of bone volume and the number of remaining natural teeth present. During the planning phase a decision will have been made about the type of prosthesis that is going to be feasible based on the above parameters and how the prosthesis is to be retained on the fixtures. This restorative driven decision also helps determine the number of fixtures that need to be placed during surgery and the sites in which they are to be placed, with fewer fixtures being needed for a removable prosthesis than for a fixed prosthesis. Due to the differences in bone quality, the mandible usually requires fewer fixtures compared to the maxilla for either type of prosthesis (fixed or removable), e.g. an implant-retained complete denture in the maxilla requires four fixtures to support it as opposed to two needed in the mandible. There are different ways in which the removable and fixed prosthesis can be connected into the implant fixtures.

Removable prostheses

The use of implants to support dentures became an accepted method of treatment following the acceptance of osseointegration as a predictable phenomenon at the Toronto conference in 1982. A number of different retaining devices (attachments) have been used and these primarily help retain the prosthesis, but may also provide some occlusal support and stabilisation to the prosthesis. The devices come as connecting male and female components, with the male component usually inserted into the fixture and the female into the denture. When the denture is then worn the female component locks into the component in the fixture thus providing the required retention. For these retaining devices to be used, it is crucial that there is adequate space to accommodate these two components. The types of devices used for implant retained removable prosthesis fall into the following categories.

- **Bars:** the original concept of using bars for supporting dentures was based on the necessity to connect the fixtures so that maximum rigidity was provided to the prosthesis. The bar is soldered onto the abutment, which is screwed into the fixture. Due to the precise location of the bar on the abutment, the fixtures need to be well aligned. The retaining female component is housed in the denture and is normally in the form of a clip (either gold or plastic), which, due to the wear and tear, will need replacing with time. The construction of a bar-retained prosthesis needs considerable interocclusal space to ensure that the height of the bar as well as the denture thickness and the height of the clips can be accommodated. The bars are more technically demanding to construct and require additional clinical time and are also more challenging for patients to clean.

- **Studs:** these are usually available in the form of ball and socket attachments. The ball is screwed into the fixture and the denture houses the female component which can either be an 'O' ring or a plastic resin clip. The earlier designs were cumbersome and bulky, but they have been replaced with smaller versions. The advantage of the studs over bars is that construction of the denture is less technically demanding and they are easier for patients to clean. This option therefore has more durability and is often advantageous in patients with manual dexterity problems.

Other systems have also been used, including magnetic attachments made from rare earth alloys. However, these are not widely used as they can only resist limited levels of shear loads, hence they are not ideal for denture wearers where larger amounts of lateral loads can be transmitted. In recent years, locators that function on a similar principle to the studs have gained wide popularity due to their size (smaller than studs); they provide retention by the use of replaceable plastic resin inserts which fit within the female housing placed inside the denture. Because the height of the locator abutment is minimal, the corresponding hole needed in the denture is smaller, thereby minimising the weak areas within the denture. The locators also allow for some small degree of movement thus providing flexibility in the alignment of the fixtures.

With all systems, wear and tear of the female retaining components housed in the denture will occur and will need replacement depending on the usage of the dentures by the patient. The oral hygiene around these devices is crucial to ensure health of the gingival tissues, and the patient will need to remove the dentures for cleaning after every meal, ensuring that they use the appropriate devices to clean around the male attachments on the fixtures. A removable prosthesis is mainly used when there has been extensive soft tissue loss or there has been severe bone loss compromising the patient's ability to wear conventional dentures successfully.

Fixed prostheses

A fixed prosthesis can be either a single crown or a bridge. The prosthesis can either be:

- **screw retained:** a screw is used to connect the prosthesis (either a crown or bridge) to the fixtures. The screw-retained crown can be one piece, where the abutment and crown are linked and connected to the fixture as one piece, or it can be constructed in two parts, where the abutment connects to the fixture with an abutment screw first and is sealed prior to the crown/bridge being screwed into the abutment using a prosthetic screw. The access hole then has to be sealed off using an interim cement

- **cement retained:** the abutment is screwed into the fixture and tightened (a process called **torquing**). The access hole is sealed off and the crown/bridge is then cemented onto the abutment using a specialised cement such that the restoration can be retrieved.

The choice between the two will depend on the complexity of the prosthesis and the aesthetic zone. The screw-retained prosthesis is easier to remove in the event of problems. If the cement-retained crown needs removal and cannot be taken out in one piece, then the crown would have to be cut off. In both cases the abutment screws and the prosthetic screws will need to be tightened (torqued) by a specified amount, depending on the system used, with the aid of special devices called **torque drivers**. Most patients prefer fixed as opposed to removable restorations as these replicate their natural teeth. It is important, however, that the patient maintains the restorations with regular and effective cleaning and appropriate professional reviews.

Fixed restorations are technically more demanding and challenging for all the teams involved in the provision of the prosthesis; however, they continue to be challenging for patients in terms of the maintenance requirement. Any lapse in the cleaning or occlusal stability can lead to inflammation and bone loss, which may ultimately cause loss of the prosthesis. Smoking is a key risk factor that compromises implant survival and success.

Recommended tasks

(1) Imagine you are discussing the prosthetic replacement options that are possible for the patient who is being planned for implants. Explain the options that you have available.
(2) You need to phone the laboratory for a patient who has had impressions taken for a single crown. The work for the next phase has not arrived. What will you ask the laboratory?

Maintenance and monitoring of dental implants

The long-term success of an implant-retained prosthesis is dependent on how well the fixtures are maintained. The outcome of implant reconstructions is determined either by survival (the proportion of implants in place at a certain time even if they are of no clinical value or have complications) or success, as determined by the stability of the marginal bone and the immobility of the implant. A failed implant is one that has to be removed.

Criteria for success

Criteria for determining the success remain challenging and the following are the recommended guidelines. The fixture (implant):

- does not cause allergic, toxic or gross infectious reactions either locally or systemically
- offers anchorage to a functional prosthesis
- does not show signs of fracture or bending
- does not show any mobility when individually tested by tapping or rocking using a hand instrument, or when using an electronic instrument does not reach the defined values of rigidity
- does not show any signs of radiolucency on an intra-oral radiograph using a paralleling technique
- shows no marginal bone loss and/or attachment loss (probing depth + recession).

The parameters described above do not include any subjective criteria of what the patient's belief is about the psychological benefits and aesthetic outcome of such treatment. Nevertheless, for the individual patient, depending on their risk analysis undertaken at the time of planning, the maintenance of the implant-retained prosthesis will remain key to a long-term successful outcome.

Oral hygiene

The bacterial flora around the implant crevice in health resembles that around the natural tooth crevice in health. The change in the bacterial flora around an implant is similar to that seen around teeth when plaque is not removed effectively. When the cleaning around implants is not optimised, local inflammation of the marginal gingival tissues occurs, known as **peri-implant mucositis**. As with gingivitis this is reversible, as no bone loss occurs providing efficient cleaning is initiated. However, when loss of bone occurs the situation becomes irreversible, a condition known as **peri-implantitis**. As there is no periodontal ligament to protect the osseointegrated surface of the fixture, the bone loss can be quite rapid and no intervention to stop this can lead to loss of the fixture. Smoking has been reported to play a key role in exacerbating implant failure. The aetiology of peri-implantitis is open to debate, with some believing it has a bacterial aetiology and others believing it is mediated by occlusal overload. It is most likely that it is a combination of the two that occurs as there is evidence to show that the associated bacteria are similar to that associated with periodontitis.

To ensure a successful outcome the dental team plays multiple roles, while the patient plays the key role. It is crucial that the patient is able to show optimal levels of plaque control with high standards of oral hygiene. Depending on the type of implant-retained prosthesis they have, the patient must use appropriate cleaning aids, such as interdental brushes, floss and chlorhexidine (if appropriate), and ensure that they are cleaning as effectively as possible around the implants to keep the bacterial flora under control.

During the maintenance phase the patient will be seen regularly either by the dentist or the hygienist. The time intervals over which the patient is recalled are customised to the patient and usually the first recall is after three months. At this visit the patient's oral hygiene is assessed and the state of the gingival condition evaluated. The patient's own cleaning technique is checked and any removal of supragingival plaque is undertaken. At this time the fit of the prosthesis is also checked. Screw-retained prosthetic units should be removed by the clinician, and the underlying abutments and stability of the fixtures checked prior to reconnecting the prosthesis. Radiographs of the bone levels around the implants are taken (usually at 12–18 months) to check the marginal bone. The prosthesis should be designed such that an optimal level of plaque control can be achieved by the patient.

Indices used to monitor health

The indices used to monitor health around implants are the same as those used around natural teeth.

- **Visual inspection:** check for any redness, swelling, loss of stippling and colour.

- **Palpation:** assess the mobility.

■ **Plaque score:** while this is used as a measure of compliance, it is not a reliable indicator to monitor disease as the patient could have easily cleaned just before attending for their appointment.

■ **Bleeding on probing:** this will help ascertain the presence of inflammation and tends to be a better parameter or marker of disease than the plaque score. The bleeding is assessed by carefully inserting a periodontal probe into the gingival crevice. Immediate bleeding on probing is indicative of inflammation.

■ **Probing depth:** while the use of probing remains controversial, this is a simple way of monitoring a change around the implants. For the probing readings to be meaningful, the implant site must be probed at multiple areas after the fit of the prosthesis. This reading will form the baseline against which any changes noted during the monitoring phase should be evaluated.

■ **Bone levels:** radiographs should be taken at periodic intervals (usually annually) to show any changes in the bone. If there is bone loss this should be assessed against the previous baseline radiographs taken immediately after the prosthesis had been fitted. The severity of the bone loss will determine whether or not intervention is required.

Follow-up regime

In the event that inflammation and/or bone loss is noted the following steps should be followed by the clinician.

■ Oral hygiene checked and corrected if inadequate.
■ Following debridement using plastic curettes of the fixtures, irrigation with chlorhexidine should be undertaken.
■ If there is pus discharge or swelling with tenderness then the use of antimicrobials should be advocated.
■ The superstructure should be removed and the implant stability assessed.
■ Once the inflammation is controlled then the need for correcting the underlying bone defect, if there is a defect, should be considered.
■ Check if the patient has any complaints.

Failing implants do not always cause pain and if connected into a fixed reconstruction may be missed if the steps detailed above are not followed carefully. There are some common features associated with failing implants, which are:

■ horizontal mobility of greater than 0.5 mm or any clinically observed vertical movement
■ rapid progressive bone loss regardless of stress reduction and peri-implant therapy
■ pain during function or percussion
■ continued uncontrolled exudates in spite of surgical attempts at correction

- more than half of the surrounding bone is lost around an implant
- increasing probing depths greater than 5 mm
- implants inserted in a poor position.

Failing implants can be distressing for the clinician as well as for the patient, but with early intervention followed by careful maintenance loss can be prevented. If the patient contacts the surgery with any of the complaints listed above an urgent appointment should be arranged. Patients will often call in a panic saying that their implant has come out. Usually the nurse will take such a call and will have to try and ascertain from an anxious patient what has happened. More often than not it is either the healing abutments or the screws that have come loose; however, the patient will describe this as their implant being loose. Hence the nurse should be aware of the types of things that can go wrong to help pacify and reassure the patient until such time as they can be seen in the surgery.

Recommended tasks

(1) A patient telephones and then attends complaining of a bad taste around an implant-retained prosthesis. What would you tell the patient and what investigations would the clinician need to carry out?
(2) What is the difference between peri-implant mucositis and peri-implantitis? How do these conditions relate to a failing implant?
(3) What does a typical maintenance visit involve?
(4) A patient phones in a panic and is convinced that their implant has fallen out. Make a list of things that you would need to be aware of so that you can handle the call effectively.

Implant stock control

Implant treatment can be demanding and time-consuming both for the dental nurse and the operator. The ordering and organisation of the equipment and materials needed is usually the responsibility of the dental nurse. The nurse should be aware of:

- the type of implants being used (i.e. the implant system)
- the components required
- the type of surgery and procedure planned
- the suppliers of the products and where to order them.

For these reasons it is essential that the nurse has good organisational and inter-personal skills and is able to communicate openly with the clinician. To be responsible for an efficient procedure the nurse must ensure the following.

Prior to the start of the procedure (at least one week before)

- Have a knowledge of the planned procedure and what the clinician is intending to do.
- Have a knowledge of the implant system and set-up that is going to be used.
- Have the details of the products that need to be used, i.e. the implant sizes and code numbers; any augmentation materials.
- Liaise with the clinician to ensure that all the required components have been ordered and are available for the day of the surgery.
- Discuss with the clinician the number of implants being placed and the estimated time required.
- Have a knowledge of whether or not the clinician is going to graft at the time of surgery and whether additional equipment for the grafting procedure will be required.
- If there is a stock of implants/products kept in the surgery, then it is important that this stock is used on a rotational basis and stored correctly maintaining the sterility according to the manufacturers' recommendations.
- Ensure that all the required equipment is in working order.
- Ensure that any laboratory work, including stents, is ready for the surgery and is available.

During the procedure

- Ensure that all required materials are available for the surgery.
- Ensure that implant packaging is not opened until the clinician is ready to place the implants.
- If only one nurse is assisting then they will have to plan how the required products will be opened; it will also be necessary to have another pair of sterile gloves available so that they can re-glove once the product has been opened.
- Ensure all other augmentation materials and equipment needed are available and ready for use so that clinical time is not wasted looking for them. Ensure that all used drills are kept in saline once used to prevent blood congealing on the drills.
- If there are two scrubbed nurses assisting then one should focus on assisting the clinician and the second should focus on the exchange of the implant drills and also ensure these are cleaned and kept in saline.

After the procedure

- A count of all the drills used must be undertaken.
- The surgical kit must be cleaned and if using multi-use drills then it is important that the number of times the drill has been used is noted on the record sheet. This will help track when the drills will need to be replaced.
- The reference code with the lot number of the implants that have been inserted must be noted in the patient's records, as well as the surgical book and the stock log along with the patient details. This should be undertaken for all devices inserted including grafting materials.

- A surgical log diary should be kept which makes a note of all the patients who have had surgery undertaken. This will help track the devices used.
- The instruments must be cleaned as per a clinical protocol and any damaged or worn drills must be replaced.

The lot numbers are used to track the device in the event of a failure or any harm that may occur as a result of the device being placed in the patient's mouth. The device tracking should be undertaken by recording the lot number in the patient's records, the surgical book as well as on the consignment stock take.

Maintenance of instruments

The longevity of instruments is ensured if the instruments are used and cleaned properly. The following points will help to achieve this.

- Ensure that if the drills are single-use they are discarded after the case is complete. For multiple-use drills it is important to keep a track of the number of times they are used. Most drills can be used for up to 10 sites and should be replaced after this. However, if they have been used in dense bone (Type 1 or 2) then they may need to be replaced sooner.
- During the surgery, the blood should be wiped off the drills immediately after use and the drills then immersed in saline. This will make cleaning much easier after the surgery.
- Always make a note of and report any missing instruments, and replace them as soon as possible.
- Always follow the recommended protocols for the cleaning of the equipment as this will help maximise its life.
- Ensure that there is a clear sterilisation protocol that is always followed to ensure effective infection control.

Check lists should be an integral part of the nurse's day-to-day routine to ensure that the appropriate sequence is followed. This list is often of great benefit for other staff who may have to provide nursing cover.

Recommended tasks

(1) Why is it important to have a stock of the implants?
(2) Make a check list of everything that you should check prior to the surgical placement of implants.

Medico-legal aspects

As implant treatment is becoming the norm and demands for this treatment are increasing, the medico-legal aspects of providing this treatment have become equally important. The dental nurse, who is an important member of the dental team, must also be aware of the medico-legal implications of this type of treatment, especially as patients may seek advice or help from the nurse, particularly if they are nervous. Since the registration of dental nurses, they are equally responsible for the patients they are involved with as other team members and are as much at risk medico-legally as the clinician.

Confidentiality

All aspects of patient care must be considered confidential and should not be disclosed to a third party or any companies. The duty of confidentiality lies with all staff and it is important that all staff are aware of what this means, which is that all aspects of the patient's care inside or outside the surgery must remain confidential. If the patient therefore rings to enquire about a procedure, the nurse should ensure that they are taking the call where someone cannot hear them discussing the patient's treatment or concerns. Sometimes confidentiality can be breached inadvertently when:

- answering a phone call
- via the internet, e.g. sending emails on an unsecured site
- on answer phones
- on video screens.

The contents of all patients' records are protected by the **Data Protection Act** of 1998. This act gives the patient the right to access their records within 40 days of the request being made in writing. It also states that records in general should not be disclosed to a third party without the patient's permission.

Case records

The accurate documentation of case records cannot be emphasised enough. High-quality care cannot be delivered without good record keeping. This would include all radiographs, study casts, photographs and correspondence over and above the clinical notes kept of any communication that takes place with the patient. This accuracy is important for all types of records, whether they are manually stored or computerised. To minimise time spent looking for casts and records, the nurse may play a role with the reception team to devise a simple storing system that enables ease of access for the required casts.

The need to ensure that all lot numbers of devices are documented as described earlier and that all documentation that is recorded is stored in a location with restricted access is important. While the operator retains the responsibility to ensure that the notes are accurately written up, the dental nurse can help by reminding the clinician to do this and also ensuring that the lot numbers are logged effectively. If the nurse is asked to write the records for the clinician they must ensure the accuracy of the information being recorded. The records should be:

- clear and easily readable
- signed and dated
- accurate
- errors must not be obliterated, e.g. by masking ink. Any errors in the notes should be crossed out
- comprehensive.

Case records are often needed in the context of litigation which can arise long after the event that has caused the concern.

Informed consent

Consent is an integral part of any patient care. The clinician has a duty to ensure that the patient has fully understood the treatment that is being proposed along with the risks and benefits of the treatment. While many assumptions can be made about consent, it is important that the patient has fully understood the treatment that has been proposed, including the alternative options. Normally patients should have at least 24 hours and preferably longer to assimilate the information they have been given about treatment so that they can make an informed choice about what they wish to do. For patients undergoing implant treatment the following points are essential to ensure that the consent given is valid.

- Information given to the patient is up to date and accurate.
- The person agreeing to the procedure is able to fully understand what is being proposed.
- Written confirmation of any proposed treatment will help to ensure that the patient has understood the proposed treatment and is able to come to a reasoned decision. The information sheets given to the patient must also be customised to the patient during their consultation and will help towards the patient's understanding of the planned treatment.

As the demand for implant treatment increases, the need for ensuring valid consent is critical. As an increasing amount of implant treatment is being undertaken, more and more patients are involved in litigation against dentists who they feel have not given them the appropriate information during the planning of their implant treatment or where the treatment provided has not met their expectation. This is further compounded by the fact that implant treatment is a high-cost treatment. While implied consent is acceptable, due to the type and complexity of implant treatment it is prudent to confirm any discussions in writing.

Recommended tasks

(1)   Why is consent important and what specific aspects should you consider?
(2)   How would you support the consent process for the patient?

References and further reading

Brånemark PI, Adell R, Breine U, Hansson BO, Lindström J and Ohlsson A (1969) Intra-osseous anchorage of dental prostheses. I. Experimental studies. *Scand J Plast Reconstr Surg* **3**(2): 81–100.

Darbar UR, Morkus S and Miller M (2008) *Implant Dental Nursing*. Oxford: Blackwell Munksgaard.

Prieskel HW (1996) *Overdentures Made Easy*. London: Quintessence Publishing.

van Steenberghe D (1997) Outcomes and their measurement in clinical trials of endoooseous oral implants. *Annals of Periodontology* **2**: 291–298.

7 The Future

Robert S. Ireland and Janet Goodwin

Future development in training and education

This is an exciting time in the development and training of dental nurses. National Vocational Qualifications (NVQs) have now been introduced and are proving to be a very successful alternative training pathway to the NEBDN National Certificate. The General Dental Council's (GDC) regulatory remit has been expanded to include dental nurses so that there is a single DCP Register for professionals complementary to dentistry. Clearly defined curricula and ethical guidance govern membership of the Register, rather than having lists of permitted duties as was the case in the past.

In the past, if the GDC wanted to change the clinical remit of hygienists or therapists it had to seek parliamentary approval. As can be appreciated, this process was very time-consuming and frustrating. If there had been no change in the law, this procedure would have also applied to dental nurses as soon as they were included on the DCP Register. Fortunately the law has been changed such that the various DCPs are now permitted to undertake clinical tasks for which they have received appropriate training and have been able to demonstrate competence. This has improved the flexibility of training because the GDC is able to amend the duties of any DCP by amending the curricula guidelines without recourse to Parliament, thereby considerably speeding up the process. It is important to remember, of course, that training will need to be appropriate to the change in remit. It will not be sufficient to meet the GDC requirements for a dental nurse to read an article in a magazine or spend a few minutes over a cup of coffee with their dentist. As the remit for dental nurses expands, appropriate training courses will be established with post-course assessment so that competence can be demonstrated. It is likely that these courses will be directed at the more specialised areas of primary care which are becoming more widely developed, such as implantology.

Modern apprenticeship

The government would like all work-based learning to be under the umbrella of a modern apprenticeship and the dental nurse NVQ qualification has been embraced within this concept. This development will allow training organisations to obtain funding for the training of dental nursing (if aged between 16 and 25) and also place the dental nurse qualification within the **National Framework of Education**. The modern apprenticeship comprises an NVQ level 3 certificate covering the occupational standards, a portfolio of evidence put together by the trainee, a technical certificate known as a VRQ in England, Ireland and Wales, and a PDA (Professional Development Award) in Scotland, to confirm the level of knowledge and key skills, which will include numeracy, literacy, communication, problem solving and working with others.

Accredited prior learning

Training is now becoming much more module based. This fits in well with undertaking further training in today's busy clinics and practices while at the same time not discontinuing current employment. It contributes to the principle of lifelong learning. It also helps to address the issue of cost, since some courses can be quite expensive and might be prohibitive if there was no employment income. Some of the skills, knowledge and understanding can be duplicated in different courses and it is possible therefore that credit in the form of accredited prior learning (APL) may be given when undertaking a new course. This could have the advantage of gaining exemption from part of the course. For example, it might be possible in the future for someone who has obtained the NEBDN Orthodontic Nursing Certificate to obtain some APL on one of the new orthodontic therapist courses. This might make attendance on the course more attractive and more practicable.

The acceptance of APL is not widely developed at the present time. If a DCP wanted to embark on the undergraduate Bachelor of Dental Surgery (BDS) course, for example, it is currently necessary to start at the same point as a student coming straight from secondary school. This makes the training programme to graduation as a dentist dauntingly long for a dental nurse, and although it has been achieved in a number of cases it is undoubtedly a significant deterrent. However, considerable development is taking place in the undergraduate curriculum in that most dental schools have moved part of the undergraduate course into outreach clinics where the dental students can work as members of the dental team being supported by dental nurses, hygienists and therapists. This enables them to understand and appreciate the roles of all the PCDs and how they can work together to improve the quality of care delivered. This has demanded a re-evaluation of the curriculum requirements defined in the GDCs document *The First Five Years*. The modularisation of the undergraduate course is probably still some way from a reality, but its development would improve the opportunities for all PCDs, including dental nurses, who wish to follow a flexible pathway leading to qualification as a dentist.

Information technology development

Technological change and development are heavily influencing the whole of life to the extent that it becomes a challenge to keep up to date with the rapid rate of progress. This is particularly so in the area of information technology (IT) and computers. The dental practice or clinic is no exception. It is worth pausing for a while to look to the future to see how this might influence, for better or worse, the work pattern of the dental nurse in the clinical environment.

Information technology and the NHS

It is estimated that almost 100% of practices are routinely using computers for either clinical record keeping or administrative purposes and over 6,000 practices (14,500 dentists) transmit data electronically to the Dental Practice Division of the Business Services Authority over an Electronic Data Interchange (EDI) link. One of the key aims of the Department of Health is to have all NHS dental practices computerised and linked to the rest of the NHS through broadband. It aims to pilot the integration of dentistry within the National Programme for Information Technology with a view to enabling dental practices and community clinics to benefit from an NHS care records service, electronic patient appointment booking, an electronic prescription service, the National Library for Health, and the NHS Connecting for Health Picture Archiving and Communications System (PACS).

There are, however, additional IT needs in dentistry that need to be addressed. It is estimated that about 60% of dentists using computerised dental practice systems employ full electronic records, and a major problem with these systems is that at a clinical level, patient records cannot be transferred between different software systems – which means that when a patient moves to a new practice or their dental practitioner retires, the patient's clinical history cannot be transferred electronically with them to the new clinic. This is because there has so far been no national information technology programme for dentistry in the UK that allows this detailed level of data interchange.

The Department of Health target of having all dental practices computerised and all branches of dentistry linked and using a standardised electronic patient record by 2005 has not been achieved and it will require considerable input from the dental software companies as well as financial support from the NHS if it is to be achieved in the foreseeable future. If or when it is achieved it would provide a powerful stimulus for practices and clinics to transfer all patient records into an electronic format and dispense with paper-based systems. Most of the software companies provide training to use their systems when they are installed. At first this new input process can seem quite daunting, but soon becomes easier to manage than a paper-based system.

Recording clinical data

In the future, it is likely that chairside computerised systems will be routinely used for the capture of all relevant clinical information including text, radiographs, photographs and even sound files. One of the tasks of the dental nurse is to help the clinical members of the dental team to keep accurate and up-to-date clinical patient records. Where records are computerised, this is usually done by inputting data via a keyboard. While this may take no longer and be just as accurate as using paper-based records, it can still use up valuable clinical time. It also presents some infection control problems when undertaken in the surgery.

The most efficient and popular way for humans to communicate is by speech, as is evidenced by the enormous growth in the use of mobile phones. Therefore it could be argued that to be able to talk to the computer would be a logical development for the dental surgery. Technology should speak our language. It would improve efficiency, overcome potential infection problems and free up the dental nurse to undertake other tasks more appropriate to their skills. It would also help to remove some of the clutter that computers generate in the surgery, which does nothing to reduce the anxiety of patients. Unfortunately effective speech recognition software has not yet been developed in dentistry on a commercial basis, possibly because of the large financial investment required in a relatively small market and the need to extensively modify all existing systems. Hopefully dentistry can take advantage of developments in this and other fields and adapt them to the dental practice of the future.

Clinical governance

The Department of Health is already introducing policies to enhance patient-centred treatment, which not only includes employing qualified, occupationally competent staff participating in continuing professional development (CPD) but also clinical governance. Clinical governance is defined by the Department of Health as 'the system through which NHS organisations are accountable for continuously improving the quality of their services and safeguarding high standards by creating an environment in which excellence in clinical care will flourish'. Clinical governance does, however, also apply to dental care provided outside the NHS. It may be stated more simply as ensuring that patients and their carers get the best possible deal out of the healthcare service provided.

Quality care

Clinical governance is all about providing quality care and quality management, but it is important to remember that it doesn't happen by accident, it has to be planned. Clinical governance should include:

■ clear lines of responsibility and accountability for the quality of clinical care
■ a comprehensive programme which improves quality
■ a means by which all members of the dental team can be involved in the development of good practice
■ a means by which patients can be involved in the development of dental care services as well as being appropriately informed about their proposed treatment
■ clear policies for managing risk
■ procedures for all members of the dental team to identify and remedy poor performance
■ a programme of continual quality improvement including CPD and audit.

There was a time when healthcare was delivered with little or no reference to the patient. The dentist decided what treatment should be provided without any discussion with the patient either before or during treatment. Times have changed radically and it is now an ethical responsibility placed on the dental team to obtain informed consent from a patient prior to undertaking any treatment. In addition, patients not only want value for money they want quality for money. However, it is important to be able to prove not only to patients but also to all members of the dental team and healthcare providers such as the NHS that quality issues are being addressed. This involves being able to answer the following questions.

■ Do the dental team understand the practice quality policy?
■ Have the entire dental team been consulted?
■ Have reasonable, measurable and achievable performance standards been set?
■ Do these standards relate to patient needs?
■ Is training provided?
■ Is there a monitoring system in place?
■ Is corrective action taken when necessary?

As can be seen, these questions address issues that are relevant to all members of the dental team. Some practical examples of clinical governance are:

■ Criteria for extraction of wisdom teeth
■ Patient satisfaction surveys
■ Criteria for taking radiographs
■ Criteria for infection control within the clinical environment
■ Clinical examination, record keeping standards and protocols.

Standards

There are three important areas to be considered.

Setting standards

Self-regulation
This is undertaken by the GDC, which is responsible for the protection of the patient by setting standards of both clinical care and education of those members of the dental team registered or enrolled with the GDC. The GDC has undergone a considerable modernisation process. In the NHS Plan for England, the government set out minimum requirements for the modernisation of regulatory bodies. It stated that 'they must be smaller with much greater patient and public representation, have faster, more transparent procedures and develop accountability to the public and the Health Service' (cited in Beecham, 2000). The GDC has committed itself to this modernisation and the structure has now been radically changed to include a much greater lay representation. The changes also include a new look at the education, training and development of the dental team.

National Institute for Health and Clinical Excellence (NICE)
The role of NICE is to provide clinical guidelines based on clinical and cost-effectiveness and to advise on clinical methodology and information on best practice. It has so far had a limited input into dentistry but has produced guidance on the extraction of wisdom teeth, recall examination intervals and the use of prophylactic antibiotics prior to invasive dental treatment.

National Service Framework
This body advises on the organisation of services within the NHS to meet specific health problems and advises on the standards that these services will have to meet.

Delivering standards

Quality improvement
This includes reviewing one's own clinical practice and then measuring it against a recognised standard (**audit**), undertaking evidence-based practice and using clinical indicators as an external measure of clinical performance. Examples of clinical indicators in dentistry are the number of teeth present, the number of carious teeth and the Basic Periodontal Examination (BPE) score. Since these indicators can now be recorded electronically as part of routine clinical record keeping, it makes it easier to monitor the effects of clinical advice or treatment on the dental health of a patient or group of patients.

Continuing professional development
CPD is dealt with in more detail in Chapter 1.

Clinical risk management

It is necessary to have a means of recording adverse effects as a result of using a drug, material or technique, as well as having mechanisms for recognising and dealing with poor performance. These include:

- identification of risks
- risk assessment
- risk reduction, elimination and transfer
- reporting and recording adverse events.

Complaints handling

The procedures for dealing with patient complaints should be defined and made known to the patients. For patients receiving treatment within the NHS, the procedure has been well established. However, in response to a government initiate, a Patients Complaints Service was established in 2007 to deal specifically with complaints from patients receiving treatment on a private payment basis; details about this service are available from the GDC website (www.gdc-uk.org/).

Compliance with Health and Safety regulations

Protocols should be developed, followed and observed by all members of the dental team with appropriate training where necessary. Every practice or clinic should have an infection control policy. Advice sheets on both health and safety and infection control are available from the British Dental Association (www.bda-dentistry.org.uk) and the British Association for Dental Nurses (www.badn.org.uk).

Monitoring standards

Commission for Health Improvement/Healthcare Commission

This body was set up by the NHS in 2000 to independently guarantee quality in the NHS and undertake rolling reviews of NHS trusts. On 31 March 2004 the Commission for Health Improvement (CHI) ceased operating. All its functions were taken over by the Healthcare Commission. The Healthcare Commission was responsible for reviewing complaints about the NHS and independent healthcare services in England that had not been resolved locally. The Healthcare Commission fulfilled its role in promoting quality in healthcare through providing an independent assessment of the standards of services provided by the NHS, private healthcare and voluntary organisations. It achieved this by:

- regulating and inspecting NHS, private and voluntary healthcare providers
- reviewing formal complaints about the NHS that have not been resolved
- handling complaints about private and voluntary healthcare service providers
- investigating serious failures in NHS, private and voluntary services.

The Health and Social Care Act (2008) has replaced the Healthcare Commission with the Care Quality Commission, which came into operation in April 2009.

National Performance Frameworks

These have been established to judge how well each part of the NHS delivers quality services. They measure performance from a patient's point of view and look at such issues as:

- health improvement gained, i.e. the outcome of healthcare provided
- access to care facilities, i.e. what are the facilities available, are they what the patient needs and are they easy for the patient to get to?
- the efficiency of the services provided
- the experiences (both positive and negative) of the patient or carer.

Annual national patient surveys

These can give an overview of patient opinion on many aspects of patient care in different parts of the country. They can also be undertaken on a local basis in the clinic or practice as part of an audit programme or research project.

Research in primary care

Much has been written both in this book and elsewhere about clinical governance. Undertaking a research project is a natural progression of this, but most people think that this is solely the province of academic institutions such as universities. Unfortunately, for many years this has been largely true and has resulted in the criticism that many of the research papers and articles published in journals have little relevance to general dental practice. It must be remembered, however, that the vast majority of dental treatment provided in the UK involves the relief of pain and restoration of function and aesthetics, and can be described as treatment at a primary care level. In addition to which, it is undertaken in a primary care environment – that is to say in general practice or community clinics. Therefore, not only is most of the information or data available in practices or clinics but any study of it will be potentially more relevant to clinical practice than if the study were undertaken in much more controlled conditions in a hospital or university setting. Fortunately, researchers and funding agencies such as the NHS are starting to see the enormous potential of undertaking research in primary care as is evidenced by the increasing number of publications and journals in this area.

It is important that research is undertaken in clinical practice so that the quality of care can be constantly improved. There is no reason why any member of the dental team should not be involved in a research project, after all, primary medical care practice teams have been undertaking successful research for some time and many of the team leaders have been practice nurses. In a very busy dental practice or clinic, it is realistically very difficult to find the time to undertake a research project. Time needs to be allocated for it. It is not something that can be squeezed in during a busy routine treatment session.

It is a big step up from clinical governance or clinical audit and should not be embarked on without first understanding the principles of what is involved. Failure to do so could result in a considerable amount of wasted time and nothing to show for it. One of the first areas to understand is the concept of evidence-based dentistry.

Evidence-based dentistry

How often have we attended a meeting or trade exhibition and overheard one of our colleagues saying something like, 'We tried that material in the practice last week and it didn't work so we decided not to use it again.' This is hardly a rational basis for making a decision that could affect the quality of treatment provided for a patient, but most, if not all, of us have been guilty at some time of this sort of reasoning. Much has been written recently in the dental press about evidence-based dentistry, so what is it? Evidence-based dentistry put simply is an approach to decision making in which the person making the decision uses the best evidence available, and where appropriate in consultation with the patient, to decide on the option that suits that patient best. This can be illustrated using an example such as 'Should protective gloves be worn when treating a patient?' Many might consider that not wearing gloves is more comfortable for both the operator and the patient and would save on cost. However, research evidence indicates that the wearing of gloves makes an important contribution to infection control for the benefit of both the operator and the patient. The evidence is considered to be sufficiently strong as to over-ride any issues of comfort or cost, so we have to be guided by this evidence and gloves are now worn routinely. Of course, it would be important to check the patient's medical history for latex allergy because the research has also indicated that a latex allergic patient can experience a severe reaction to latex gloves. This is why it is important that the clinical decision takes into account the individual patient. The evidence in effect provides a decision support process. It does, however, raise many issues over the quality of the evidence available.

In searching for and finding the evidence it is important to understand and make sense of it and reject it if it is poor. The statement at the start of this section is an example of poor evidence. Some dental companies quote 'in-house' unpublished data to back up claims for their products. This is another example of poor evidence. Nowadays a quick and easy option is to search the internet, but again while this will uncover a mass of information, the quality of it can be very suspect. Searching for the best evidence can be a time-consuming process, but adopting an evidence-based approach will have a profound effect on the way treatment is undertaken in the future and will impact on every member of the dental team.

The research team

Research can be very rewarding, particularly when published, and any member of the dental team could form part of a research team. Each member will bring specific skills to the project which will add to its ultimate success. It is important, however, that advice is sought from someone who has had experience of undertaking primary care research and can advise on the many issues that will need to be considered, such as planning, funding, statistical analysis, writing up and publishing. It is beyond the scope of this book to provide a comprehensive guide to undertaking research. It is intended only to give a brief outline of the research process and some of the important issues involved. There are many books and articles on undertaking research in general practice and the reader is directed to those listed under Further reading. A useful review paper is Burke *et al.* (2002).

The research process

What is the question?

The first stage of any research project is to turn a problem into an answerable question. This is perhaps best illustrated by using an example. Many practices and clinics are now using computers in the surgery to record the clinical charting of patients. This is introducing a number of new problems that haven't been encountered before. The sort of questions that a dental nurse might be asking are: 'Is it quicker or more accurate to capture the clinical charting data on computer in comparison to the more traditional method of using a paper-based system?'

After all, if we knew the answer it might have a considerable bearing on whether we introduced such technology into the surgery. Speed and accuracy, although linked, are in fact two different research questions. How would one go about answering these questions?

Literature review

We would probably think first of asking a colleague or the computer supplier. However, even if they could come up with an answer, on what evidence would that answer be based? Usually it is a personal opinion which could be heavily influenced by fears or enthusiasm for computers or even the desire to sell a system. After all, the computer salesperson is unlikely to provide a negative answer! The first stage is to find out if any studies have been undertaken to answer the research question. This involves a study of all published information by looking in textbooks, journals, review articles and electronically via the internet – but with over 700 dental journals alone published every year, this is a mammoth task. Many researchers use electronic databases on the internet as a starting point. The largest and most readily available is **MEDLINE**, which can be accessed free of charge at the PubMed website (www.ncbi.nlm.nih.gov/PubMed). MEDLINE contains over 11 million citations dating back to 1966. It must be remembered, however, that a MEDLINE search will only identify about half of all the relevant papers on a topic.

Carrying out the study

Having decided on the research question and established as far as possible that the study has not been undertaken before, it is necessary to plan how the study is going to be carried out. This requires a basic understanding of study method and statistics. One could take two nurses and ask them to input the clinical data for 10 patients each using both paper and electronic methods and then compare the results. Would this provide an answer to the question? It may be found that there is no statistical difference between the two methods but this may be because too few nurses or two few patient records have been used. Sometimes it is necessary to undertake an **initial pilot study** in order to decide on the numbers, in this case nurses or patient records, needed to produce a statistically significant answer. This is where the help of a statistical expert is necessary. It highlights the importance of having this advice before starting the study and possibly not wasting both time and money on a project that might ultimately prove nothing.

Funding

As has been stated, carrying out a research project will always involve additional time and time costs money. It is always more encouraging to have research time and materials funded, although it will probably never be funded excessively. There are a number of bodies such as the NHS, the British Dental Association and the Faculty of General Dental Practice (FGDP) that are keen to offer funding for research carried out in a primary dental care setting. To obtain funding it is necessary to write up and submit a proposal or protocol detailing all the stages of the project. This in itself can be a very time-consuming and skilful process with no guarantee that funding will be achieved. It is estimated that only about one in every 10 projects is approved for funding and this applies to experienced researchers as well as those wanting to undertake research for the first time. Failure to obtain funding doesn't necessarily mean that the project is in some way flawed. It may be because the funds available are insufficient for the number of projects submitted or the research area is not relevant or of interest to the funding body. It is wise therefore not to approach a funding body without first having obtained advice from an experienced colleague.

Recording the results

The results of a study can be recorded in the form of numbers such as age, weight, DMF, etc., usually represented by tables or graphs. This is known as a **quantitative study** as would be the case with the computer example above. On the other hand, the study may involve the recording of non-numerical values such as sex, social class, opinions or comments. This is known as a **qualitative study**. A satisfaction questionnaire asking for patients' opinions would be an example of a qualitative study. The results of a study need to be recorded in a format that is quick, easy and meaningful for the reader to understand.

Publishing the results

The ultimate goal of any study is to get it published. The whole purpose of publishing is so that others will be able to benefit from what has been found out and be able to apply it in their clinical practice, hopefully thereby improving the quality of care provision. The better quality journals such as the *British Dental Journal* and *Dental Update* will always send submitted papers for **peer review** prior to considering them for publication. The independent peer reviewers will be experts in their own field and will advise the editor as to whether the paper should be published. Peer-reviewed papers will normally have this stated at the start of the paper. Invariably the reviewers will recommend some modification prior to publication. The peer-review process helps to improve the quality of papers published but it doesn't guarantee that a study has drawn an accurate or correct conclusion. Not all dental journals or magazines adopt a peer-review process and therefore research published in these journals must be interpreted with even greater caution.

Critical appraisal

There is a great tendency to adopt the view that if a research project is published, the conclusions drawn must be true. However, almost all scientific studies are flawed in some way because it is almost impossible to design and undertake the perfect study. There are many examples of different studies investigating the same problem and coming to completely different conclusions. This is frequently because a study will look at only a small sample of the population and not the whole population. For example, a study looking at the effects of water fluoridation on children's teeth in the Birmingham area will not be able to include all the children in that locality and will therefore endeavour to take a representative sample. However, this sample may not represent the whole population, and two or more studies looking at different samples may come to different conclusions. It is important therefore to develop the skill of critical appraisal. This doesn't involve being an expert, but it does require the reader to acquire some skills and to be able to ask important questions, such as the following.

- What were the findings of the study?
- Are the aims clearly stated and have they been achieved?
- Have the results been interpreted correctly?
- Have some results been ignored?
- What are the conclusions of the authors?
- Are the authors' conclusions relevant to my patients?

As evidence-based dentistry becomes more a part of routine clinical practice it is very important that every member of the dental team becomes proficient at critically appraising the literature.

References and further reading

Beecham J (2000) UK to set up new regulatory bodies. *BMJ* **321**: 404.
Burke FJT, Crisp RJ and McCord JF (2002) Research in dental practice: a SWOT analysis. *Dent Update* **29**: 80–97.

Davis JPL and Crombie IK (2003) The why and how of critical appraisal. In: Clarkson J. *et al.* (eds) *Evidence-based Dentistry for Effective Practice*. London: Martin Dunitz.

Department of Health (2002) *NHS Dentistry: options for change*. London: Department of Health.

Department of Health (1998) *Information for Health*. London: Department of Health.

Faculty of General Dental Practitioners (UK) (2003) *Research in General Dental Practice (Study Guides)*. London: Faculty of General Dental Practitioners.

General Dental Council (2002) *The First Five Years. A framework for Undergraduate Dental Education* (2e). London: General Dental Council.

Information Technology and Dentistry: Department of Health website: www.dh.gov.uk/en/Aboutus/Chiefprofessionalofficers/Chiefdentalofficer/DH_4138825

Abbreviations

ACTH	adrenocorticotrophic hormone
ADH	anti-diuretic hormone
ADHD	attention deficit hyperactivity disorder
AIDS	acquired human immunodeficiency syndrome
ALS	Advanced Life Support
ANUG	acute necrotising ulcerative gingivitis
AOB	anterior open bite
APL	accredited prior learning
ASA	American Society of Anesthesiologists
ASD	atrial septal defect; autism spectrum disorder
AV	atrioventricular (node)
BADN	British Association of Dental Nurses
BDA	British Dental Association
BDRA	British Dental Receptionists Association
BFS	British Fluoridation Society
BLS	Basic Life Support
BNF	British National Formulary
BOS	British Orthodontic Society
BP	blood pressure
BSE	bovine spongiform encephalopathy
CABG	coronary artery bypass graft
CAL	computer-assisted learning
CAPD	continuous ambulatory peritoneal dialysis
CCD	charge coupled device
CD	controlled drug
CDS	Community Dental Service
CHD	congenital heart defect
CHI	Commission for Health Improvement
CJD	Creutzfeld-Jakob disease
CL/P	cleft lip/palate
CNS	central nervous system
CO_2	carbon dioxide

COSHH	Control of Substances Hazardous to Health
CP	cerebral palsy
CPD	continuing professional development
CPR	cardiopulmonary resuscitation
CVA	cerebrovascular accident
DMF	decayed, missing, filled (permanent teeth)
dmf	decayed, missing, filled (deciduous teeth)
DPB	Dental Practice Board
DPMA	Dental Practice Managers Association
DVT	deep vein thrombosis
ECG	electrocardiogram
ECT	electroconvulsive therapy
EMLA	eutectic mixture of local anaesthetics
EOA	extra-oral anchorage
EOT	extra-oral traction
ERV	expiratory reserve volume
FDI	Fédération Dentaire Internationale (World Dental Federation)
FGDP	Faculty of General Dental Practice (UK)
FMPA	Frankfort mandibular plane angle
GA	general anaesthesia
GABA	gamma-amino-butyric acid
GDC	General Dental Council
GDS	General Dental Services
GIC	glass ionomer cement
GORD	gastro-oesophageal reflux disease
GTN	glyceryl trinitrite
Hg	mercury
HIV	human immunodeficiency virus
HRT	hormone replacement therapy
ICON	Index of Complexity Outcome and Need
ICP	inter-cuspal position
IM	intramuscular
IMCA	independent mental capacity advocate
INR	International Normalised Ratio
IOTN	Index of Orthodontic Treatment Need
IRV	inspiratory reserve volume
IS	inhalation sedation
IUL	intra-uterine life
IV	intravenous
LA	local anaesthesia
LFH	lower face height
MAC	minimum alveolar concentration
MBT	McLaughlin, Bennett and Trevesi
MCA	Mental Capacity Act

MDAS	Modified Dental Anxiety Scale
MG	myasthenia gravis
MI	myocardial infarction
MS	multiple sclerosis
MVP	mitral valve prolapse
NAI	non-accidental injury
NEBDN	National Examining Board for Dental Nurses
NHS	National Health Service
NICE	National Institute for Health and Clinical Effectiveness
NiTi	nickel titanium
NME	non-milk extrinsic (sugars)
NPSA	National Patient Safety Agency
NSAID	non-steroidal anti-inflammatory drug
NVQ	National Vocational Qualification
OPCS	Office of Population Census and Surveys
OPG/OPT	orthopantomograph
PAR	Peer Assessment Rating
PCD	professionals complementary to dentistry
PCO_2	partial pressure of carbon dioxide
PCT	primary care trust
PDA	patent ductus arteriosus
PDS	Personal Dental Service
PEG	percutaneous endoscopic gastrostomy
PO_2	partial pressure of oxygen
PTH	parathyroid hormone
RA	relative analgesia
RCP	retruded contact position
RCT	randomised controlled trial
RSA	root surface area
RV	residual volume
SA	sinoatrial (node)
SaO_2	arterial oxygen saturation
SARME	surgically assisted rapid maxillary expansion
SDS	salaried dental service
SMART	**S**pecific, **M**easurable, **A**chievable, **R**ealistic, **T**ime-related
SMO	standard midline occlusal
SMOG	Simple Measure of Gobbledegook
TB	tuberculosis
TCA	tricyclic antidepressant
TIA	transient ischaemic attack
TMA	titanium-molybdenum alloy
TMD	temporomandibular joint disorders
TMJ	temporomandibular joint
TV	tidal volume

URA	upper removable appliance
UTI	urinary tract infection
VC	vital capacity
VME	vertical maxillary excess
VRQ	vocationally related qualification
VSD	ventriculo-septal defect
WEL	workplace exposure limits
WHO	World Health Organization

Index